Infusion Therapy

made Incredibly Easy!

Fifth Edition

Clinical Editor
Lynn Hadaway, MEd, RN-BC, CRNI
President
Lynn Hadaway Associates, Inc.
Milner, Georgia

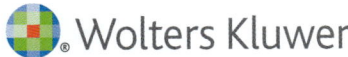

Philadelphia • Baltimore • New York • London
Buenos Aires • Hong Kong • Sydney • Tokyo

Executive Editor: Nicole Dernoski
Development Editors: Kathleen Scogna & Maria M. McAvey
Editorial Coordinators: Maria M. McAvey and Lindsay Ries
Production Project Manager: David Saltzberg
Design Coordinator: Elaine Kasmer
Manufacturing Coordinator: Kathleen Brown
Marketing Manager: Linda Wetmore
Prepress Vendor: SPi Global

5th edition

Copyright © 2018 Wolters Kluwer

All rights reserved. This book is protected by copyright. No part of this book may be reproduced or transmitted in any form or by any means, including as photocopies or scanned-in or other electronic copies, or utilized by any information storage and retrieval system without written permission from the copyright owner, except for brief quotations embodied in critical articles and reviews. Materials appearing in this book prepared by individuals as part of their official duties as U.S. government employees are not covered by the above-mentioned copyright. To request permission, please contact Wolters Kluwer at Two Commerce Square, 2001 Market Street, Philadelphia, PA 19103, via email at permissions@lww.com, or via our website at lww.com (products and services).

9 8 7 6 5 4 3 2 1

Printed in China (or the United States of America)

Library of Congress Cataloging-in-Publication Data
Names: Hadaway, Lynn C., editor.
Title: Infusion therapy made incredibly easy! / clinical editor, Lynn Hadaway.
Other titles: I.V. therapy made incredibly easy!
Description: Fifth edition. | Philadelphia : Wolters Kluwer Health, [2018] |
   Preceded by I.V. therapy made incredibly easy!. 4th ed. c2010. | Includes bibliographical references and index.
Identifiers: LCCN 2017034935 | ISBN 9781496355010
Subjects: | MESH: Infusions, Parenteral | Nurses' Instruction
Classification: LCC RM170 | NLM WB 354 | DDC 615/.6--dc23 LC record available at https://lccn.loc.gov/2017034935

This work is provided "as is," and the publisher disclaims any and all warranties, express or implied, including any warranties as to accuracy, comprehensiveness, or currency of the content of this work.

This work is no substitute for individual patient assessment based upon healthcare professionals' examination of each patient and consideration of, among other things, age, weight, gender, current or prior medical conditions, medication history, laboratory data and other factors unique to the patient. The publisher does not provide medical advice or guidance and this work is merely a reference tool. Healthcare professionals, and not the publisher, are solely responsible for the use of this work including all medical judgments and for any resulting diagnosis and treatments.

Given continuous, rapid advances in medical science and health information, independent professional verification of medical diagnoses, indications, appropriate pharmaceutical selections and dosages, and treatment options should be made and healthcare professionals should consult a variety of sources. When prescribing medication, healthcare professionals are advised to consult the product information sheet (the manufacturer's package insert) accompanying each drug to verify, among other things, conditions of use, warnings and side effects and identify any changes in dosage schedule or contraindications, particularly if the medication to be administered is new, infrequently used or has a narrow therapeutic range. To the maximum extent permitted under applicable law, no responsibility is assumed by the publisher for any injury and/or damage to persons or property, as a matter of products liability, negligence law or otherwise, or from any reference to or use by any person of this work.

LWW.com

Dedication

In memory of my parents, Carl and Gladys Hadaway, who taught me I could achieve anything I set my mind to.

Lynn Hadaway

Contributors

Catherine B. Amero, MSN/Ed, CRNI, LNC
Infusion Education Coordinator
Milford Regional Medical Center
Milford, Massachusetts

Patti Jo Carruth, MSN, RN, OCN, CRNI
Clinical Research Nurse
City of Hope Comprehensive Cancer Center
Duarte, California

Lynda Cook, MSN, RN, CRNI
Vascular Access Specialist
3M Critical and Chronic Care Solutions Division
Greensboro, North Carolina

Beth Fabian, BA, RN, CRNI
Manager, Oncology Infusion
Ascension/St. John Hospital & Medical Center
Outpatient Infusion Centers
Detroit, Michigan

Anne Marie Frey, BSN, RN, CRNI, VA-BC
Clinical Expert, Neonatal and Pediatric Vascular Access
The Children's Hospital of Philadelphia
Philadelphia, Pennsylvania

Sheila Hale, BSN, RN, CRNI, VA-BC
Senior Vascular Access Specialist
Seton Healthcare Family
Austin, Texas

Karen Laforet, RN, MCISc, IIWCC, VA-BC, CVAA
Director, Clinical Services
Calea
Mississauga, Ontario, Canada

Donna Scemons, RN, MSN, MA, FNP-C, CNS
Assistant Professor
California State University School of Nursing
Los Angeles, California
Family Nurse Practitioner

Angelia Sims, RN, CRNI, OCN
Nursing Services Manager
Compass Oncology
Portland, Oregon

Allison J. Terry, RN, MSN, PhD
Assistant Dean
College of Nursing and Health Sciences
Auburn University at Montgomery
Montgomery, Alabama

Previous Edition Contributors

Catherine B. Amero, MSN/Ed, CRNI, LNC

Jane Banton, RN, BSN

Sandra J. Hamilton, RN, BSN, MEd, CRNI

Susan K. Poole, RN, BSN, MS, CRNI, CNSN

Donna Scemons, RN, MSN, MA, FNP-C, CNS

Ruth K. Seignemartin, MOL, CRNI, CNAA

Angelia Sims, RN, CRNI, OCN

Denise Stefancyk, RN, BSN, CCRC

Allison J. Terry, RN, MSN, PhD

Foreword

If you're like me, you're too busy caring for your patients to have the time to wade through a foreword that uses pretentious terms and umpteen dull paragraphs to get to the point. So let's cut right to the chase! Here's why this book is so terrific:
1. It will teach you all the important things you need to know about infusion therapy. (And it will leave out all the fluff that wastes your time.)
2. It will help you remember what you've learned.
3. It will make you smile as it enhances your knowledge and skills.
   Don't believe me? Try these recurring logos on for size:

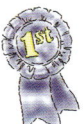

Best practice—Provides evidence-based standards for administering and monitoring infusion therapy

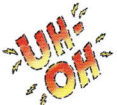

Warning—Alerts about possible risks or complications

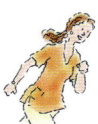

Running smoothly—Offers pointers on how to ensure that the patient and his equipment remain problem free

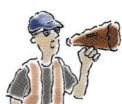

That's a wrap!—Contains a succinct summary of key chapter information for a quick review

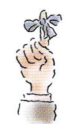

Memory jogger—Reinforces learning through easy-to-remember anecdotes and mnemonics

See? I told you! And that's not all. Look for me and my friends in the margins throughout this book. We'll be there to explain key concepts, provide important care reminders, and offer reassurance. Oh, and if you don't mind, we'll be spicing up the pages with a bit of humor along the way, to teach and entertain in a way that no other resource can.

I hope you find this book helpful. Best of luck throughout your career!

Contents

1	**Introduction to infusion therapy** Karen Laforet, RN, MCISc, IIWCC, VA-BC, CVAA	1
2	**Infusion therapy using peripheral veins** Angelia Sims, RN, CRNI, OCN	53
3	**Infusion therapy requiring central venous access** Sheila Hale, BSN, RN, CRNI, VA-BC	119
4	**Infusion fluids and medications** Catherine B. Amero, MSN/Ed., CRNI, LNC	193
5	**Transfusions** Lynda Cook, MSN, RN, CRNI	238
6	**Antineoplastic therapy** Allison J. Terry, RN, MSN, PhD	269
7	**Biologic therapy** Patti Jo Carruth, MSN, RN, OCN, CRNI	305
8	**Parenteral nutrition** Donna Scemons, RN, MSN, MA, FNP-C, CNS	326
9	**Infusion therapy in pediatrics** Anne Marie Frey, BSN, RN, CRNI, VA-BC	357
10	**Infusion therapy in older adults** Beth Fabian, BA, RN, CRNI	389

Appendices — 415

Practice makes perfect	416
Checklist for prevention of central line-associated bloodstream infections	434
Glossary	436
Index	445

Chapter 1

Introduction to infusion therapy

Just the facts

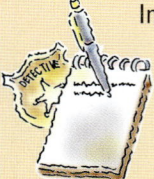

In this chapter, you'll learn:
- ♦ purposes of infusion therapy
- ♦ normal fluid and electrolyte balance
- ♦ infusion delivery methods
- ♦ infusion flow rates
- ♦ professional standards for infusion therapy
- ♦ patient education regarding infusion therapy
- ♦ documentation for infusion therapy.

A look at infusion therapy

Infusion therapy is one of the most common interventions in health care, with more than 90% of hospitalized patients receiving some form of infusion therapy during the course of their care. Intraosseous infusion is now the recommended route for emergency situations when the intravenous (I.V.) route cannot be obtained quickly. Subcutaneous infusion is used for home, palliative, and long-term care, while intraspinal infusion is used in a number of settings for short- and long-term needs. Clinicians need to know the standards and guidelines that determine responsibilities associated with infusion therapy. As the professional administering infusion therapy, you are accountable for the outcome of your decisions and interventions.

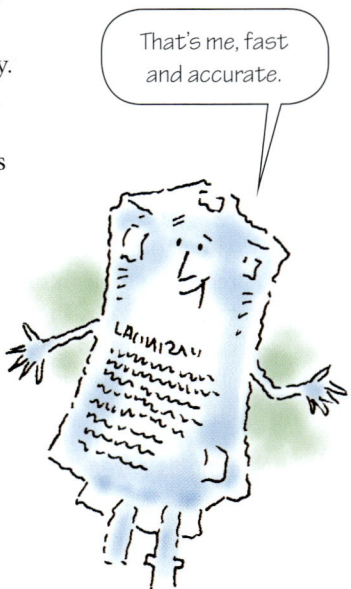

That's me, fast and accurate.

What is infusion therapy?

In its most simplified terms, liquid solutions such as fluids, medications, and blood products are introduced directly into the bloodstream or another anatomical space with easy absorption into the bloodstream.

Infusion therapy is used to:
- restore and/or maintain fluid and electrolyte balance
- administer medications

- transfuse blood and blood components
- provide parenteral nutrition.

Benefits of infusion therapy

Infusion therapy has a number of benefits. When the patient cannot or should not rely on oral administration of medication, infusion is the best alternative. The effect of the infused solution is seen quickly. Medication reaches the bloodstream immediately, without reliance on absorption from the muscle or the gastrointestinal tract.

Risks of infusion therapy

Like other invasive procedures, infusion therapy has its downside. While infusion therapy is commonly used in a variety of settings, clinicians need to proceed with caution; since it is an invasive procedure, it carries risk. These risks include:
- bleeding or air emboli from accidental disconnection at the catheter hub or inadvertent catheter removal
- blood vessel damage caused by medications and catheter insertion and manipulation
- fluid overload
- overdose because medication effect is more rapid
- allergic and other adverse responses to the infused substance(s), such as hearing loss or kidney damage
- incompatibility caused when some drugs and I.V. solutions are in contact with each other
- many complications associated with the catheter such as infiltration and extravasation, phlebitis and thrombophlebitis, nerve injury, and infection.

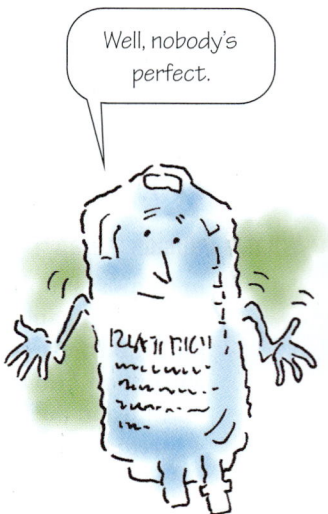

Well, nobody's perfect.

Strings attached

The patient's activities of daily living can be compromised while receiving their infusion. Simple tasks like chair transfers, driving a car, or taking a shower may be complicated or not possible when coping with an infusion pump, the I.V. administration set, the vascular access device (VAD), and necessary methods for stabilizing and dressing.

No such thing as a free lunch—or infusion!

Finally, infusion therapy may seem more costly than oral or intramuscular methods of delivering medications. The overall cost of safe infusion therapy is balanced with the needs for timeliness and effectiveness of the treatment.

Fluids, electrolytes, and infusion therapy

Fluid and electrolyte balance is the fundamental basis for infusion therapy. An overview of the fluid compartments and fluid and electrolyte regulation will increase your understanding of how all of this works together.

We're all wet (well, mostly)
Body fluid (water) makes up 50% to 75% of total body weight (or mass) of the human body. Age and gender determine the percentage of water weight. Babies tend toward 75%, the average adult male around 60%, and an elderly man approximately 50%.

Of solvents and solutes
Body fluids are composed of water (a solvent) and dissolved substances (solutes). The solutes in body fluids include electrolytes (such as sodium) and nonelectrolytes (such as proteins).

Fluid functions
What functions do body fluids provide? They:
- help regulate body temperature
- transport nutrients and gases throughout the body
- carry cellular waste products to excretion sites.

Understanding body fluid distribution
Body fluid is distributed between two main compartments — extracellular and intracellular. Extracellular fluid (ECF) has two components — interstitial fluid (ISF) and intravascular fluid (plasma). This illustration shows body fluid distribution for a 155-lb (70.5-kg) adult.

ECF
About 19 L (20% of body weight)

ISF
About 15 L (20% of body weight)

Intravascular fluid (plasma)
About 3.5 L (5% of body weight)

Intracellular fluid
About 23 L (40% of body weight)

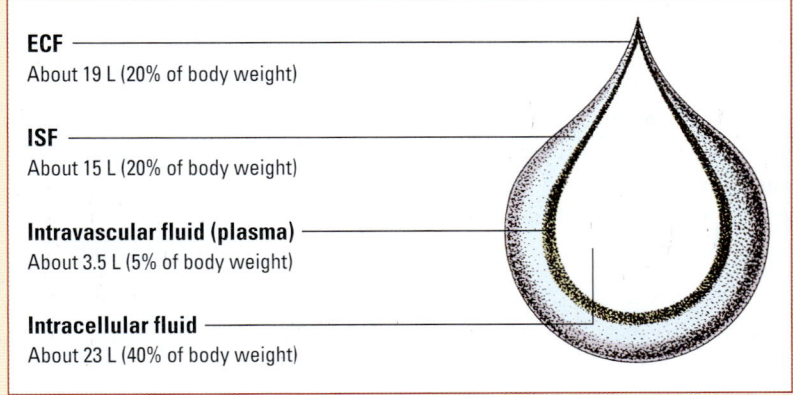

4 Introduction to infusion therapy

Aim for the optimum

When fluid levels are optimal, the body performs swimmingly; however, when fluid levels deviate from the acceptable range, organs and systems can quickly become congested or depleted.

Inside and outside

Body fluids are divided among functional spaces or compartments — intracellular fluid (ICF) or inside the millions of cells in the human body, extracellular fluid (ECF) or outside the cells, and transcellular such as GI fluid and urine. ICF accounts for about two-thirds of the total body fluid and about 40% of total body weight. ECF includes plasma and interstitial fluid for a total of about 20% of body weight. The two compartments are separated by the cell membranes. Intracellular fluids are high in potassium and magnesium, while ECF fluids are high in sodium and chloride. Normally, the distribution of fluids between the two compartments is constant. (See *Understanding body fluid distribution*.)

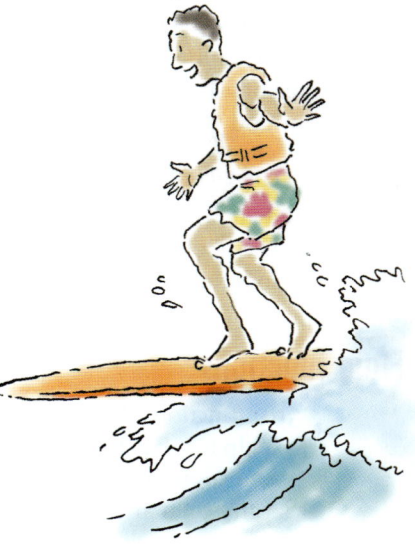

With optimal fluid levels, you're riding a wave of good health!

The ABCs of ECF

The two key components of the ECF are interstitial fluid (ISF) and intravascular fluid (plasma). Interstitial fluid lies in the spaces between cells and outside the blood vessels bathing cells with fluid. The ISF is the conduit between plasma and the intercellular fluid enabling the bidirectional flow of nutrients, wastes, gases, enzymes, and messengers (this will be discussed in more detail in the section titled "Fluid movement"). Intravascular fluid is the liquid component of blood and is the only real fluid collection that totally exists in one location. It surrounds red blood cells (RBCs) and accounts for most of the blood volume.

Transcellular fluid is part of the ECF and is produced by cellular metabolism. Cerebrospinal and lymphatic fluid, urine and gastrointestinal fluid, and secretions from the salivary glands, pancreas, liver, and sweat glands are transcellular fluid that are frequently examined to determine what replacement fluid and electrolytes are needed.

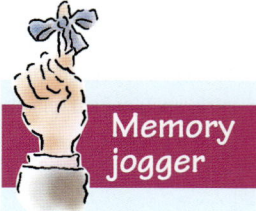

Memory jogger

Remember, when it comes to body fluids, two i's make an e. The two i's (intravascular and interstitial fluid) are part of the e (extracellular fluid) not the i (intracellular fluid).

Daily fluid gains and losses

Each day the body gains and loses fluid through several different processes. The illustration at right shows the main sites involved. The amounts shown apply to adults; infants exchange a greater amount of fluid than adults.

Note: Gastric, intestinal, pancreatic, and biliary secretions total about 8,200 mL. However, because they're almost completely reabsorbed, they aren't usually counted in daily fluid gains and losses.

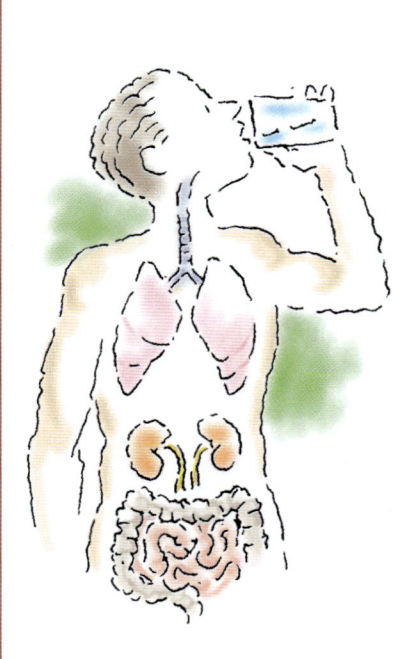

Daily total intake
- Liquids
  – 1,000 to 1,500 mL
- Water in solid foods
  – 800 to 1,000 mL
- Water of oxidation (combined water and oxygen in the respiratory system)
  – 300 to 400 mL

Daily total output for an average healthy adult
– 2,500 mL
- Lungs (respiration)
  – 300 mL
- Skin (perspiration)
  – 100 to 600 mL, but could be as high as 1 or 2 L in hot conditions or with exercise
- Kidneys (urine)
  – 1,400 to 1,800 mL
- Intestines (feces)
  – 100 to 200 mL

Balancing act

Maintaining fluid balance in the body involves the kidneys, heart, liver, adrenal, and pituitary glands. An imbalance in either of these elements may be life threatening. It is a clinician's responsibility to monitor fluid intake and output as well as recognize early signs and symptoms of imbalance. This balancing act is affected by:
- fluid volume
- distribution of fluids in the body
- concentration of solutes in the fluid.

You gain some, you lose some

Every day, the body gains and loses fluid. To maintain fluid balance, the gains must equal the losses. (See *Daily fluid gains and losses.*)

Hormones at work

Total body fluid volume is controlled through a number of mechanisms responding to changes in intravascular volume and the osmolality. (See *Osmolality vs osmolarity: what's the difference*, page 6.) Water balance is regulated by the secretion of antidiuretic hormone (ADH) and the thirst mechanism. Aldosterone, primarily responsible for serum sodium concentration, also has a role in maintaining fluid balance.

ADH, known as the water-conserving hormone and secreted by the pituitary gland, regulates water balance by its effect on the kidneys. It's secreted when plasma osmolarity increases or circulating blood volume decreases and blood pressure drops. When ADH is released, more water is reabsorbed into the cells.

Hormonal regulation of sodium balance is mediated by aldosterone from the adrenal glands. Aldosterone regulates blood pressure through monitoring blood volume, serum sodium, and potassium levels. When circulating blood volume is reduced or there is an imbalance in sodium or potassium serum levels, aldosterone is released.

Thirst quencher

The thirst mechanism (awareness of the desire to drink) is a major process for maintaining fluid and electrolyte balance. Feeling thirsty indicates that total fluid volume is low and stimulates water drinking. Hyperosmolarity, a drop in intravascular volume, or dry mouth triggers osmoreceptors in the hypothalamus resulting in the person feeling thirsty. Drinking water restores plasma volume and reduces ECF osmolarity by dilution.

Osmolality vs osmolarity: What's the difference?

Osmolality and osmolarity are measures of the solute concentration of a solution, and both terms are often used interchangeably even though they refer to different units of measurement, one by volume and one by weight.
- Osmolarity measures the volume of both fluids and dissolved particles, expressed as mOsm per liter, a unit measuring volume. This is used more frequently for measuring fluids outside the body.
- Osmolality measures the weight of the fluids, expressed in mOsm per kilogram, a unit measuring weight, and used most commonly for fluids inside the body.

The term *osmolarity* and osmolality are used interchangeably because 1 liter of water weighs 1 kilogram.

Picking out the baseline

Clinicians need to anticipate changes in fluid balance that can occur during infusion therapy. A baseline fluid status is needed prior to starting fluid replacement therapy. During infusion therapy, changes in fluid status alert impending fluid imbalances. (See *Identifying fluid imbalances*.)

Identifying fluid imbalances

By carefully assessing a patient before and during infusion therapy, you can identify fluid imbalances early — before serious complications develop. The following assessment findings and test results indicate fluid deficit or excess.

Table 1-1 Identifying fluid imbalances

Signs and symptoms	Fluid deficit	Fluid excess
Clinical observations	Dry mucous membranes; sunken eyes; pale; skin cool to touch; ↓ perspiration; longitudinal furrows in tongue	Periorbital edema; puffy eyelids
Urine output	↓ < 30 mL/hour	↑, polyuria
Heart rate	↑ at rest; thready	Bounding pulse
Respiratory	↑ rate	↑ rate; dyspnea; moist crackles or rales (indicative of >1 L excess fluid)
Blood pressure	↓ by 10 mm Hg; orthostatic hypotension	May be elevated
Central venous pressure CVP	↓; flat neck veins in supine position	↑; Distended internal jugular at 30°
Vascular	Capillary refill greater than 2 seconds; slow filling of hand veins when arm lowered	↓ emptying of hand veins when arms elevated
Skin integrity	Lack of moisture in axillae and groin; ↓ skin turgor (nonspecific in elderly)	Dependent edema; generalized edema (anasarca); pitting dependent edema
Mental status	Status changes	Headache; lethargy; weakness; seizures
Patient symptoms	Thirst; dry mouth; weakness,	Cramps; nausea; vomiting
Serum levels		
Hematocrit	↑	↓
Electrolytes	↑ serum sodium	↓ serum sodium
Renal status	↑ urine specific gravity greater than 1.010; ↑ urine osmolarity	↓ urine specific gravity less than 1.010; ↓ urine osmolarity
BUN (urea)	↑	↓
Osmolarity	↑	↓

Electrolytes

Electrolytes are a major component of body fluids and play a vital role in maintaining homeostasis including fluid balance, acid-base balance, and neurological and cardiovascular regulation. There are six major electrolytes: sodium, potassium, calcium, chloride, phosphorus, and magnesium.

You'll get a charge outta this

As the name implies, electrolytes are associated with electricity. These vital substances are chemical compounds that dissociate in solution into electrically charged particles called *ions*. Like wiring for the body, the electrical charges of ions generate electricity to move fluids and water within the body, contract muscles and other activities needed for normal cell function (See *Understanding electrolytes*.)

> Electrolytes are chemical compounds that separate in solution into electrically charged particles called ions — anions for those with a negative electrical charge and cations for those with a positive electrical charge.

Understanding electrolytes

Electrolyte concentrations may be expressed in a number of ways:
- Milliequivalents per liter (mEq/L) is the chemical combining power of ions. This measure is based on the principle that anions and cations combine milliequivalent for milliequivalent.
- Milligrams per 100 mL (deciliter) — expresses the weight of the solute per unit volume.
- Millimole per liter — one mole (mol) of a substance is defined as the atomic (molecular) weight of the substance in grams. For example, a mole of potassium is equivalent to 3.5 g as the atomic weight of potassium is 3.5. A millimole is one-thousandth of a mole and the atomic (molecular) weight is expressed as mmol/L. The Système International d'Unités (SI units) is used internationally and is included in the table below.

(Text continues on page 10)

Table 1-2 Understanding electrolytes

Electrolyte	Principal functions	Signs and symptoms of imbalance
Sodium (Na^+) • Chief cation in ECF • Plasma level: 135–145 mEq/L 135–145 mmol/L	• Controls distribution of water throughout body • Maintains normal fluid balance • Affects concentration, excretion, and absorption of potassium and chloride • Helps regulate acid-base balance • Essential for electrical activity of neurons and muscle cells	*Hyponatremia:* apprehension, abdominal cramps, muscle twitching, diarrhea, decreased skin turgor, headache, confusion, tremor, seizures, coma *Hypernatremia:* intense thirst, fever, flushed skin, oliguria, disorientation, excitement, dry, sticky mucous membranes
Potassium (K^+) • Major cation in intracellular fluid (ICF) • Normal serum level: 3.5–5.0 mEq/L 3.5–5.1 mmol/L (adult)	• Major cation in ICF • Necessary for cell function • Essential for electrical activity of neurons and all muscle cells • Maintains cell electroneutrality • Plays a major role in acid-base balance	*Hypokalemia:* decreased reflexes (muscle atony); apathy; muscular cramps; postural hypotension; decreased blood pressure; decreased bowel motility; paralytic ileus *Hyperkalemia:* cardiac arrhythmias; decreased tendon reflexes; muscle weakness; peaked and elevated T waves on ECG; abdominal cramping; paresthesias; apathy; confusion
Calcium (Ca^{++}) • Major cation in ECF • Normal serum level: total: 8.4–10.6 mg/dL 2.1–2.5 mmol/L	• Vital function for formation and function of bones and teeth • Necessary for cell membrane structure, function, and permeability • Maintains normal excitability of neurons and muscle cells • Essential for blood clotting • Activates serum complement in immune system function	*Hypocalcemia:* muscle tremors and cramps; Trousseau's sign (earliest most sensitive sign) where an inflated BP cuff produces muscle spasms of the forearm; hyperreflexia; bleeding, excessive irritability; numbness or tingling in the fingers, toes, and area surrounding the mouth *Hypercalcemia:* lethargy; fatigue; constipation; anorexia; excessive amounts of urine (polyuria); excessive thirst (polydipsia); depressed reflexes; cardiac arrhythmias and ECG changes (shortened QT interval and widened T wave)
Chloride (Cl^-) • Chief anion in ECF • Normal serum level: 96–106 mEq/L 96–106 mmol/L	• Provides electroneutrality particularly with sodium (the positive and negative charges are equal) • Helps regulate osmotic pressure • Combines with major cations to create important compounds, such as sodium chloride ($NaCl$), hydrogen chloride (HCl), potassium chloride (KCl), and calcium chloride ($CaCl_2$)	*Hypochloremia:* deficiency in chloride leads to deficiency in potassium; muscle twitching; sweating; shallow depressed breathing; tetany; high fever *Hyperchloremia:* dehydration; fluid loss; stupor; Kussmaul's breathing (rapid and deep breathing); muscle weakness; diminished cognitive ability; coma

(continued)

Table 1-2 Understanding electrolytes *(continued)*

Electrolyte	Principal functions	Signs and symptoms of imbalance
Phosphorus (HPO$_4^-$) • Chief anion in ICF (85% in bones/teeth) • Normal serum phosphate level: 3–4.5 mg/dL 1.0–1.5 mmol/L	• Helps maintain bones and teeth • Major role in acid-base balance (as a urinary buffer) • Building block for cell membranes, DNA, RNA, ATP, and phospholipids • Plays essential role in muscle, red blood cell, and neurologic function	*Hypophosphatemia:* irritability; confusion; coma; paresthesias (circumoral and peripheral), lethargy, speech defects (such as stuttering or stammering), muscle dysfunction and weakness including respiratory failure, cardiomyopathies *Hyperphosphatemia:* muscle cramps and spasms, neuroexcitability to tetany and seizures; prolonged state results in calcification of soft tissues (lungs, kidneys, joints)
Magnesium (Mg^{++}) • Major cation found in ICF (closely related to Ca^{++} and P) • Normal serum level: 1.3–2.1 mg/dL 0.65–1.05 mmol/L	• 50% found in bone • Primary role in enzyme activity • Metabolizes carbohydrates and proteins • Essential for ATP production and activity of neurons and muscle cells • Facilitates Na$^+$ and K$^+$ movement across all membranes • Influences Ca^{++} levels	*Hypomagnesemia:* common imbalance in critically ill patients; neuromuscular irritability; increased reflexes; nystagmus; tetany; leg and foot cramps; disorientation; mood changes *Hypermagnesemia:* muscle weakness; drowsiness; lethargy; coma; arrhythmias; slow weak pulse; hypotension; vague neuromuscular changes (such as tremor); vague GI symptoms (such as nausea); peripheral vasodilatation

Fluid and electrolyte balance

Where infusion therapy is concerned, fluid and electrolytes are generally discussed in tandem due to their interdependence. Any change in one alters the other, and any I.V. solution given affects a patient's fluid and electrolyte balance.

Electrolyte balance

Earlier, we identified the three principle fluids in the body: (1) the intravascular and (2) interstitial fluid that comprises the extracellular fluid (ECF) and the (3) intracellular fluid (ICF). We also discussed the ion concentrations that differ depending on where they are located. (See *Understanding Body Fluid Distribution,* page 5.) The reason for the difference is due to cell membrane selective permeability: only certain ions can cross the cell membrane and at certain times. Although ICF and ECF contain different solutes, the concentration levels of the two fluids are about equal when balance is maintained.

Extra(cellular) credit

The two ECF components — the intravascular and interstitial fluids — have identical electrolyte components: the most abundant cation is sodium (Na^+) and the most abundant anion is chloride (Cl^-). The intracellular fluid's most abundant cation is potassium (K^+), with phosphorus (HPO_4^-) the major anion. Pores in the capillary walls allow electrolytes to move freely between the two components and plasma, allowing for equal distribution of electrolytes in both substances. (See *Understanding body fluid distribution*, page 5.) Both the ICF and the intravascular fluids contain proteins, mainly albumin, globulin, and fibrinogen. Interstitial fluid however does not contain proteins because protein molecules are too large to pass through capillary walls. Intravascular pressure, mainly in the capillaries, comes from these plasma proteins preventing fluid from the plasma from leaking into the interstitial fluid.

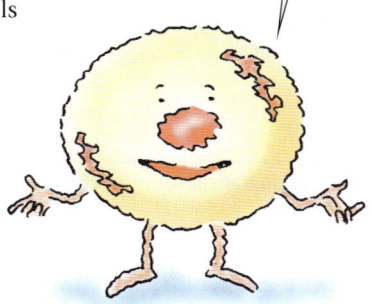

I practice selective permeability. Some electrolytes get through my membranes and some don't.

Fluid movement

Fluid movement is major mechanism that regulates fluid and electrolyte balance.

Ebb and flow

Body fluids are in constant motion. Although separated by membranes, they continually move between the ECF and ICF and within the ECF. The distribution of water, nutrients, gases, and waste products as well as electrolyte balance is accomplished through various mechanisms of transport across a semipermeable membrane, such as the cell wall. Passive transport does not require expenditure of energy, while active transport does require energy. The energy is in the form of adenosine triphosphate (ATP). Here, molecules are moved back and forth using physiologic pumps, similar to the sodium-potassium pump that keeps the higher amounts of potassium inside the cell and sodium outside the cell. In this case, sodium ions are moved from the ICF to the ECF and potassium is moved from the ECF to the ICF — basically an ion exchange balancing the concentrations for both molecules. Balance is maintained as solutes, and fluid molecules are evenly distributed on each side of the membrane.

Mechanisms of transport

Method	What is moving	From	To
Passive transport—osmosis	Water Example: water moving out of the endothelial cells lining a vein to dilute a highly concentrated solution (e.g., 3% sodium chloride)	Area of low solute concentration	Area of high solute concentration
Passive transport — diffusion	Molecules and ions Example: oxygen and carbon dioxide moving between the pulmonary capillary and alveoli in the lungs	Area of higher concentration	Area of lower concentration
Passive transport — filtration	Water and solutes Example: fluids, nutrients, and waste products in the capillary bed	Area of higher pressure	Area of lower pressure
Active transport	Any molecule Example: sodium-potassium pump	Area of lower concentration	Area of higher concentration

Notice that different particles move by different mechanisms. Most of the time, this involves a concentration gradient moving from higher to lower or down the gradient. With filtration, pressure causes the movement from higher to lower areas of concentration. In osmosis, water is moving for the purpose of diluting the area with the highest concentration.

Three major forces control this distribution and movement of fluids across the cell membrane:
- cell membrane permeability
- osmotic pressure
- hydrostatic pressure.

The cell membrane's job is to protect what is inside the cell, so this membrane is very selective about what it allows to pass through. The rate of passage or permeability of the cell membrane depends upon the number of layers in the membrane; the amount of protein, lipids, and sugar inside the cell; and by changes in other properties of the membrane that allows passage. Water, oxygen, and other small molecules without an electrical charge move freely across the cell membrane. Large molecules and those with an electrical charge require a little extra help from various proteins on the cell surface.

Fluids, electrolytes, and infusion therapy

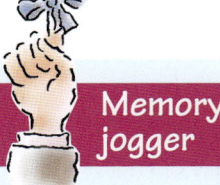

Memory jogger

Remember, diffusion is a descender; active transport is an ascender.

Diffusion descends (high to low)

In **diffusion**, molecules **descend** the concentration gradient. Movement is from an area of **higher** concentration to one of **lower** concentration.

Active transport ascends (low to high)

In **active transport**, molecules **ascend** against the gradient. Movement is from an area of **lower** concentration to an area of **higher** concentration, as if **a**scending.

Oh, osmosis

In osmosis, water is moving across the membrane. The rate of this movement depends upon the number of dissolved solutes, with a higher amount of solutes causing faster osmosis. Water creates pressure, known as osmotic pressure. A greater amount of water moving means a higher osmotic pressure. Oncotic pressure, also known as colloid osmotic pressure, is a form of osmotic pressure that comes from protein, primarily albumin, in the blood or interstitial fluid.

Opposing forces

Hydrostatic pressure opposes oncotic pressure. As the heart pumps blood, it exerts pressure against blood vessel walls. Arteries get smaller as they move away from the heart, becoming arterioles and even smaller capillaries. The capillary bed is where the exchange of nutrients and cellular waste products occur. The arteriole side of the capillary bed exerts hydrostatic pressure (the same as arterial blood pressure) to move nutrients and water out of the bloodstream and into the interstitial fluid by filtration. In the capillary, osmotic pressure remains steady. On the venous side of the capillary, hydrostatic pressure allows fluid and molecules to move from the interstitial space back into the bloodstream.

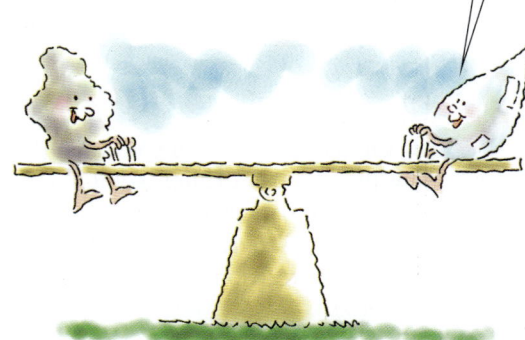

We maintain balance by crossing cell membranes as needed.

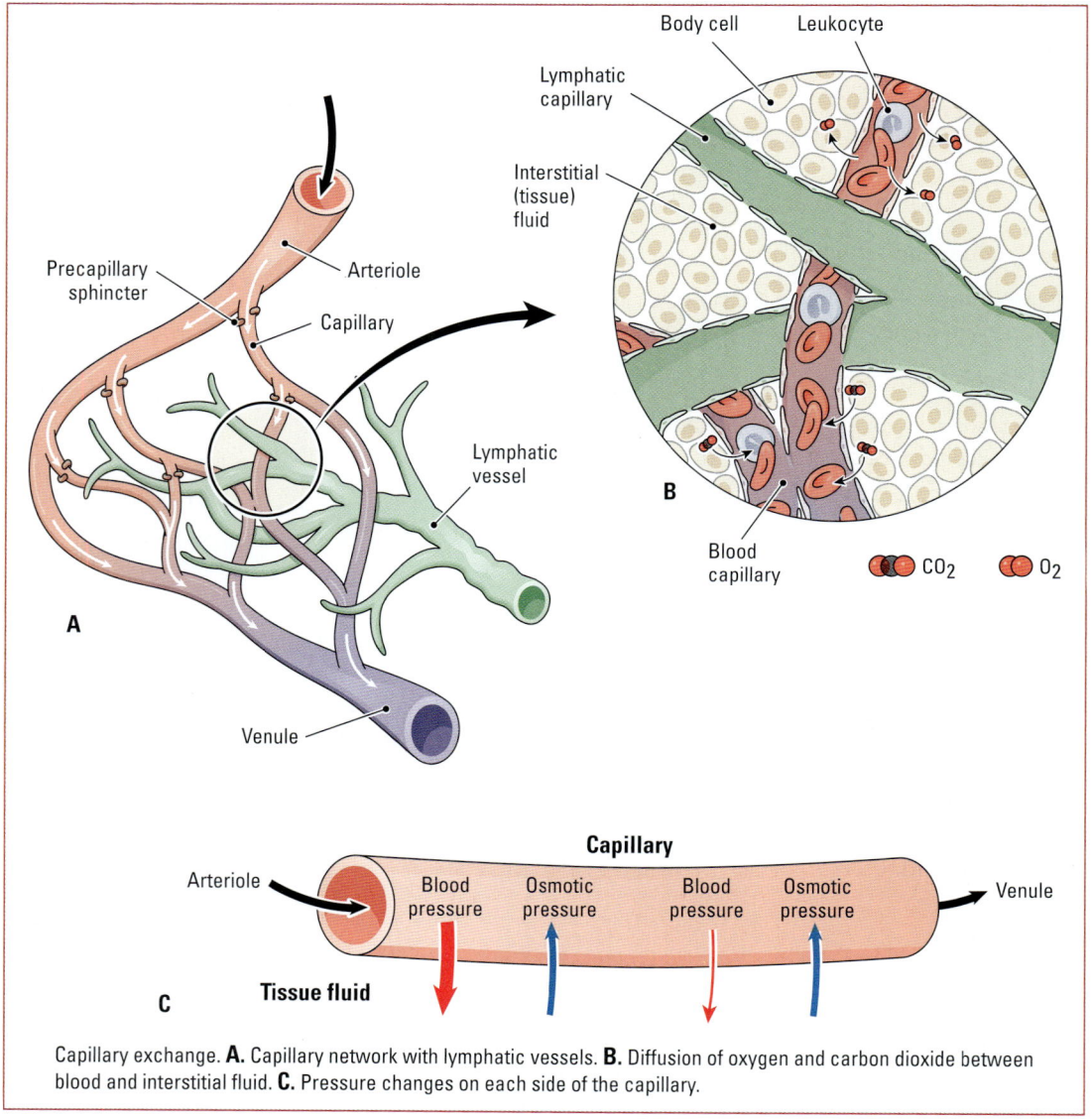

Capillary exchange. **A.** Capillary network with lymphatic vessels. **B.** Diffusion of oxygen and carbon dioxide between blood and interstitial fluid. **C.** Pressure changes on each side of the capillary.

Up against the capillary wall

The capillaries are the only vessel in the vascular system that have walls thin enough to allow solutes to pass. These solutes and water cross the capillary walls by two opposing forces:
1. Capillary filtration
2. Capillary reabsorption

Opposing forces

The net movement of fluid is based on the pressure gradient as the plasma flows from the arterial to the venous end of the capillary. How does this work? At the arterial end of the capillary, the hydrostatic pressure inside the small arteriole is approximately 35 mm Hg. The oncotic pressure exerted by the proteins stays relatively constant at approximately 25 mm Hg because proteins do not normally cross the capillary membrane. At this point, the hydrostatic pressure exceeds oncotic pressure, and it is sufficient to push water across the capillary membrane into the interstitial fluid. Left unchecked, capillary filtration would cause plasma to move in only one direction — out of the capillary. The result would cause severe hypovolemia and shock.

Reabsorption to the rescue

As mentioned earlier, pressure gradients are responsible for the egress and ingress of fluid. As long as capillary hydrostatic pressure exceeds the oncotic pressure, fluids and solutes filter out into the interstitial space. Near the venule end, there's a shift in pressure. The capillary oncotic pressure (stable at 25 mm Hg) exceeds hydrostatic pressure which has dropped to approximately 15 mm Hg. Fluids are attracted back (reabsorbed) into the capillary.

May the force be with you

In any capillary, blood pressure normally exceeds colloid osmotic pressure up to the vessel's midpoint and then falls below colloid osmotic pressure along the rest of the vessel. That's why capillary filtration takes place along the first half of a capillary and reabsorption occurs along the second half. Fortunately, capillary reabsorption keeps capillary filtration in check.

The integrity of the capillary membrane is critical to this balance.

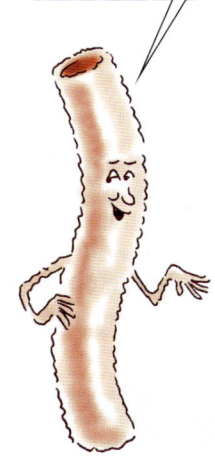

Correcting imbalances

Having spent time understanding how the body maintains fluid and electrolyte balance, let's briefly explore the role of infusion therapy. The effect an I.V. solution has on fluid compartments depends on the solution's osmolarity compared with serum osmolarity

Osmolarity at parity?

Normally, plasma has the same osmolarity as other body fluids: approximately 290 mOsm/L. A lower serum osmolarity suggests overhydration, while an elevated serum osmolarity suggests dehydration. (*See Osmolality vs osmolarity: what's the difference.*)

I.V. fluids are measured by their tonicity, which is the tension of the osmotic pressure of the solutions against the cell wall. I.V. solutions contain solutes such as dextrose that will not pass through the cell wall. These solutes create the force that causes water to move into or out of cells, thus changing their size.

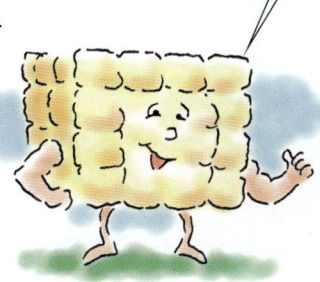

There are three basic types of I.V. solutions:
- isotonic
- hypotonic
- hypertonic. (See *Understanding I.V. solutions,* page 17.)

A few common solutions can be used to illustrate the role of I.V. therapy in restoring and maintaining fluid and electrolyte balance. (See Chapter 4, *Quick guide to I.V. solutions,* for more discussion about composition and characteristics of specific I.V. solutions.)

Isotonic solutions

An isotonic solution has the same osmolarity (or tonicity) as serum and other body fluids. Because the solution doesn't alter serum osmolarity, it stays where it's infused — inside the blood vessel (the intravascular compartment). The solution expands this compartment without pulling fluid from other compartments.

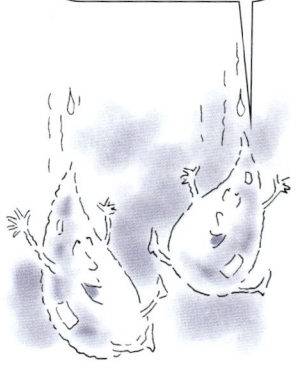

An isotonic solution stays where it's infused — inside the blood vessel.

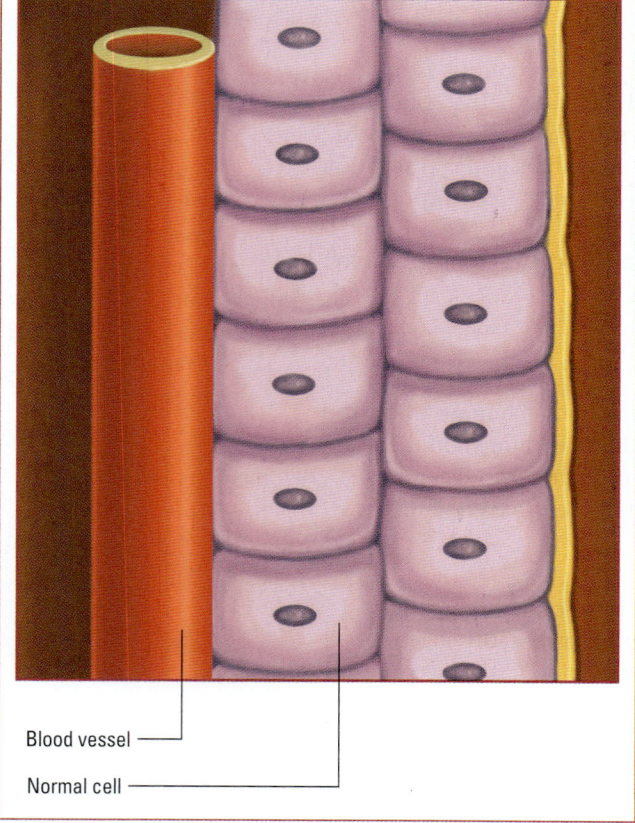

Blood vessel
Normal cell

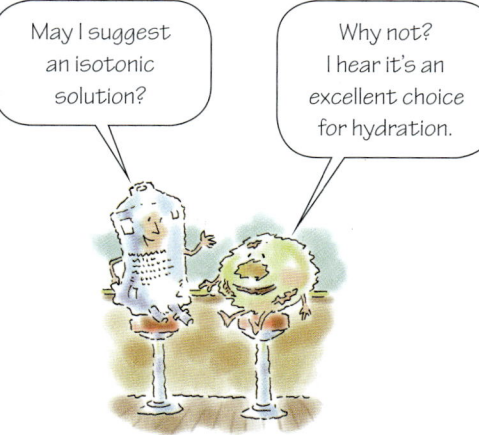

May I suggest an isotonic solution?

Why not? I hear it's an excellent choice for hydration.

That's right. An isotonic solution maintains body fluid balance.

Order up lactated Ringer's for me; we could all use some balance.

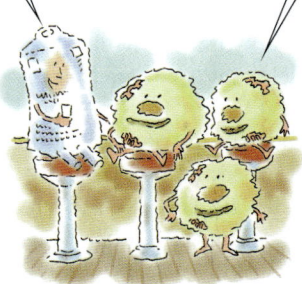

Understanding I.V. solutions

Solutions used for I.V. therapy may be isotonic, hypotonic, or hypertonic. The type you give a patient depends on whether you want to change or maintain his body fluid status.

Isotonic solution

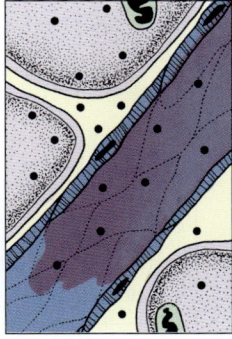

Hypotonic solution

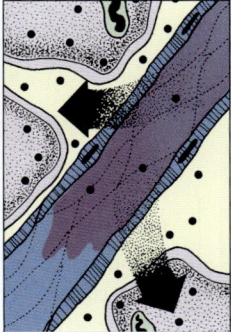

Hypertonic solution

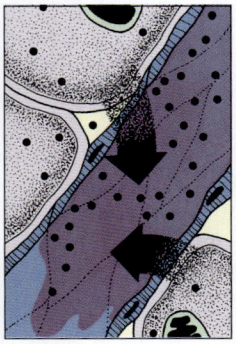

An isotonic solution has an osmolarity about equal to that of serum. Fluid stays in the intravascular space, expanding the intravascular compartment.

A hypotonic solution has an osmolarity lower than that of serum. It shifts fluid out of the intravascular compartment, hydrating the cells and the interstitial compartments.

A hypertonic solution has an osmolarity higher than that of serum. It draws fluid into the intravascular compartment from the cells and the interstitial compartments.

Hypertonic solutions

A hypertonic solution has an osmolarity higher than serum osmolarity. When a patient receives a hypertonic I.V. solution, serum osmolarity initially increases, causing fluid to be pulled from the interstitial and intracellular compartments into the blood vessels.

Introduction to infusion therapy

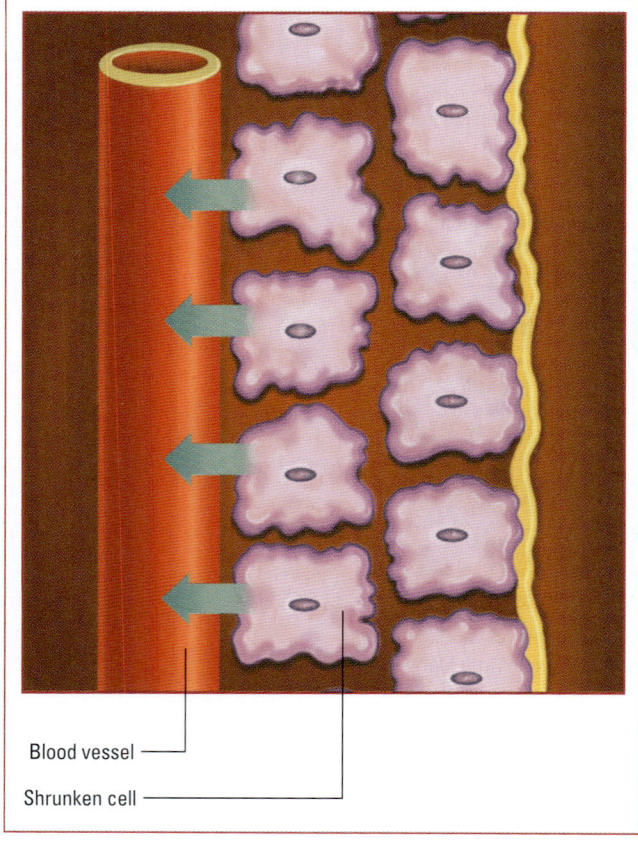

Blood vessel
Shrunken cell

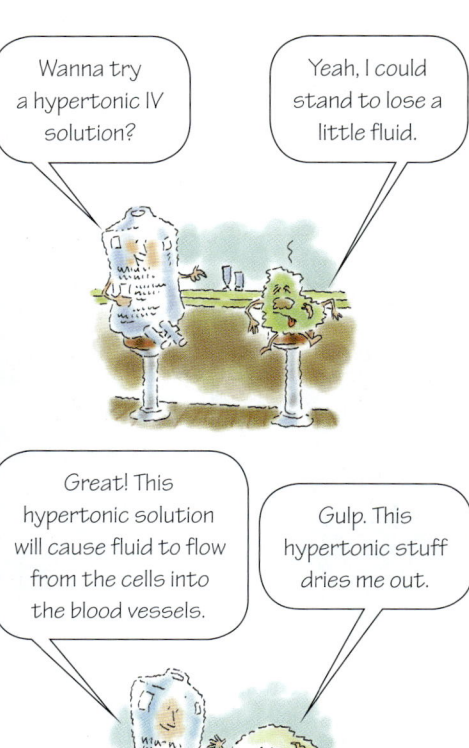

When, why, and how to get hyper

Hypertonic solutions may be ordered for patients postoperatively because the shift of fluid into the blood vessels caused by a hypertonic solution has several beneficial effects for these patients. For example, it:
- reduces the risk of edema
- stabilizes blood pressure
- regulates urine output.

Hypotonic solutions

A hypotonic solution has an osmolarity lower than serum osmolarity. When a patient receives a hypotonic solution, fluid shifts out of the blood vessels and into the cells and interstitial spaces, where osmolarity is higher. A hypotonic solution hydrates cells while reducing fluid in the circulatory system.

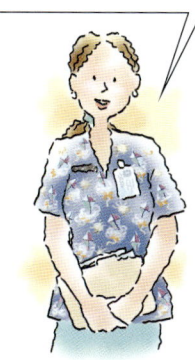

A hypertonic solution causes fluid to be pulled from the interstitial and intracellular compartments into the blood vessels.

Fluids, electrolytes, and infusion therapy

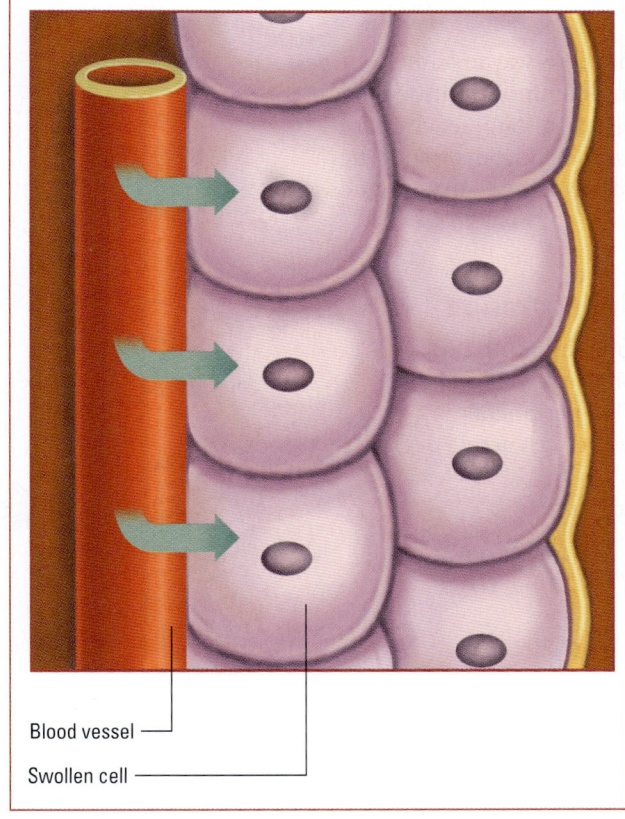

Blood vessel
Swollen cell

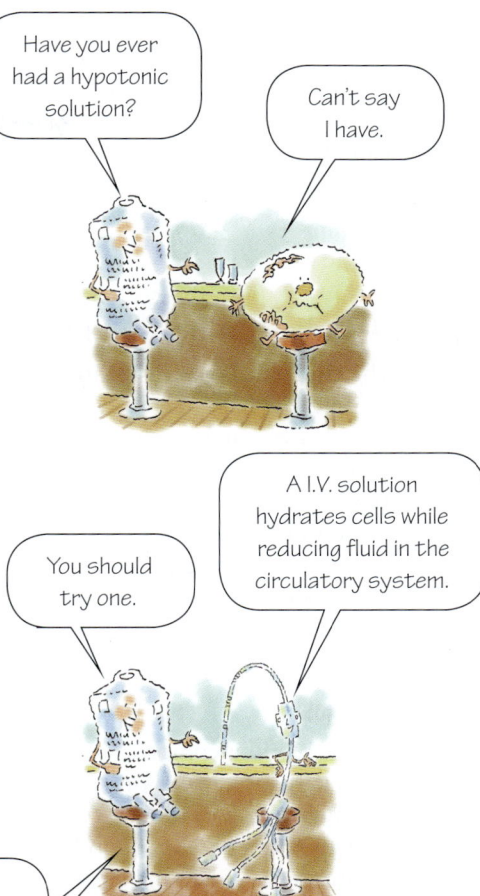

Flood warning
Because hypotonic solutions flood cells, certain patients shouldn't receive them. For example, patients with cerebral edema or increased intracranial pressure shouldn't receive hypotonic solutions because the increased ECF can cause further edema and tissue damage.

Additional types of infusion therapy

Drug administration
The parenteral route enables the administration of medications (see Chapter 4, *Infusion fluids and medication*, page 193), transfusion of blood and blood components (see Chapter 5, *Transfusions*, page 238),

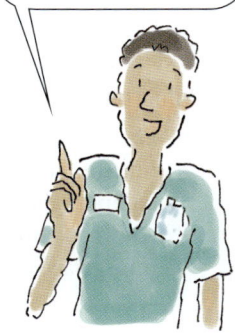

and the delivery of parenteral nutrition (see Chapter 8, *Parenteral nutrition*, page 326).

The I.V. route provides a rapid and efficacious way to administer medications. Depending on the care setting, commonly infused medications may include antibiotics, thrombolytics, histamine receptor antagonists, antineoplastic, cardiovascular, and anticonvulsant drugs delivered as a single dose, intermittently, or as a long-term continuous infusion.

Blood and blood component administration

The clinician's responsibilities may include initiating and monitoring patients receiving transfusion therapy. Blood and blood components may be given through a peripheral vascular access device (PVAD) or a central venous access device (CVAD) to:
- restore and maintain adequate circulatory volume
- prevent cardiogenic shock
- increase the blood's oxygen-carrying capacity
- maintain hemostasis.

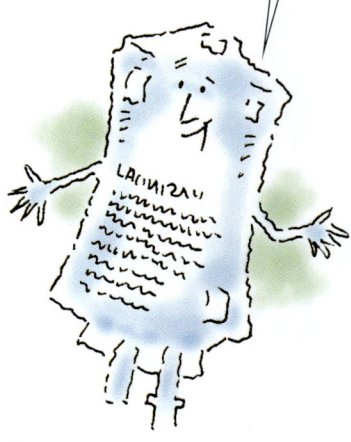

Talk about useful. I'm great for administering drugs, blood and blood products, and parenteral nutrition, too.

Parts of the whole

Whole blood is composed of cellular elements and plasma, packaged separately for transfusion. Cellular elements include:
- erythrocytes or RBCs
- leukocytes or white blood cells (WBCs)
- thrombocytes or platelets
- plasma or plasma derivatives.

Parenteral nutrition

Parenteral nutrition (PN) provides necessary nutrients and calories that are the essence of a balanced diet. If the gastrointestinal tract is working normally, enteral nutrition is best. Parenteral nutrition is indicated when the gastrointestinal tract cannot or should not be used.

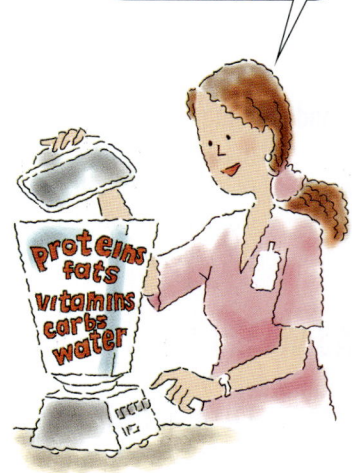

PN is a customized blend that provides all of a patient's energy and nutrient requirements.

It isn't gourmet, but it has all you need…

PN is customized for each patient based on a comprehensive nutritional assessment, their clinical status, fluid and electrolyte balance, and specific goals for PN. The solution will include a combination of proteins, carbohydrates, fats, electrolytes, vitamins, trace elements, and water.

Infusion delivery

Typically, infusion therapy is delivered into a vein, either a peripheral vein of the upper extremity in adults or a central vein in the thorax. Currently, other routes are being used for specific indications:
- Intraosseous (IO) infusion is needed for rapid access in emergent, life-threatening situations when there is no time to locate a peripheral vein. It is also useful for short-term infusion in patients with difficult venous access. The IO device can remain in place for 24 hours, while a more appropriate type of vascular access device is planned and inserted. (See Chapter 2, pages 74–75.)
- Subcutaneous (SC) infusion can be used for continuous administration of isotonic fluids to treat dehydration or for certain medications such as morphine or immune globulins. This route is useful in hospice and palliative care patients when locating and inserting an I.V. catheter may be difficult and painful. Patients receiving intermittent medications by this route may be in home care or other alternative settings. (See Chapter 2, pages 75–76.)
- Intraspinal infusion may be into the epidural space, intrathecal directly in contact with the spinal cord, and intraventricular into the ventricular cerebrospinal fluid.
- Other routes include intra-arterial, intraperitoneal, and intrapleural.

Know where each infusion is going! Don't assume all catheters are infusing into a vein.

Peripheral or central vein?

Intravenous infusion therapy may be delivered through one of two routes: peripheral or central veins. The national standard is selection of the least invasive vascular access device (VAD), with the smallest outer diameter and the fewest number of lumens for the therapy prescribed. The decision is based on a careful decision-making process after a thorough assessment including:
- the current prescribed type(s) of infusion therapy
- the length of infusion therapy and any anticipated changes such as extension or changes of antibiotics after culture results are known
- the patient's age, current medical diagnosis, and other chronic conditions
- the patient's history of vascular access and changes to the vascular anatomy and blood flow due to disease, trauma, and surgical alterations

- the care setting and the ability of staff and/or patient (that is, home care) to administer the infusion therapy and care for the VAD.

Inappropriate use of CVADs can be a significant problem as they are more invasive and associated with a greater risk of more severe complications. Indications for their use includes:
- solutions with an osmolarity greater than 900 mOsm/L
- episodic antineoplastic treatment greater than 3-month duration
- continuous infusion therapy such as PN and certain medications such as inotropic agents or high concentrations of potassium chloride
- long-term intermittent infusion therapy (for example, anti-infective drugs)
- pulmonary arterial monitoring
- history of failed or difficult peripheral venous access, especially if use of ultrasound guidance has failed.

(See Chapter 2, *Infusion Therapy Using Peripheral Veins* and Chapter 3, *Infusion Therapy Requiring Central Venous Access*.)

Delivery methods

There are three basic methods for delivering infusion therapy that are used alone or in combination:
- Continuous infusion therapy provides a carefully regulated amount of fluid infusing constantly over an extended period of time (for example, days or even weeks for some patients).
- Intermittent infusions are medications (for example, antibiotic) given over a short infusion time (for example, 30 to 120 minutes) at set intervals like every 6, 8, or 12 hours.
- Push injection is a manual injection of a medication from a syringe connected to the VAD.

"I.V. bolus" is often used interchangeably with these terms; however, this should refer to any solution given rapidly over a short period of time. This could be a 2- to 3-mL dose of a medication injected over a few seconds or a liter of I.V. fluid infused over 10 to 15 minutes.

Veins used in infusion therapy

This illustration shows the veins commonly used for peripheral and central venous access.

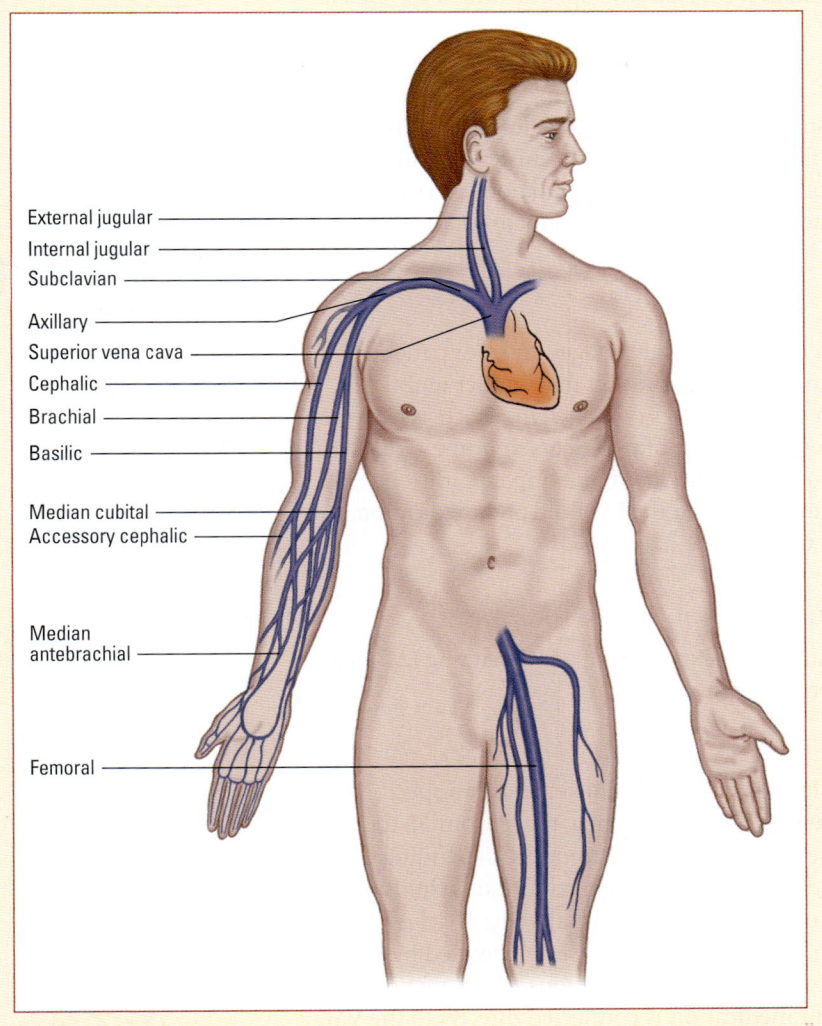

Continuous infusion

Continuous infusion provides a constant and steady infusion of fluids, electrolytes, and/or medications. The goal may be to ensure a consistent infusion of fluid and electrolytes to correct a serious imbalance or to maintain a constant therapeutic drug level such as heparin.

Upside...

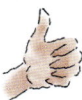

The advantages of continuous infusion include less time to initiate and monitor the fluid flow instead of administering multiple intermittent medications. The risk of contamination is less because all connections on the entire system should remain intact without manipulation.

...and downside

Continuous infusion has some disadvantages, too. For patients, the infusion pump and administration set may hinder mobility and interfere with other activities of daily living such as early ambulation in the hospital or work for patients in home care. If an electronic infusion pump is not used, the drip rate must be carefully monitored to ensure that the I.V. fluid and medication don't infuse too rapidly or too slowly.

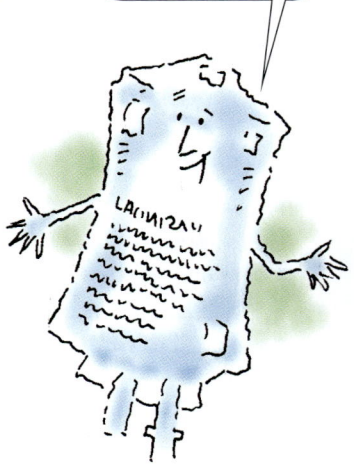

Don't disconnect me until it is time to change the administration set!

Intermittent infusion

The most common and flexible method of administering I.V. medications is by intermittent infusion.

On again, off again

In intermittent infusion, drugs are administered over a specified period at varying intervals. The volume may range from 50 to 250 mL and are usually delivered over 30 to 120 minutes, depending on the medication's required infusion rate. When continuous fluids are infusing, the intermittent medication is usually piggybacked into the primary line for both gravity flow and infusion regulated by an electronic infusion device (EID). When continuous fluids are not being given, the intermittent medication is connected directly to the VAD hub or a short extension set attached to the hub.

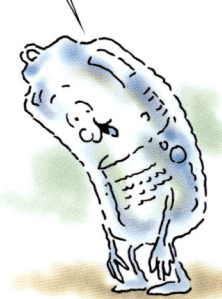

I can be flexible. Use intermittent infusion to administer drugs over short periods at varying intervals.

Push or direct injection

An I.V. push is used for direct manual administration of a medication from a syringe. The medication may be connected to any peripheral or central VAD that has been locked with an appropriate locking solution such as saline or heparin. Or it may be administered using an injection port on the administration set of a continuous infusion. When administering I.V. push medications this way, use the injection port closest (proximal) to the patient unless it is contraindicated or not available such as during a sterile procedure.

The infusion system

The complete infusion system begins with the solution container and includes the correct administration set, necessary add-on devices, and a flow control device.

Start at the top — the solution container

Solution containers include flexible plastic bags, semirigid plastic bottles, glass bottles, and syringes. Plastic bags are the most common container used today; they are a collapsible closed container and do not require venting and have less breakage and weight; and disposal is easier. There is concern about chemicals added to some types of plastics. These chemicals, known as Di[2-ethylhexyl] phthalate (DEHP), soften the plastic, making it more flexible and durable. But they are known to increase risk for some patients, especially neonates and pediatrics, when the chemical leaches from the container into the solution.

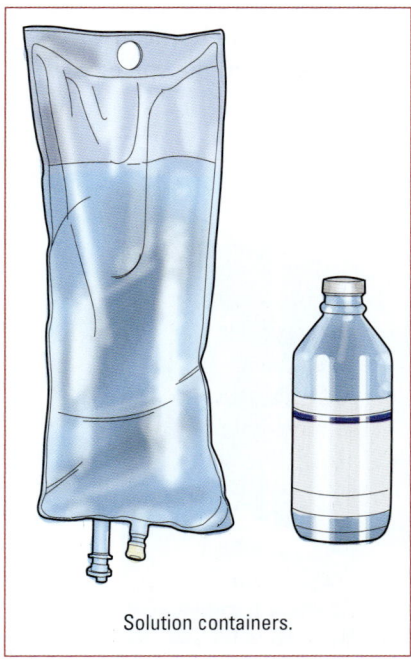

Solution containers.

Glass bottles are used when the solution is incompatible with plastic such as some I.V. fat emulsions. Glass and semirigid plastic bottles require venting making them an open container with an increased risk of contamination from the air entering the container. When using a glass or semirigid solution container, the administration set must have a vent, which is a filtered port near the spike that allows air to enter and displace fluid.

A syringe is used to hold the drug for a manual I.V. push or may be loaded into a syringe pump. Syringes, with their limited volume capacity, is the vehicle of choice for neonatology, pediatrics, and in some adult settings where delivery of low volumes of solution are required.

Administration sets

Administration sets are attached to the solution container by a long spike pushed through a designated port on the container. Sets come in a wide variety of configurations such as the length of the set, the size of the drop known as the drop factor, and the number of injection ports. A macrodrop set may provide 10, 15, or 20 drops per mL, while a microdrop set provides 60 drops per mL. Some infusion pumps require an administration set designed exclusively for that pump, while others allow for the use of any administration set. If infusing from a glass or semirigid bottle, use only an administration set with a vent located between the spike and the drip chamber.

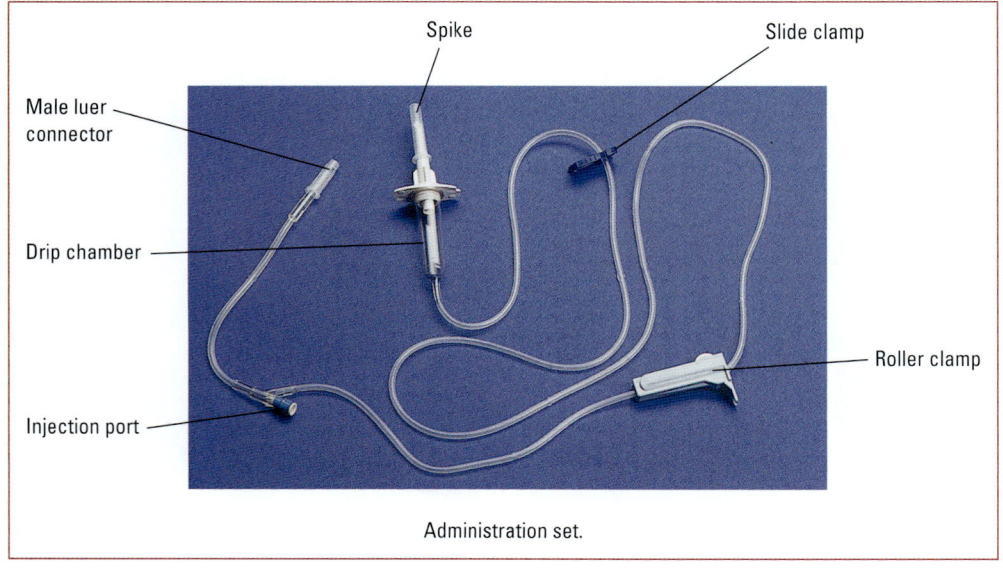

Administration set.

All connections on the infusion system are required to be a luer-locking design. The center portion of the male tip is pushed into female side of the catheter hub, and then a locking collar is tightened around the catheter hub. This type of connection reduces the risk of accidental disconnections, which would increase the risk of organisms and air to enter the lumen or bleeding from the catheter lumen.

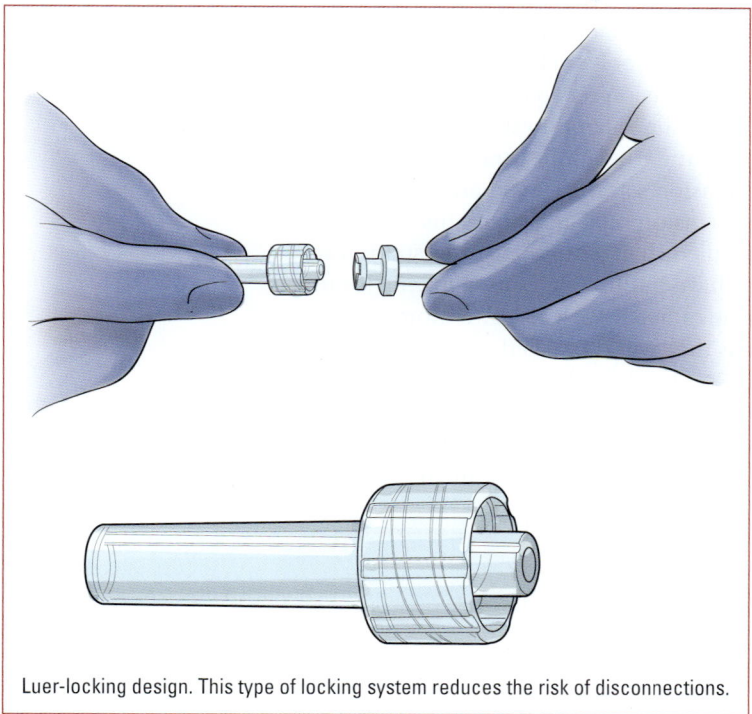

Luer-locking design. This type of locking system reduces the risk of disconnections.

Some components of the administration set are sterile and some are not. Inspect the set as you open the package to ensure that the caps on both ends are secure. The spike and the male luer end of the set are sterile along with the internal fluid pathway, but the outside of the set is not sterile.

Make the right connection

Administration sets used for all types of infusions have the same luer-locking connection as many other types of tubing, such as oxygen tubing and blood pressure cuffs. Mistakes when making connections have been documented to pose a tremendous risk for patients. Frequent disconnection of continuous administration sets not only increases the risk of contamination and infection but it also could mean that the set is not reconnected correctly. Anytime disconnection and reconnection is required, always trace the set from the VAD to the fluid container, and read all labels to ensure the correct connection.

Add-on devices

This group of devices includes a wide variety of extension sets, filters, and stopcocks and serves many patient needs. Adding these devices to the administration set adds risk of contamination because there are additional points of connection in the system, allowing for greater manipulation and increasing the risk of contamination. It is better to use an administration set of the desired length and with the additional devices built into the set rather than adding these pieces.

Extension sets may be needed for extra length. Care for a short peripheral catheter with an extension set attached to its hub will be easier. The extension set has a slide clamp to stop the backflow of blood and reduce your exposure. The administration set is connected at the distal end of the extension set, reducing manipulation of the catheter in the vein. The extension set usually remains on the peripheral catheter making scheduled changes of the administration set easier. Extension sets may have multiple lumens, allowing for multiple infusions through one catheter. Pay close attention to compatibility of these solutions as they will mix together inside the catheter lumen. A longer extension set may be added to a midline or peripherally inserted central catheter for home care patients. This allows the patient to hold the extension set hub while connecting the syringes and administration set for self-administration of medication.

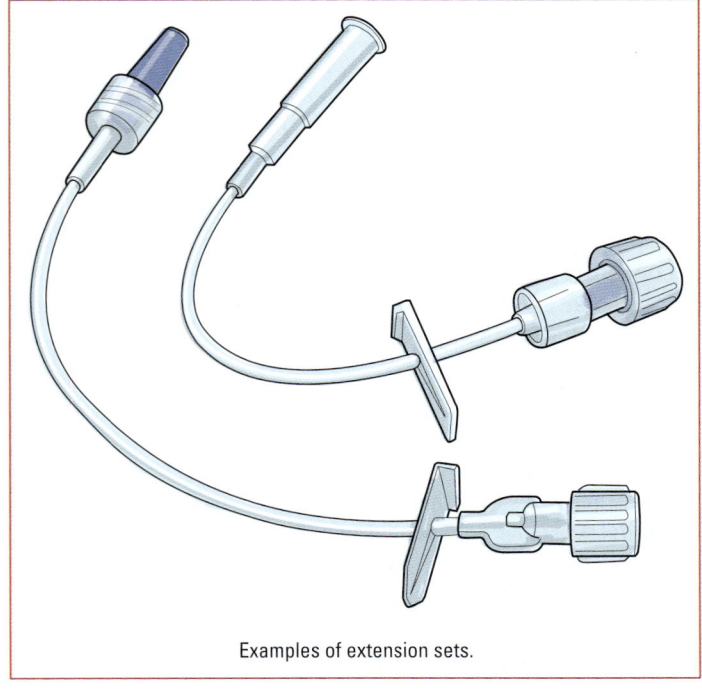

Examples of extension sets.

Stopcocks are used for connecting multiple infusions to the catheter and to direct the fluid flow from one infusion at a time. When the administration set or syringe is detached from the stopcock, they remain an open port and require covering with a new sterile cap. Frequently, the lumen remains open making stopcocks a known risk for contamination and subsequent bloodstream infection. New designs of stopcocks have a needleless connector bonded to each port, closing each side when the set or syringe is disconnected. The use of stopcocks are often seen in operating rooms and critical care and trauma settings but should be removed from the infusion system as soon as possible.

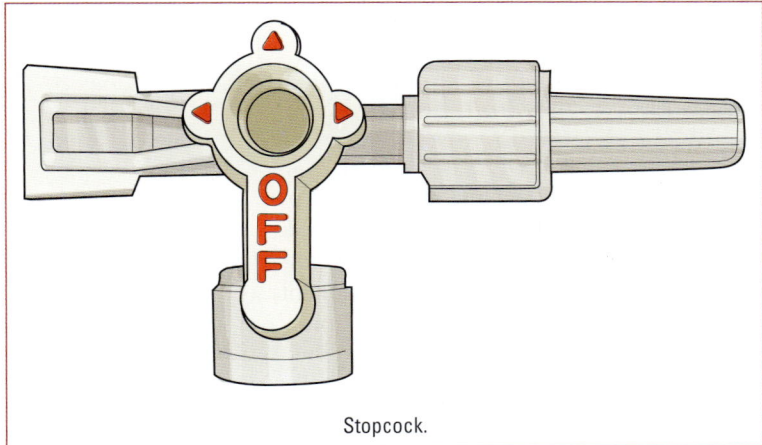

Stopcock.

In-line filters

In-line filters may be built into the administration set or be a device added to the set. In-line filters remove pathogens, air, and particles, thus potentially reducing the risk of infection and other complications. Air escapes through venting in the filter housing. Filters are needed with certain fluid infusions such as parenteral nutrition and I.V. fat emulsion. (*See more in* Chapter 8, *Parenteral Nutrition*.) Some medications require filtration during preparation in the pharmacy or during infusion; however, in-line filters are not currently used for the majority of fluids and medications. Some medications will not pass through the filter, and very small medication volumes may also be trapped in the filter, preventing the patient from receiving the medication. The use of an in-line filter should also be considered in critically ill patients as this has been associated with a decrease in complications. In pediatric patients, the use of an in-line filter has been associated with a decrease in systemic inflammatory response syndrome (SIRS). Follow instructions provided on the fluid or medication label or contact the pharmacy if you have questions about filter use.

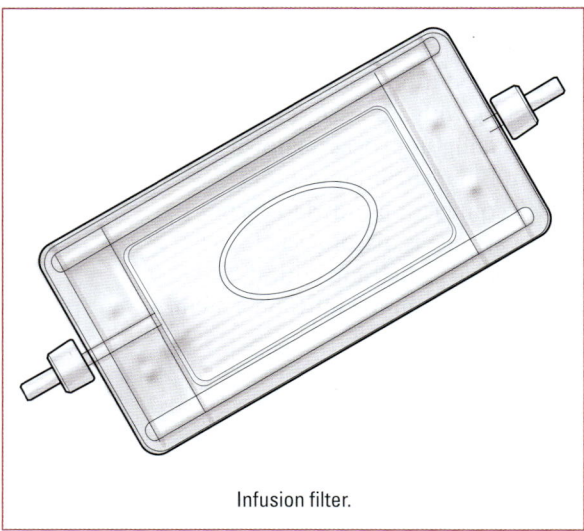

Infusion filter.

The filter is labeled by the size of the pore openings and prevents particles larger than this size from passing through. Common sizes include 0.2 micron, 1.2 microns, and 5 microns; thus, the size of the drug molecule directs what filter size may be used. Blood and blood components require filtration; however, the pore sizes for blood filters ranges from 170 to 260 microns. (See Chapter 5, *Transfusions*.)

Follow your facility's guidelines for using in-line filters and remember these additional points:
- Most in-line filters can be used with an infusion pump, but make sure that it can withstand the pump's infusion pressure.
- When added to the administration set, the filter should be located close to the patient.
- Carefully prime the in-line filter to eliminate all the air from it, following the manufacturer's directions.

Needleless connectors

Needleless connectors (NCs) attach to the female hub of vascular access device (VAD) or extension set to allow easy intermittent access to the system. They are also built onto all injection ports of the administration set. Their purpose is to eliminate the use of needles and protect clinicians from needlestick injuries. The downside is that they are a source for contamination due to a variety of design issues, but there is no evidence about which design poses the least risk for contamination. Strict disinfection protocols are needed to reduce the patient's risk of infection. Current evidence and practice standards require disinfection by thoroughly scrubbing the connection surface before each entry into the system.

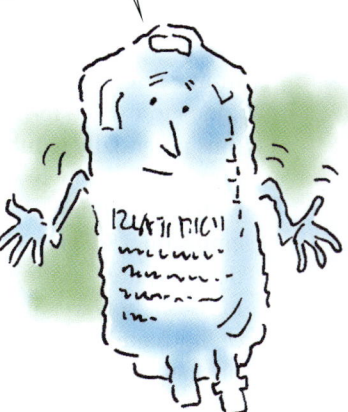

I don't like pathogens and particles. That's why I hooked up with an in-line filter.

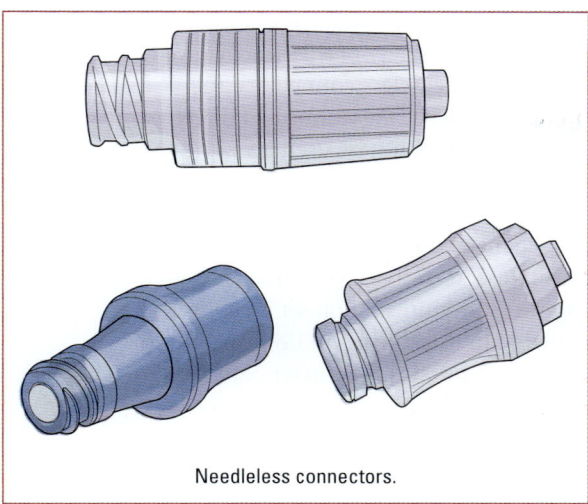

Needleless connectors.

Disinfection can be accomplished by manual and passive methods. Manual disinfection involves using a pad with 70% isopropyl alcohol, povidone-iodine, or alcoholic chlorhexidine and vigorously scrubbing the connection surface. The length of scrub time varies between 5 and 60 seconds, depending on the NC being used. Follow your facility's policy and procedures.

Passive disinfection involves the use of a plastic cap containing alcohol. This cap is placed on the needleless connector immediately after each use. The alcohol bathes all surfaces to disinfect it and protect from body fluids, skin oils, and other contaminants in the area. When the next intermittent medication is to be administered, this cap is removed and discarded. At this point, the needleless connector can be safely entered without additional scrubbing; however, each subsequent entry requires manual disinfection. Therefore, it is necessary to scrub between the saline flush, the medication administration, and the additional flushing and locking solutions.

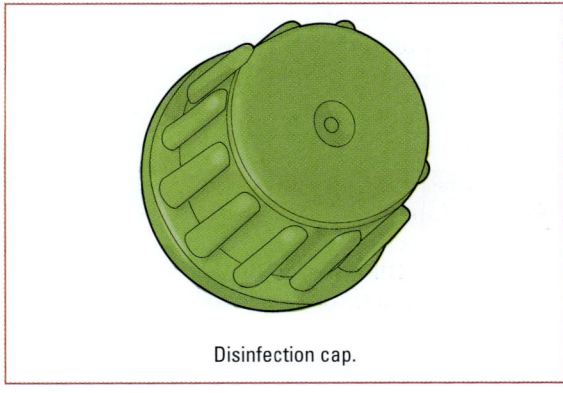

Disinfection cap.

Attaching a needleless connector directly to the VAD hub for continuous infusion is a controversial issue. The safety of this practice is unknown. Prior to the introduction of needleless connectors, the male luer-locking end of the administration set was connected directly to the VAD hub. Needleless connectors should not be used for rapid infusion of I.V. solutions or when red blood cells are being transfused as they slow down the infusion rate.

Needleless connectors are to be changed no more frequently than every 96 hours. If they are placed on the VAD hub for continuous infusion, they must be changed when the I.V. administration set is changed.

Needleless connectors are available in three different designs, and when you close the clamp is critical to maintaining catheter patency. Just looking at the device will not provide the information you need about how the device works, so check the manufacturer's instructions for use and your facility's policy and procedures.

- Negative fluid displacement NC causes blood to reflux back into the catheter lumen when the syringe is disconnected. Continue to hold pressure on the syringe plunger, then close the clamp on the catheter or extension set, then disconnect the syringe.
- Positive fluid displacement NC holds a small volume of extra fluid inside. When the syringe is disconnected, the internal mechanism moves this fluid toward the catheter lumen, thus moving any blood out of the catheter lumen and back into the bloodstream. For this type, give the flushing and locking solution, disconnect the final syringe allowing time for this fluid displacement to occur, and then close the clamp on the catheter or extension set.
- Neutral displacement NCs are designed to reduce the backflow of blood into the catheter lumen. With this type, you can clamp and disconnect in any sequence.

Most NCs have an open internal fluid pathway, while the administration set is attached to it, allowing blood to move into the catheter lumen. As soon as the intermittent infusion is complete, the set should be removed and the VAD flushed and locked. Another type of NC is known as an antireflux valve that works by a pressure-sensitive mechanism. As soon as the solution container is empty, pressure from infusing fluid is no longer present. This device automatically closes preventing blood from moving into the catheter lumen although the administration set is still attached.

Infusion flow rates

A key aspect of administering infusions is maintaining accurate flow rates for the prescribed solutions. If an infusion runs too fast or too slow, your patient may suffer complications like circulatory overload and adverse drug reactions. Flow control devices and the correct administration set help prevent such complications.

Many factors may affect fluid flow including the inner diameter and length of the VAD, a change in the VAD's position in the vein, size of the vein lumen, infusion pressure and solution temperature that can produce vasoconstriction, length of administration set, and height of the solution container.

Flow control devices include manual, mechanical, and electronic methods.

- Manual devices are slide clamps, roller clamps, and flow regulators. The slide clamp can stop or start the flow but can't regulate the rate. Roller clamps and flow regulators are the least accurate device with rates varying by + or −25%. Flow with these devices depends upon gravity, and the solution container should be 3 to 4 feet above the patient.
- Mechanical devices include elastomeric balloon, spring-based, and negative-pressure pumps used for low risk infusions primarily in home care. Flow rates are controlled by mechanical means such as the size of the opening between the fluid container and the attached administration set.
- Electronic infusion devices (EID) include infusion pumps of all types. Large, pole-mounted pumps use precise technology to measure and regulate fluid volume and flow rate. Syringe pumps are included in this category along with smaller ambulatory EIDs more frequently seen in home care. Many EIDs include dose error reduction software for reduction of medication administration errors.

The decision about which type of flow control is best for your patient is determined by the patient's age, the characteristics of the infusion therapy, and the care setting. Follow your facility's policy and procedure to ensure correct selection for flow control.

Gravity flow rate calculation

When gravity flow will be regulated by a manual device such as a roller clamp, the flow rate must be calculated. You must know the drop factor for the administration set to be used — macrodrop and microdrop. Each set delivers a specific number of drops per milliliter (gtt/mL). Macrodrop sets deliver 10, 15, or 20 gtt/mL, and microdrop sets deliver 60 gtt/mL.

Regardless of the type of administration set used, the same formula is used to calculate the flow rate for administering the infusion solution by gravity flow. (See *Calculating flow rates,* page 34.)

Calculating flow rates

When calculating the I.V. solution flow rate (drops per minute), remember that the number of drops required to deliver 1 mL is dependent on the manufacturer's design and the type of administration set:
- Administration sets are of two types — macrodrip (the standard type) and microdrip. Macrodrip delivers 10, 15, or 20 gtt/mL; microdrip usually delivers 60 gtt/mL (see illustrations).
- Manufacturers calibrate their devices differently, so be sure to look for the "drop factor" — expressed in drops per milliliter or gtt/mL as indicated on the packaging.

This packaging also has crucial information about such things as special infusions and blood transfusions.

Once the device's drop factor is known, use the following formula to calculate specific flow rates:
Formula for calculating the flow rate using **macrodrip tubing**:

$$\text{gtt/min} = \frac{\text{gtt/mL (drop factor) of set} \times \text{total hourly volume (mL)}}{60 \text{ minutes}}$$

Calculating flow rate using **microdrip tubing**.

For microdrip tubing, the **number of gtts per minute equals the number of mL/hour.**

After you calculate the flow rate for the set to be used, take a watch and place it next to the drip chamber to count the drops and the seconds at the same time. Adjust the clamp to achieve the ordered flow rate and count the drops for **one full minute**. Readjust the clamp as necessary and count the drops for another minute. Keep adjusting the clamp and counting the drops until the correct rate is established.

Macrodrip 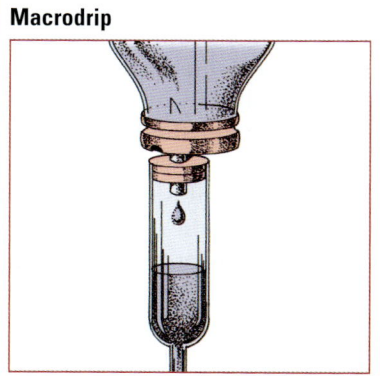 **Microdrip**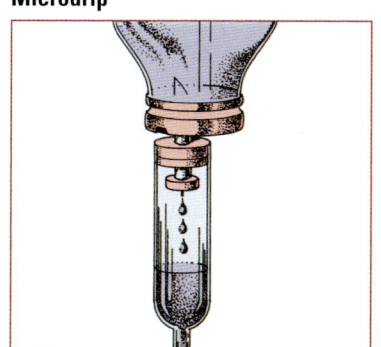

Passive disinfection device for a needleless connector.

Regulating flow rates

After calculating the flow rate for a gravity infusion, the roller clamp or flow regulator is used to adjust the fluid flow. For the roller clamp, it is best to close it completely and slowly roll it upward while counting the drops per minute. When the correct flow rate is verified, leave the roller clamp is in that position. For a manual flow regulator, do not rely on the numbers printed on the dial; counting drops per minute is still necessary to ensure the flow rate is as close to accurate as possible. Changing the distance between the patient's VAD and the fluid container can alter these set flow rates, so the patient may need assistance for getting out of bed or ambulating. Also, move the roller clamp as high as possible on the administration set so that patient movement will have the least impact on the roller clamp's position.

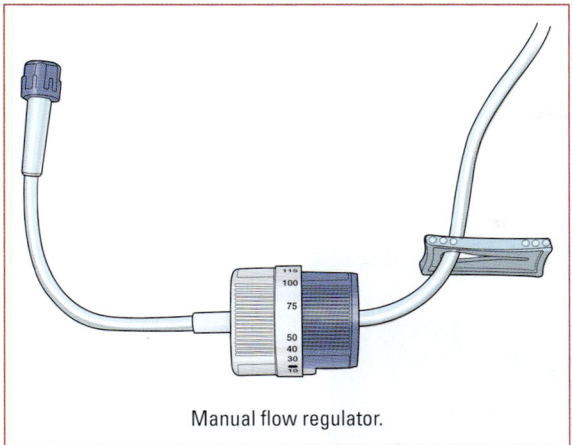
Manual flow regulator.

When using a mechanical pump, know the specific mechanism of how the device works. For most of them, simply opening the clamp on the attached I.V. administration set is all that is needed. Elastomeric balloon pumps contain a collapsed balloon inside the hard outer case. The prescribed medication is added to expand the balloon to its full capacity. The administration set is permanently attached to the device. Fluid flow rate is regulated to the size of the opening where the set is attached to the balloon and the collapsing balloon provides the force to cause infusion. The patient or family caregiver only has to attach the set to the VAD hub and open the clamp, making this an easy device for home infusion.

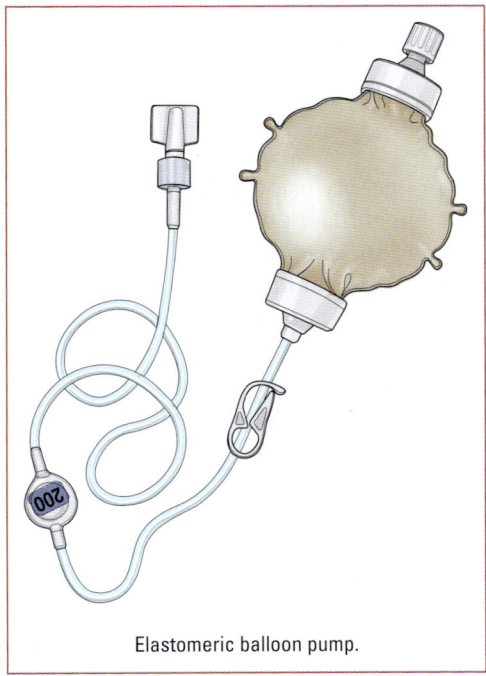
Elastomeric balloon pump.

EIDs are regularly used in a number of facilities to closely control fluid volumes. There should always be an anti-free flow mechanism to stop the fluid flow when the pump door is opened and/or the set is removed from the pumping mechanism. Usually, the set can be regulated manually if necessary while it is out of the pump.

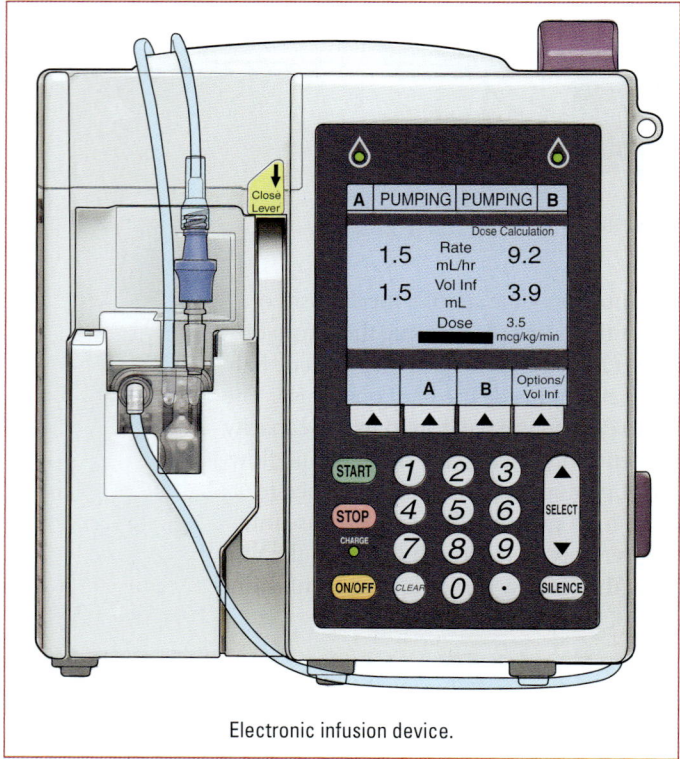

Electronic infusion device.

Alarms on these pumps include air-in-line, occlusion, infusion complete, and low battery. But remember that none of these alarms will indicate the exact fluid pathway, so assess the VAD and surrounding site to rule out infiltration. The pump may also allow automatic programming that will ramp up or taper off flow rates over time. Infusion pumps with dose-error reduction software are commonly called "smart pumps." The software contains drug libraries, preset in conjunction with the facility's pharmacy to reduce risk of error. The drug libraries include minimum and maximum rates for infusion for each drug, clinician information, and lockout features to prevent clinicians from inventing ways to work around these safeguards.

When programming an EID, you will need to enter the rate of infusion in mL/hour and the volume to be infused which is usually the amount of fluid in the solution container. Some EIDs allow for control of multiple infusion simultaneously so you may be entering this information for the primary fluid and the secondary medication. Smart pumps may also allow entering medications doses in milligrams per hour or some other metric. Ensure that you have a thorough understanding of how to program the pump you are using. While counting drops is not necessary, you should still frequently assess the volume of fluid remaining in the container as a check on the accuracy of the infusion pump.

Technological advances result in new and more advanced pumps available for clinician's use. Professional practice responsibilities require clinicians to attend all training sessions to gain confidence and competence in using EIDs and to keep instruction and resource manuals handy. A best practice is to secure an instruction manual to the device wherever possible. Maintaining the infusion involves planning and delivering care to prevent problems, plus frequent assessment of the patient to identify complications and treat them early.

mL/hour or gtt/minute?

When regulating an I.V. flow rate with a roller clamp, the rate is usually measured in drops per minute (gtt/minute). The numbers printed on a flow regulator represent milliliters per hour, but counting drops per minute is also required. Flow rate for an EID is programmed into the pump as milliliters per hour (mL/hour). Always verify how the flow rate is calculated on any device or administration set that will be used.

Infusion orders

Lastly, familiarize yourself with all of the information in the orders from the licensed independent practitioner (LIP) and be able to identify incomplete or incorrectly written infusion therapy orders. Fluid flow rate for continuous infusion is required in the LIP written order. An order that simply state "keep vein open" or KVO is not sufficient because there is no magic rate of flow that will ensure the catheter will remain open and patent (see *Reading an I.V. order*).

Orders for infusion therapy may be standardized for different illnesses and therapies or written for each patient. Patient care should be individualized; however, standing patient order sets or an approved written protocol are acceptable methods for some infusion therapy orders. Some facility policies dictate an automatic stop order for infusions (for example, I.V. fluids are in effect for 24 hours from the time they're written, unless otherwise specified).

Reading an infusion order

It's complete when the following is included:
- route (remember not all infusion therapy is given through a vein)
- type and amount of solution
- rate in mL/hour or a specific volume over a specific number of hours
- any medications with specific dose to be added to the solution (for example, 10 mEq potassium chloride in 500 mL 5% dextrose in water).

For intermittent infusion medication orders, look for:
- medication name, preferably generic or both generic and trade name
- route
- dose.
- Frequency of administration

The dilution of each medication and the rate of administration are usually determined by the pharmacy based on drug manufacturer instructions. So don't expect to see this information in the order unless there is a special circumstance.

When it isn't complete
If the LIP's order is incomplete, or if the clinician determines the I.V. order is inappropriate for the patient's condition, consult with the LIP. You may first need to review the literature on the specific drug and/or consult with the pharmacy for more information.

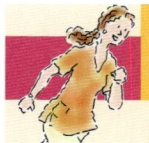

Running smoothly

Using I.V. clamps

A roller clamp may be used to regulate the flow of a solution. With this type of clamp, a wheel increases or decreases the flow rate through the administration site. A slide clamp moves horizontally to open and close the I.V. line. It can stop and start the flow but doesn't allow adjustments for drop regulation. The illustrations below show both types of clamps, with arrows to indicate the direction you turn or push to open the clamp.

Roller clamp

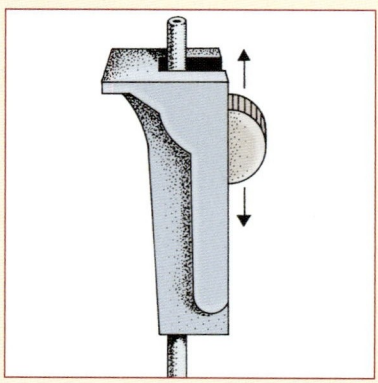

Slide clamp

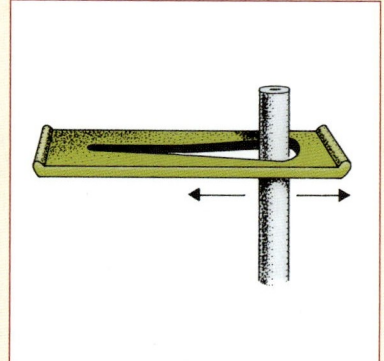

Factor these in

Flow rate must be monitored closely and adjusted as needed for all methods of flow control. Such factors as vein spasm, vein pressure changes, patient movement, manipulations of the clamp, and bent or kinked set can cause the rate to vary markedly. For easy monitoring, use a time tape, which marks the prescribed solution level at hourly intervals. (See *Using a time tape,* page 40.) The frequency of flow rate checks depends on the patient's condition and age and the solution or medication being administered.

I'll be back soon!

Many clinicians check the I.V. flow rate every time they're in a patient's room and after each position change. There are different risk factors for infusion through a short peripheral catheter versus a central VAD. Frequent assessment of infusion through a short peripheral catheter is necessary to protect patients by early identification of complications. Toward that end, the Infusion Nurses Society recommends the following frequency for site assessment which includes the entire infusion system and flow rate:
- for patients who are alert and oriented and receiving nonirritating and nonvesicant infusions — a minimum of every 4 hours
- for critically ill patients, those receiving sedatives or have cognitive alteration, and infusion sites at areas of joint flexion — every 1 to 2 hours
- for neonates and pediatrics — every hour
- for patients receiving vesicant medications — every 5 to 10 minutes. For these types of infusion, the clinician should encourage insertion of a central VAD.

Start at one end and work to the other

Assessment requires checking all aspects of the system. Inspect and palpate the I.V. insertion site, and ask the patient how it feels. Check the integrity of the VAD dressing and all signs and symptoms of complications. Work up the entire infusion system, checking all connections, the flow control device, and the solution container for correct flow rate and fluid level. Check all labels for when the container, set, and dressing should be changed.

Minor (not major) adjustments

The use of EIDs for flow control is now very prevalent among health care facilities of all types. They provide a more accurate rate of infusion and reduce risk associated with over or under infusion. Roller clamps and other manual flow regulators are simply not as accurate and require frequent assessment of the fluid level in the container and counting drops to ensure on-time delivery. A situation of having to catch up or slow down the infusion should always be prevented.

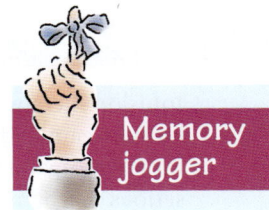

Memory jogger

To remind yourself of the need to check and adjust flow rates, remember the following tongue twister:

Fight fickle flow with frequent follow-up.

Professional and legal standards

Infusion therapy can be a risky business! Placing a catheter into the bloodstream and infusing solutions and medications create a conduit for microorganisms along with the fluid. The catheter can produce serious mechanical complications depending upon the insertion site, placement techniques, and the routine maintenance to care for the catheter. Medications are associated with significant adverse reactions, both local and systemic.

Know your responsibility

Health professionals have a legal and ethical responsibility to their patients. As technology and knowledge advance and health care environments change, the clinician is still required to adhere to standards of care, defined as reasonable and prudent patient care based on the specific circumstances. The standard of care has four characteristics:
- It must be a reasonable expectation given the level of knowledge and skill of the clinician. For example, a beginning clinician would not be responsible for insertion of a peripherally inserted central catheter (PICC); however, using the PICC to administer fluid and medication plus appropriate dressing changes would be part of the job for a new clinician after your competency is documented.
- Care provided is measurable based on evaluation of the individual's performance.
- Care is appropriate based on where the care is provided. There are state-based variations in rules and regulations for some aspects of infusion therapy.
- It must be based on the current state of knowledge. Practice evolves because research provides new evidence.

Follow the rules!

Health care practice is governed by numerous federal and state/province laws and agencies.

Federal regulations

In the United States, the federal government issues regulations and establishes policies related to infusion therapy administration. For example, the Occupational Safety and Health Administration (OSHA) established standards to protect all health care workers from bloodborne pathogens by requiring use of safety engineered devices that reduce needlestick injury and blood exposure. The Food and Drug Administration (FDA) regulates the drugs and devices that can

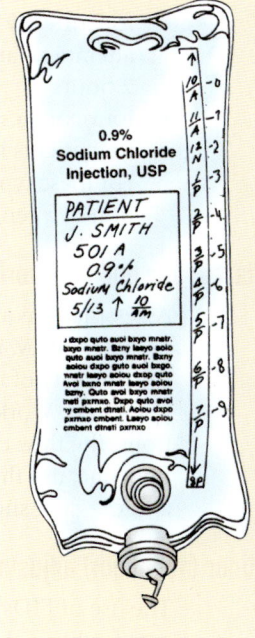

Using a time tape

Here's a simple way to monitor I.V. flow rate: Attach a piece of tape or a preprinted strip to the solution container; then write hourly times on the tape or strip beginning with the time you hung the solution.

Compare the actual time with the label time to quickly see if the rate is accurate.

Don't write directly on the plastic fluid container as the ink could move through the plastic and into the fluid.

be sold in the United States along with mandating that hospitals, long-term care facilities, and other ambulatory care centers report events where a device contributed to a patient's injury, illness, or death. Centers for Medicare and Medicare Services (CMS) sets standards for health care providers who received payments caring for patients eligible for Medicare or Medicaid. Finally, the Centers for Disease Control and Prevention establish guidelines for providing care such as hand hygiene and preventing intravascular related infections.

In other countries, health care regulations and funding models are different. Regulatory agencies have different names, depending on the country. Regulations may or may not be present to protect health care workers. Requirements for selling a specific device in each country will also vary. Some countries have accreditation organizations that survey hospital and community care to ensure quality patient outcomes. Infusion therapy practice is provided according to required operating procedures (R.O.P) in each facility.

Nurse practice acts (NPA)

Each state, province, or country has a law that establishes the regulatory body that governs the nursing profession. This law defines the profession, requirements for entry into practice, and the legal scope of practice for the professional. Most US state boards of nursing use scope of practice decision trees to guide decisions about specific practice questions. There are variations in the NPA between states, and each nurse is responsible for knowing the law and regulations where they practice. One example of these differences is the requirements for licensed practical/vocational nurses to perform I.V. infusions. In the United States, some states require these nurses to attend additional education courses before they can perform infusion therapy, while registered nurses have no similar requirements.

For other types of professionals, regulations may come from other regulatory agencies and/or professional organizations such as the American Society of Radiologic Technologists. Each clinician is responsible for knowing how and who regulates practice, understanding boundaries for their legal scope of practice, and practicing within those boundaries.

Know your legal limits

Every clinician is expected to care for patients within defined limits. If a clinician goes beyond their scope of practice, he or she becomes vulnerable to charges of violating the state practice act. Contact your state/province or country's professional regulatory agency for a copy of the specific act for your profession.

Professional organizations

In addition to the legal agencies and their laws, professional standards of practice are written by members of the same profession or specialty. For instance, the American Nurses Association writes standards that apply to all nursing practice. Specialty organizations write standards and guidelines with a focus on their area of expertise. A "standard" is defined as an authoritative statement expressed and disseminated by the profession for the purpose the judging the quality of practice, service, and education. Regarding infusion therapy, the list of organizations is lengthy. These organizations work collaboratively to reduce conflicting statements and ensure the most recent evidence is used for writing these documents.

- The Infusion Nurses Society (INS) developed the *Infusion Nursing Standards of Practice* more than 30 years ago. In 2016, INS revised the standards and changed the title to *Infusion Therapy Standards of Practice* to reflect the interdisciplinary nature of infusion therapy and the evolving role of health professionals. The goals of these standards are to protect the patient and clinician who administers infusion therapy. These standards address all aspects of infusion therapy practice and apply to all settings where infusion therapy is provided. More information is available at *www.ins1.org*.
- The American Society of Health-Systems Pharmacists (ASHP) is a pharmacy-based organization establishing safe practice for medication management.
- The Oncology Nursing Society (ONS) writes the *Chemotherapy and Biotherapy Guidelines and Recommendations for Practice*.
- The American Society for Parenteral and Enteral Nutrition (ASPEN) produces standards and guidelines about nutrition for nurses, pharmacists, dieticians, and physicians.
- The Association of Practitioners in Infection Control and Epidemiology produces resources on all aspects of preventing infection in health care.
- The American Association of Blood Banks (AABB) produces numerous guidelines, textbooks and other resources for the blood banking industry which includes administration of blood and blood components.
- The Society for Healthcare Epidemiology of America and the Infectious Disease Society of America publishes guidelines on the prevention, diagnosis, and management of VAD-related infections.

Other organizations

The Joint Commission (TJC) is a nongovernmental accrediting organization that sets standards for hospitals, home care, long-term care, and ambulatory care.

The Institute for Safe Medication Practices is a nonprofit agency focusing on medication errors, understanding their systems-based causes, and disseminating practice improvement recommendations for health care providers, consumers, and the pharmaceutical industry.

Facility policies and procedures

Every health care facility needs infusion therapy policies and procedures in place. All of the governmental, nongovernmental, and professional organizations listed above have evidence-based resources that serve as the foundation for writing policies and procedures for your facility. The increased focus on patient safety and evidence-based practice has placed greater emphasis on using these valuable resources. Infusion therapy carries a high risk to both patients and clinicians if not performed within the standards.

Knowledge of facility policy, procedures, practice guidelines, approved standing orders, or protocols is important in all areas of practice. Your performance is measured by these documents. Consider a policy statement to be the "rules of the road," and there is variation between each facility and agency. For example, home health nurses need to be acutely aware of patient and family education policies as infusion systems are being used in the home 24 hours per day without the presence of full-time nursing staff. In the hospital, the policy about radiographic verification of a CVAD is critical before infusion therapy begins or when there is a question about malposition.

Competency: getting it, keeping it, and documenting it

Competency is an integration of behaviors in the work setting that demonstrates the individual's ability to perform the activities of the job. Competency is important for all aspects of a job in health care; however, it is critical for infusion therapy to protect public safety. Infusion therapy is high risk and problem prone. Certain infusion-related activities may also be low volume depending on your patient population and health care setting. For instance, a skilled nursing facility may have very few patients with a VAD, peripheral or central, making routine dressing changes a difficult task for the nursing staff.

The individual clinician bears the responsibility for obtaining and maintaining competency for all infusion-related activities within their legal scope of practice. Competency includes more than just being able to perform a task. It also includes knowledge, critical thinking skills, and your ability to use these skills for appropriate decision-making.

The health care facility or agency is responsible for assessing your competency and documenting it. Accrediting bodies like TJC look at competence as part of the process of maintaining a high-quality work force especially for areas considered high risk such as infusion therapy. Competency assessment programs validate competency when one is initially employed, when your scope of practice expands or you change jobs, and when new procedures or technology are introduced. Competency should also be assessed on a continuing basis based on the clinical outcomes and problem identification through quality improvement processes. A wide variety of assessment methods may be used including self-assessment, written tests, simulation laboratories, and observation in the work setting.

One important aspect of competency is that invasive infusion-related procedures should NEVER be performed on peers or colleagues. Physical and emotional stress has been documented with these practices.

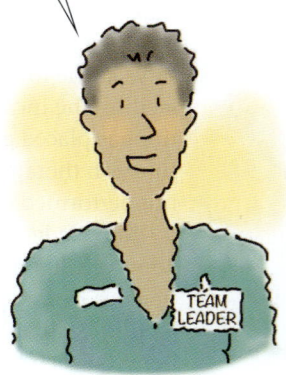

Document your I.V. care on the proper forms, such as progress notes, I.V. flow sheets, and the patient's medication sheet.

Documentation

Documentation is expected of all clinicians. Comprehensive documentation provides:
- accurate description of care that can serve as legal protection (for example, as evidence that a prescribed treatment was administered)
- mechanism for recording and retrieving information
- record of the care provided for payment of services
- communication vehicle to promote consistency and continuity of care among the health care team.

Forms, forms, forms

Infusion therapy may be documented on progress notes, a computerized chart, a special I.V. therapy flow sheet, a care plan on the patient's chart, or an intake and output sheet. Infusion therapy is also commonly recorded on the patient's medication sheet, which provides specifics regarding the medications administered. Know the proper documents to use in your facility.

Documenting initiation of infusion therapy

The components needed for comprehensive documentation include:
- patient education provided and their comprehension of the information (for example, ability to explain instructions or perform a return demonstration)
- infection prevention and safety measures used
- date and time of VAD insertion including size, length, and type of the device
- number of venipuncture attempts
- name of the person who inserted the device

- specific site location using anatomical descriptions, side of insertion, other physical landmarks, and vein name
- use of local anesthetic agents on insertion
- use of vascular visualization technology for insertion
- type of dressing and stabilization device used
- condition of the site
- if I.V. fluid started, type of solution and flow rate
- type and amount of flushing and locking solution for an intermittent VAD
- any medication(s) in the primary fluid or given intermittently including the type and volume of their dilution and rate of administration
- use of an electronic infusion device or other type of flow control device
- patient response to interventions
- patient teaching and evidence of patient understanding.

How to label a dressing

To label a new dressing over an I.V. site, include:
- date of insertion
- gauge and length of catheter
- date and time of the dressing change (if applicable)
- clinician's initials.

Label that dressing!

In addition to documenting in the patient's medical record, the dressing on the catheter insertion site also needs to be labeled. Whenever you change the dressing, label the new one. (See *How to label a dressing*.)

The fluid container also needs to have a label along with a time tape on it. In labeling the container and the set, follow your facility's policy and procedures. (See *How to label an I.V. bag*.)

The administration set should be labeled in two places:
1. Near the drip chamber with the date and time it was started or the date and time it should be changed.
2. Near the connection to the VAD with the contents of that administration set to reduce risk of misconnection.

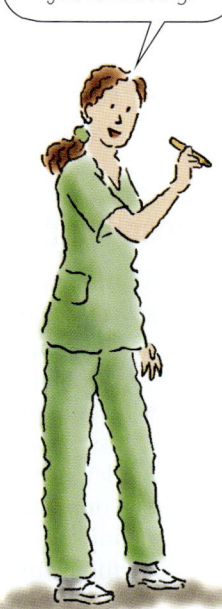

Remember to label your patient's dressing on the catheter insertion site and the I.V. bag of the solution you're infusing.

Documenting infusion therapy maintenance

When documenting infusion therapy maintenance, specify:
- condition of the site using a validated scoring system or grading scale to measure phlebitis and infiltration
- site care provided
- dressing changes
- administration set and solution changes
- patient teaching and evidence of understanding.

Flow sheets

With the advent of electronic health records (EHR), many facilities have developed flow sheets that highlight specific patient information

according to preestablished parameters of patient care. When monitoring and tracking infusion therapy, the required information for safe practice includes:
- date
- flow rate
- use of an electronic infusion device or flow control device
- type of solution including added medications
- patency of the VAD by absence of resistance to flushing and the presence of a blood return that is the color and consistency of whole blood
- condition of the vascular access site
- date and time of dressing and tubing changes.

Intake and output sheets

When documenting infusion therapy on an intake and output sheet, follow these guidelines:
- Children, critical care patients and those deemed at risk for fluid overload need to have their intake recorded every 1 to 2 hours, including: all I.V. solutions, medications, flush solutions, blood and blood products, and parenteral nutrition.
- Document the total amount of each solution and totals of all infusions periodically according to your facility policy and procedure. Monitor fluid balance by comparing intake to output. Make sure the math is correct.
- Note all output according to facility policy, LIP order, and patient's condition. Output includes urine, stool, vomitus, and gastric drainage. For an acutely ill or unstable patient, you may need to assess urine output every 15 minutes.
- Read fluid levels from the solution containers or EID to determine the amounts infused and the amounts remaining to be infused.

Documenting discontinuation of infusion therapy

All things come to an end and when that time comes in infusion therapy, record it! Documenting the discontinuation of infusion therapy needs to include:
- time and date
- reason for discontinuing therapy
- assessment of venipuncture site before and after the venous access device is removed
- complications, patient reactions, and nursing interventions
- integrity of the venous access device on removal
- follow-up actions such as heat or cold application for treating a local complication
- amount of I.V. fluid infused before discontinuing therapy.

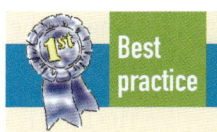

Best practice

I.V. bag label

The IV solution container needs to contain the following information (in addition to the time tape):
- patient's name, identification number, and room number
- date and time the container was hung
- any medication(s) added, the dose and date and time added
- rate at which the solution is to infuse
- expiration date and time of infusion.

When placing the label on the bag, be sure not to cover the name of the I.V. solution.

Patient teaching

Clinicians are accustomed to infusion therapy in all its form: not so for most patients. Patients may be apprehensive about the procedure and concerned that their condition has worsened. Teaching the patient and, when appropriate, members of the family will help everyone relax and take the mystery out of infusion therapy.

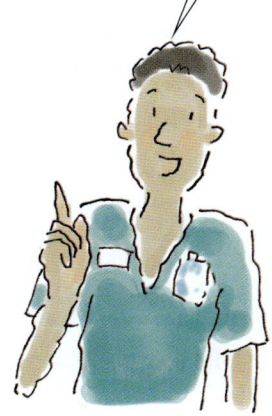

Good teaching will help infusion therapy appear less mysterious to the patient.

Based on past experience

Begin by assessing the patient's previous infusion experience, their expectations, and knowledge of venipuncture and infusion therapy. Once this is known, individualize the teaching. The minimum elements for teaching patients about their infusion therapy should include:

- Description of the procedure. Tell the patient that *I.V.* means "inside the vein" and that a plastic catheter will be placed in their vein.
- Explain that fluids containing certain nutrients or medications will flow from a bag or bottle through a length of tubing and then through the plastic tube or catheter placed in their vein.
- Tell the patient how long the catheter might stay in place, and explain that their LIP will decide how much and what type of fluid and medication is needed.

The whole story

Give the patient as much information as possible. It is important that the patient has all the information needed to provide informed consent. All patients sign a general consent on admission which includes things like insertion of a short peripheral catheter. This procedure was probably not explained when this document was signed so education about the procedure is very important. Other procedures like CVAD insertion may require a separate signed consent form. Remember — informed consent is a shared decision-making process involving education of the patient and family as appropriate. The process ends with the patient or surrogate signing the consent document after all information is understood.

Consider providing pamphlets, demonstrating with sample catheters and I.V. equipment, slides, videotapes, and other appropriate resources as appropriate for the patient's condition and the setting. Some practice areas, such as home care, use patient-teaching checklists that must be signed by the patient or their caregiver. Be sure to tell the whole story:

- Tell the patient that, although they may feel transient pain as the needle goes in, the discomfort should stop when the catheter is in place. Emphasize the need to let you know immediately if the pain is intense or extends to other locations on the extremity or does not quickly go away.

- Explain why the infusion therapy is needed and how the patient can help by holding still and not withdrawing if they feel pain when the needle is inserted.
- Explain that the I.V. solution may feel cold at first; however, the sensation should last only a few minutes.
- Instruct the patient to report any discomfort they feel after therapy begins.
- Explain activity restrictions such as those regarding bathing and ambulating.

Easing anxiety

Give the patient time to express their concerns and fears, and take the time to provide reassurance. Also, encourage the patient to use stress reduction techniques such as deep, slow breathing. Allow the patient and their family to participate in the care as much as possible.

But did they get it?

Be sure to evaluate how well the patient and their family understand the instructions. Evaluate their understanding during and after the teaching. One way is to ask frequent questions throughout the training and have them explain or demonstrate what they've been taught.

Don't forget the paperwork

Document all the teaching in the patient's records. Note what was taught as well as how well the patient understood it.

Stay out of court!

Administering medications and fluids to patients is one of the most legally significant interventions in all of health care. The majority of lawsuits are settled long before they go to court with all settlements remaining a private matter. Only those cases that get to court are a matter of public knowledge, making it impossible to determine the number of infusion-related lawsuits and the financial outcomes of settlements. Complications that frequently lead to a lawsuit include extravasation, nerve injury, air embolism, catheter damage, and medication errors. Strategies to protect your patient, your facility, and yourself are critically important:

- Take the time to become competent with all infusion-related interventions you are expected to perform. Develop your self-confidence by employing all opportunities for working with a knowledgeable preceptor.
- Follow the policies and procedures of your facility. If you have questions about their accuracy, bring this to the attention of your supervisor. In a lawsuit, your performance will be measured by the

standards and guidelines documents discussed above, so pursue getting outdated documents revised.
- Listen to your patient and their complaints about the infusion. Evaluate all comments. Don't try to explain away the problem. Common, but inappropriate, phrases include "that medicine always hurts," or "all patients complain about that site," or "it hurts only because the medicine is cold." Pain or any form of discomfort means there is a problem that requires further investigation and correction.
- Document all interventions, your thought processes leading to the decisions made, all patient complaints about their infusion, and all actions taken. Three or four years later when you are giving a deposition, your documentation will be the only reliable information to support your testimony.

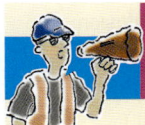

That's a wrap!

Introduction to infusion therapy review

Objectives of infusion therapy
Maintain and restore fluid and electrolyte balance
- Administer medications
- Transfuse blood and blood products
- Provide parenteral nutrition

Benefits
- Administers fluids, drugs, nutrients, and other solutions when a patient can't take oral substances
- Allows for more accurate dosing
- Allows medication to reach the bloodstream immediately

Risks
- Blood vessel damage
- Infiltration and extravasation
- Infection
- Overdose
- Incompatibility of drugs and solutions when mixed
- Adverse or allergic reactions
- May limit patient activity
- Expensive

Fluids, electrolytes, and infusion therapy
Fluid functions
- Helps regulate body temperature
- Transports nutrients and gases throughout the body
- Carries cellular waste products to excretion sites
- Includes intracellular fluid (fluid existing inside cells) and extracellular fluid, which is composed of interstitial fluid (fluid that surrounds each cell of the body) and intravascular fluid (blood plasma)

Electrolyte functions
- Conducts current that's necessary for cell function
- Includes sodium and chloride (major extracellular electrolytes), potassium and phosphorus (major intracellular electrolytes), calcium, and magnesium

Fluid and electrolyte balance
- Fluid balance involves the kidneys, heart, liver, adrenal glands, pituitary glands, and nervous system.
- Fluid volume and concentration are regulated by the interaction of antidiuretic hormone (regulates water retention) and aldosterone (retains sodium and water).
- The thirst mechanism helps regulate water volume.
- Fluid movement is influenced by membrane permeability and colloid osmotic and hydrostatic pressures.
- Water and solutes move across capillary walls by capillary filtration and reabsorption.

(continued)

Introduction to infusion therapy review *(continued)*

Infusion delivery methods
- *Continuous infusion* provides constant therapeutic drug level, fluid therapy, or parenteral nutrition.
- *Intermittent infusion* administers drugs at specific intervals over a defined time.
- *Push injection* used for a small-volume medication that is safe to manually inject.

Administration sets
- Selection depends on the type of infusion, solution container, and need for flow control device.
- Must be vented for glass or semi-rigid containers.
- Needleless connectors eliminate needles and protect health care workers from needlestick injuries.
- To reduce CLABSI, a vigorous mechanical scrub is required prior to each access.
- Use passive disinfection caps as recommended.

Infusion flow rates
- Macrodrip delivers 10, 15, or 20 gtt/mL.
- Microdrip delivers 60 gtt/mL.

Calculating flow rates
- Divide the volume of the infusion (in mL) by the time of infusion (in minutes) and then multiply this value by the drop factor (in drops per mL).

Regulating flow rates
- Choose the method of flow control safest for the patient and the setting.
- Factors affecting flow rate include vein spasm, infusion pressure changes, patient movement, manipulations of the clamp, bent or kinked tubing, height of the infusion container, type of administration set, and size and position of the vascular access device.

Checking flow rates
- Assess flow rates more frequently in patients who are critically ill, those with conditions that might be exacerbated by fluid overload, pediatric patients, elderly patients, and those receiving a vesicant drug that can cause tissue damage if infiltration occurs.

Professional and legal standards
- Professional and legal standards are defined by state nurse practice acts, federal regulations, standards and guidelines from professional organizations, and facility policy.

Documentation of I.V. therapy
- When therapy is initiated, label the dressing on the catheter insertion site and the fluid container according to facility policy and procedures.
- Document all pertinent information about VAD insertion and infusion therapy given on the correct forms in the medical record according to facility policy and procedure.
- Document each patient assessment and the routine maintenance required for the infusion therapy.
- Document patient/family teaching, evidence of comprehension, and their ability to provide self-care as indicated for home infusion.
- Document for discontinuation for fluids and medications, and LIP notification as appropriate; removal of all VADs with the reason for removal and site condition, along with any follow-up care provided.

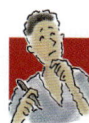

Quick quiz

1. What percentage of body weight is attributed to ECF?
    A. 5%
    B. 10%
    C. 20%
    D. 40%

Answer: C. ECF makes up about 20% of body weight.

2. Which type of solution raises serum osmolarity and pulls fluid from the intracellular and interstitial compartments into the intravascular compartment?
   A. Isotonic
   B. Solvent
   C. Hypotonic
   D. Hypertonic

Answer: D. The higher osmolarity of hypertonic solutions draws fluid into the intravascular compartment.

3. Which electrolyte is critical for the blood coagulation process?
   A. Calcium
   B. Magnesium
   C. Phosphorus
   D. Chloride

Answer: A. Calcium is essential for clotting.

4. What safety mechanism on electronic infusion devices prevents a rapid infusion?
   A. Occlusion alarm
   B. Anti–free flow mechanism
   C. Air-in-line alarm
   D. Programming for the volume to be infused

Answer: B. The anti–free flow mechanism automatically stops the fluid flow when the door is opened or the set is removed from the pump.

5. When capillary blood pressure exceeds colloid osmotic pressure:
   A. water and diffusible solutes leave the capillaries and circulate into the ISF.
   B. water and diffusible solutes return to the capillaries.
   C. there's no change.
   D. intake and output are affected.

Answer: A. When capillary blood pressure exceeds colloid osmotic pressure, water and diffusible solutes leave the capillaries and circulate into the ISF. When capillary blood pressure falls below colloid osmotic pressure, water and diffusible solutes return to the capillaries.

Scoring

★★★ If you answered all five questions correctly, congratulations! Clearly, reading this chapter has infused you with a great deal of knowledge.

★★ If you answered three or four questions correctly, good job! Whether hypertonic, hypotonic, or isotonic, you have most of the correct solutions.

★ If you answered fewer than three questions correctly, don't fret! Put this book under your pillow at night and see if you can absorb the material by osmosis.

Suggested References

Alexander, M., Corrigan, A., Gorski, L., Hankins, J., & Perucca, R. (Eds.). (2010). *Infusion nursing: An evidence-based approach* (3rd ed.). St. Louis, MO: Saunders/Elsevier.

Gorski, L., Hadaway, L., Hagle, M., McGoldrick, M., Orr, M., & Doellman, D. (2016). Infusion therapy standards of practice. *Journal of Infusion Nursing, 39*(1S), 159.

ISMP. (2015). *Safe practice guidelines for adult IV push medications.* Horsham, PA: Institute for Safe Medication Practices.

Phillips, L., & Gorski, L. (2014). *Manual of I.V. therapeutics* (6th ed.). Philadelphia, PA: FA Davis.

Weinstein, S. M., & Hagle, M. (2014). *Plumer's principals and practice of infusion therapy* (9th ed.). Philadelphia, PA: Wolters Kluwer Health.

Chapter 2

Infusion therapy using peripheral veins

Just the facts

In this chapter, you'll learn:

- ♦ the purpose of peripheral I.V. therapy
- ♦ selection and preparation of a peripheral venipuncture site
- ♦ how to insert a peripheral I.V. catheter
- ♦ peripheral infusion maintenance
- ♦ the signs and symptoms of complications of peripheral I.V. therapy and their management
- ♦ how to discontinue a peripheral infusion.

Understanding peripheral I.V. therapy

Few nursing responsibilities require more time, knowledge, and skill than administering peripheral I.V. therapy. At the bedside, you need to assemble the equipment, prepare the patient, insert the venous access device, regulate the I.V. flow rate, and monitor the patient for possible adverse effects. You also have behind-the-scenes responsibilities, such as checking the orders from the licensed independent practitioner (LIP), ordering or preparing supplies and equipment, labeling fluid and medication containers and administration set, and documenting your nursing interventions.

Practice should be performed through simulation on anatomical models and with the assistance and instruction of a knowledgeable and competent instructor. Practice should not be performed on coworkers due to the risk for injury. So, practice, practice, practice — but do so safely.

Practice, practice, practice

Perhaps the most challenging aspect of peripheral I.V. therapy is performing the venipuncture itself. You need steady hands and a sharp eye, plus lots of practice — it's worth the effort, both in terms

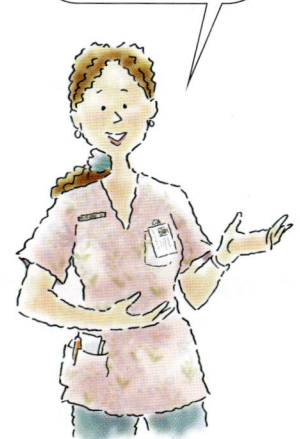

Peripheral I.V. therapy requires time, knowledge, and skill — at the bedside and behind the scenes.

of positive outcome and patient satisfaction. As you gain experience, you'll learn to perform even difficult venipunctures confidently and successfully.

Basics of peripheral I.V. therapy

Prescription of peripheral I.V. therapy means that venous access is needed, for example, when a patient requires surgery, transfusion therapy, or emergency care. You may also use peripheral I.V. therapy to maintain hydration, restore fluid and electrolyte balance, provide fluids for resuscitation, or administer I.V. drugs, blood and blood components, and some nutrients for metabolic support.

Peripheral I.V. access

Peripheral I.V. therapy offers access to the peripheral veins and allows for rapid administration of solutions, blood, and drugs. It is a basic and critical element of patient care that has become more complex over time. It requires knowledge and skill to successfully manage a patient's peripheral I.V. access, monitor for complications, and safely administer I.V. therapies. Organizations should consider using specialized teams of infusion nurses to improve the success rates for placement of peripheral I.V. devices and to decrease complications related to peripheral I.V. therapy.

Peripheral I.V. therapy concerns and cost

Peripheral I.V. therapy is an invasive vascular procedure that carries such associated risks as bleeding, infiltration, and infection. Rapid infusion of some drugs can produce hearing loss, bone marrow depression, kidney or heart damage, and other irreversible adverse effects. Finally, peripheral I.V. therapy can't be used indefinitely and costs more than oral, subcutaneous, or I.M. drug therapy.

A mainstay and crucial contributor

Despite its risks, peripheral I.V. therapy remains a mainstay of modern medicine and a crucial contribution that nurses make to their patients' well-being. The key is to do it well and that starts with preparation.

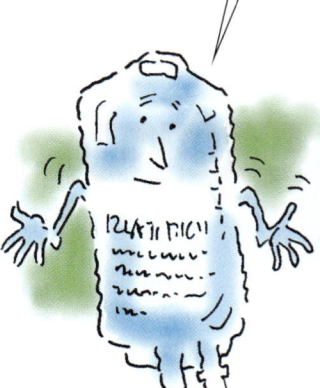

Face it. Any invasive procedure carries certain risks.

Preparing for venipuncture and infusion

Before performing venipuncture, talk with the patient, select and prepare the proper equipment, assess the patient for the best access site, and choose the best venous access device to deliver the I.V. therapy.

Preparing the patient

Before approaching the patient, check medical record for allergies, medical history, and current diagnosis and care plan. Review the LIP's orders, noting pertinent laboratory studies that might affect the administration or outcome of the prescribed therapy.

Care + confidence = a relaxed, cooperative patient

Keep in mind that the patient may be apprehensive. Among other things, this anxiety may cause vasoconstriction, making the venipuncture more difficult for you and more painful for the patient. Careful patient teaching and a confident, understanding attitude will help the patient relax and cooperate during the procedure. (See *Teaching a patient about peripheral I.V. therapy*.)

Teaching a patient about peripheral I.V. therapy

Many patients feel apprehensive about peripheral I.V. therapy. So, before you begin therapy, teach your patient what to expect before, during, and after the procedure. Thorough patient teaching can reduce his anxiety, making device placement easier and decreasing the risk of complications easier. Follow the guidelines below.

Describe the procedure

- Tell the patient that "intravenous" means inside the vein and that a plastic catheter (plastic tube) will be placed in the vein. Explain that fluids containing certain nutrients or medications will flow from an I.V. bag or bottle through a length of administration set and then through the plastic catheter into the vein.
- Tell the patient approximately how long the I.V. catheter will stay in place (if known). Explain that the LIP will decide how much and what type of fluid he needs.
- Mention that he may feel some pain during insertion but that the discomfort will stop once the catheter is in place. If the pain extends up or down the arm or causes tingling or numbness, he should let you know immediately.
- Tell him that the I.V. fluid may feel cold at first, but this sensation should last only a few minutes.

Do's and don'ts

- Tell the patient to report any discomfort after the catheter has been inserted and the fluid has begun to flow.

- Explain any restrictions, as ordered. If appropriate, tell the patient that he can walk while receiving I.V. therapy. Depending on the insertion site and the device, he may also be able to shower or take a tub bath during therapy, but you will need to cover the site to prevent it from getting wet.
- Teach the patient how to assist in the care of the I.V. system. Tell him not to pull at the insertion site or administration set and not to remove the container from the I.V. pole. Also, tell him not to kink the administration set or lie on it. Explain that he should call a nurse if the flow rate suddenly slows down or speeds up.

The worst (and it wasn't that bad) is over

- Explain that removing a peripheral I.V. line is a simple procedure. Tell the patient that pressure will be applied to the site until the bleeding stops. Reassure him that, once the device is out and the bleeding stops, he'll be able to use his arm as usual.

What goes on behind drawn curtains

After you complete your teaching, ensure the patient's privacy by asking visitors to leave and drawing the curtains around the bed. In the ambulatory setting, ensure patient privacy by performing the procedure in a private area. However, if the patient requests that his family stay during the procedure, respect his wishes. For hospital patients or those in a same-day surgery or procedure unit, have him put on a gown if not already wearing one. For patients in an ambulatory setting such as an infusion clinic, adjust any clothing such as long sleeves, and remove any jewelry from the arm where the I.V. catheter will be inserted. When the patient is ready, position him comfortably in the bed or chair. Make sure that the area is well lit and that the bed or chair is in a position that allows you to maneuver easily when inserting the device.

Selecting the equipment

Besides the venous access device, peripheral I.V. therapy requires a solution container, an administration set (sometimes with an in-line filter), and, if needed, an infusion pump (see *Chapter 1 for discussion of equipment used for I.V. therapy*).

The most frequently used I.V. administration sets are as follows:
- *Primary infusion sets* are used to infuse the main I.V. fluids, which could be given continuously for hours or even days. When no fluids are infusing, but intermittent medications are still needed, the primary set is connected during the infusion time and disconnected when the medication has infused.

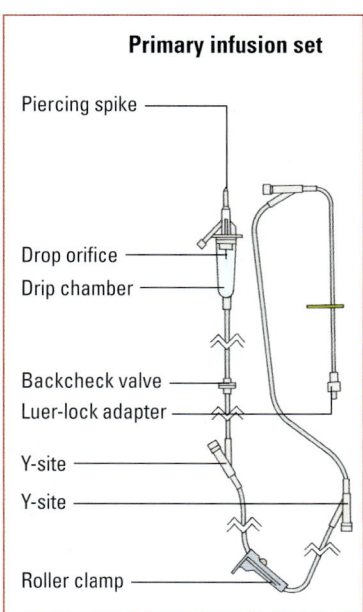

Primary infusion set

Piercing spike

Drop orifice
Drip chamber

Backcheck valve
Luer-lock adapter

Y-site
Y-site

Roller clamp

- *Secondary or piggyback sets* are used to infuse intermittent medications (every 6, 8, or 12 hours) and are attached to the primary set at one of the injection ports.

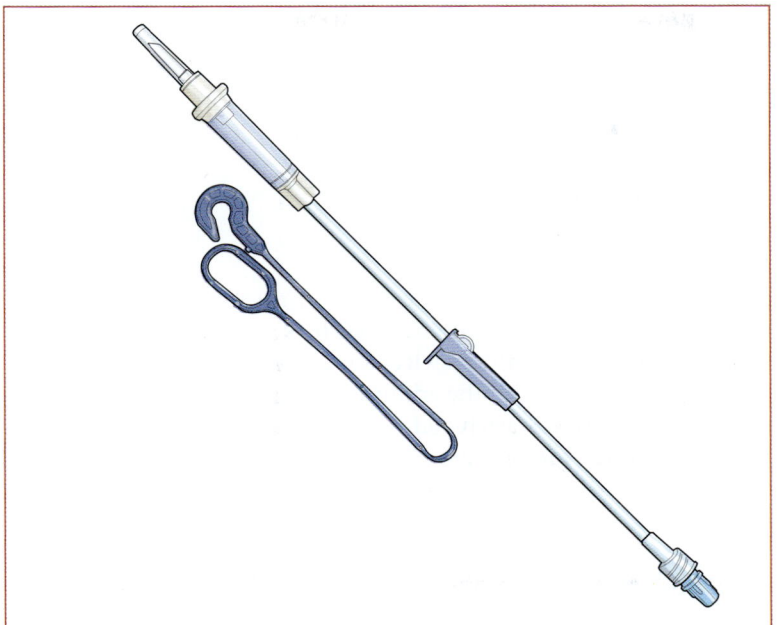

- *Volume-control sets*, also known as metered chamber sets, hold a limited amount of fluid and are primarily used for pediatric patients.

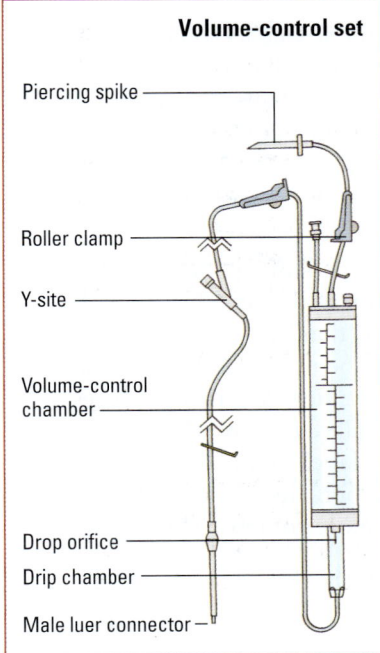

Volume-control set

- Piercing spike
- Roller clamp
- Y-site
- Volume-control chamber
- Drop orifice
- Drip chamber
- Male luer connector

Strict aseptic technique should be used when working with I.V. administration sets. The sterile components are both ends of the set covered by caps and the internal fluid pathway. Frequent disconnection increases the risk for contamination and adds to the risk of bloodstream infection in your patient. When disconnecting any administration set that is to be reconnected to the catheter, a sterile cap must be placed on the male luer end of the set. When reconnecting the administration set, the surface of the needleless connector should be properly disinfected to reduce possible contaminants from entering the system.

Add-on devices

Depending on the type of therapy ordered, you may need to supplement the administration set with other equipment, such as extension sets and needleless connectors. Add-on devices should have a luer-lock design and be compatible with the administration set. The risk of contamination increases with each add-on device, so it is recommended to limit their use. (See *Chapter 1 for more information*.)

Back to basics

Basic I.V. administration sets range from 70″ to 110″ (178 to 279 cm) long. Choosing the right length for a peripheral I.V. site is important to allow the patient enough room to move in bed or to ambulate without it being so long that it drags on the floor.

Secondary Piggyback

The backcheck valve prevents backflow of the secondary solution into the primary solution. After the secondary solution has been infused, the set automatically resumes infusing the primary one. Secondary sets are usually attached to the primary set at the injection site immediately below the backcheck valve.

Down to the milliliter

Volume-control sets — used primarily for pediatric patients — have a metered chamber located at the top of the set. This chamber is filled with a small amount of fluid (that is, 1 or 2 hours of the prescribed fluid). These sets may also be used to deliver a dose of medication by adding it to the chamber; however, this produces a labeling problem. The label should be placed on the chamber when the medication is infusing, but the label should be removed when there is no medication in the chamber. Electronic infusion pumps for precise flow control are now more common than these metered chambers.

In-line filters

In-line filters may be needed for some medications infused through a peripheral vein, but there is insufficient evidence that the routine use of filters reduces the risk of phlebitis. Blood components require filtration; however, the micron size is much greater. Don't expect to use a 0.2-micron filter if you're administering blood, blood components, or lipid emulsions; the larger particles in these solutions could clog the filter. Very-low-dose and low-volume medications could be retained on the filter, decreasing the amount that actually reaches the patient's vein. Check with the pharmacy if you have questions about what drugs should or should not be filtered. (See *Chapter 1 for additional filter information and Chapter 5 for more details on blood filtration*).

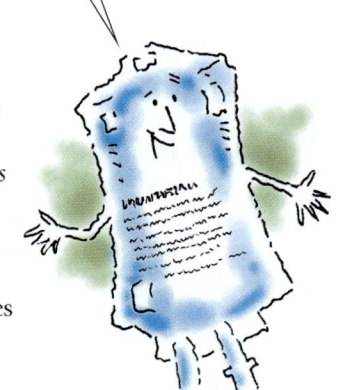

I don't like pathogens and particles. That's why I hooked up with an in-line filter.

Keeping in line with in-line filters

Most facilities have guidelines for using in-line filters; these guidelines usually include the following instructions:
- Carefully prime the in-line filter to eliminate all the air from it, usually by inverting the filter when fluid is flowing through the empty I.V. set; follow the filter manufacturer's directions.
- The filter should be changed simultaneously with the administration set. Do not open the infusion system to change the filter alone as this manipulation can increase contamination risk.
- If you suspect that the filter causes infusion problems such as slowed infusion rate or pump alarms, this could mean that the filter is doing its job! Check the medications being infused to verify the compatibility of all solutions. Particulate matter caused by contact with incompatible medications could be the cause and the filter is trapping those particles, preventing them from reaching the lungs.

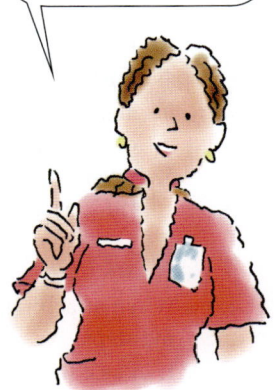

Discard a damaged or suspicious-looking I.V. container, and always use aseptic, nontouch technique when preparing to attach the container to the administration set. Better safe than sorry!

Preparing the equipment

After you select and gather the infusion equipment, you'll need to prepare it for use. Preparation involves inspecting the I.V. container and solution, verifying all manufacturer and pharmacy labels, attaching and priming the administration set, and setting up the electric infusion pump.

Inspecting the container and solution

Check that the solution is free of floating particles and is not discolored, and the type of I.V. solution is correct. Note the beyond-use date (BUD) or expiration date; discard an outdated solution.

When in doubt, throw it out

Make sure that the solution container is intact. Examine a glass container for cracks or chips and a plastic container for tears or leaks. (Plastic bags commonly come with an outer wrapper, which you must remove before inspecting the container.) Discard a damaged container, even if the solution appears clear. If the solution isn't clear, discard the container and notify the pharmacy. Solutions may vary in color, but they should never appear cloudy, turbid, or separated.

Preparing the solution

Make sure that the container is labeled with the following information: the patient's name, identification number, and room number; the date and time the container was hung; the container number (if such information is required by your facility); and your name or initials.

After the container is labeled, use aseptic, nontouch technique to remove the cap or pull tab. Be careful not to contaminate the port or the spike from the administration set.

Attaching the administration set

Make sure that the administration set is correct for the patient and the type of I.V. container and solution you're using. Also make sure that the set has no cracks, holes, or missing clamps. Glass containers have a solid stopper requiring venting from the administration set.

Glass bottle

When attaching a glass bottle to an administration set, take the following steps:
1. Place the bottle on a stable surface and remove the metal protective cap.
2. Remove the administration set from the package and close the roller clamp.
3. Remove the protective cap from the spike. Do not allow the spike to touch anything other than the stopper on the bottle.
4. Push the spike through the center of the stopper. Avoid twisting or angling the spike to prevent pieces of the stopper from breaking off and falling into the solution.
5. Invert the bottle. Hang the bottle on the I.V. pole, about 36" (91 cm) above the venipuncture site.

Plastic bag

When attaching a plastic bag to an administration set, take the following steps:
1. Place the bag on a flat, stable surface or hang it on an I.V. pole.

2. Remove the protective cap or tear the tab from the administration set insertion port.
3. Close the roller clamp.
4. Remove the protective cap from the spike preventing it from touching anything.
5. Hold the port carefully and firmly with one hand, and then, insert the spike with your other hand.
6. Hang the bag about 36″ above the venipuncture site.

Priming the administration set

Before you prime an administration set, label it with the date and time you opened it or the date and time to be changed according to organization policy and procedure. If the solution contains medications or additives, check the label for the patient's information and drug or additive information. To prime a set using an electronic infusion pump, follow the instructions included with the pump.

Basic training

When priming any set, take the following steps:
1. Close the roller clamp below the drip chamber.
2. Squeeze the drip chamber until it's half full.
3. Aim the distal end of the administration set at a receptacle.

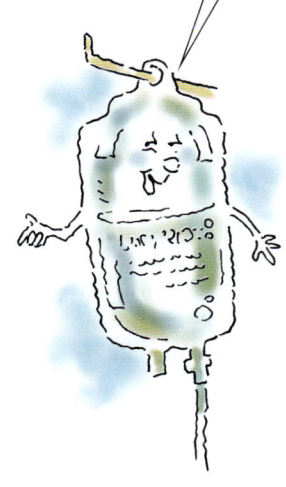

That's where I like to hang — about 36″ above the venipuncture site.

Best practice

Electronic infusion devices

An electronic infusion device, such as a pump, helps regulate the rate and volume of infusions, improving the safety and accuracy of drug and fluid administration.

Follow the pump instructions for inserting the set and priming:

Administration sets used with electronic infusion devices should have anti–free flow mechanisms to prevent gravity flow when the set is removed from the device. The anti–free flow mechanism automatically clamps the set upon removal to prevent serious patient injury or death from the infusing fluid flowing freely while the set is still connected to the patient.

When choosing an electronic infusion device, use a "smart pump" with dose error reduction software if one is available. The "smart pump" technology assists health care providers with calculating and programming infusion dose and delivery rates. Prevention of medication errors and patient harm is the goal. This technology should not replace adherence to established standards of practice for safe administration of medications. Do not attempt to bypass the correct steps to program the smart pump, as this can increase the risk of medication errors and patient harm.

4. Open the roller clamp, and allow the solution to flow through the administration set to remove the air. (Most caps on the male luer end of the set allow the solution to flow without remove it.) Areas of the backcheck valve and injection ports should be inverted and tapped to remove air bubbles.
5. Close the clamp after all the air has been purged from the system.

My sweet secondary set

Follow the same steps you would use to prime a primary set, along with these additional steps:
1. Confirm compatibility of the secondary I.V. fluid/medication with the primary I.V. fluid.
2. The primary infusion container is positioned lower than the secondary infusion container using the hook provided with the secondary set.

What about a filter?

Follow your facility's guidelines for using in-line filters and remember these additional points:
- Most in-line filters can be used with an infusion pump, but make sure that it can withstand the pump's infusion pressure. Some filters are made for use only with gravity flow and may crack and leak if the pressure exceeds a certain level.
- When added to the administration set, the filter should be located close to the patient.
- Carefully prime the in-line filter to eliminate all the air from it, following the manufacturer's directions. (See *Chapter 1 for more discussion about in-line filters.*)
- If you must add a filter to the I.V. administration set, attach it to the primed distal end of the I.V. set and follow the manufacturer's instructions for priming. Most filters are primed while holding the distal end of the administration set facing upward so the solution will wet the filter membrane completely and all air bubbles will be purged.

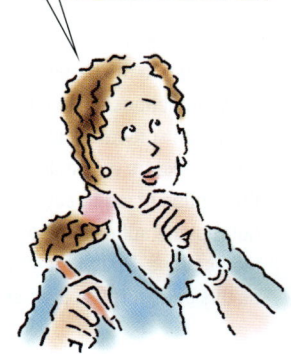

Do not rely on the infusion pump alarm to detect I.V. infiltration or extravasation. Infusion pumps do not detect or prevent I.V. infiltration or extravasation.

Setting up and monitoring an infusion pump

Infusion pumps help maintain a steady flow of liquid at a set rate over a specified period.

Determining when to use an infusion pump should include the patient's age and condition, the infusion therapy prescribed, and the setting where the therapy will be delivered. Infusion pumps are widely used in all health care settings. Infusion pumps are the standard of care in most settings due to an increasingly complex patient population, the complexity of I.V. fluids and medications being delivered, and patient safety. Make sure you know how to insert the correct set for the pump in use, how to set the infusion rate and the volume to be infused, and the alarms on the pump.

Sounding the alarm

Infusion pump alarms are meant to alert health care providers to potential problems with the pump, the infusion, or indicate completion of an infusion. Here are some basic alarms that you may encounter:
1. No flow: Administration set may be clamped or pinched.
2. High-pressure alarm: Administration set may be clamped or the catheter may be occluded.
3. Volume infused: Programmed volume to be infused has been completed.
4. Low battery: Pump has been disconnected from electrical source long enough to drain the battery.

Alarms will vary depending on the manufacturer of the pump.

While alarms are part of the safety features of the device, they do not prevent or detect infiltration or extravasation. Because so many pieces of equipment have alarms, alarm fatigue is recognized as a serious safety issue. A 2013 Sentinel Event Alert from the Joint Commission advised health care organizations to make a concentrated effort to look at and address this patient safety issue. Use of infusion pumps with alarms cannot replace good basic nursing care when providing infusion therapy to patients.

Frequently check the infusion pump to make sure that it's working properly — specifically, note the flow rate and solution volume remaining in the container. Closely monitor the catheter insertion site and surrounding area for signs and symptoms of infiltration. Pumps will continue to operate when infiltration is occurring, so patient protection is dependent upon quick detection of this complication.

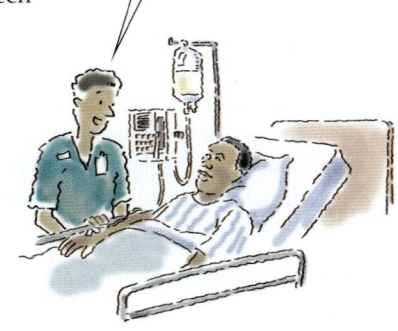

Be alert to alarm fatigue. With multiple medical devices in use that have alarm systems, health care personnel become desensitized to the alarms that may be warning of a problem.

Change the administration set

After the equipment is up and running, you'll also need to change the administration set according to the manufacturer's instructions and your facility's policy.

Selecting the insertion site

Here are general suggestions for selecting a vein for venipuncture:
- Keep in mind that the most prominent or visible veins aren't necessarily the best veins. Site selection is based on a thorough assessment of the patient's age, diagnosis, physical and vascular

Best practice

Administration set changes

Administration sets are routinely changed based on:
1. types of solution
2. whether the infusion is continuous or intermittent
3. if contamination is suspected
4. when the system or product has been compromised
5. whenever a new peripheral or central vascular access device is inserted.

Primary and secondary continuous administration sets
- Primary and secondary administration sets that have solutions running continuously should be changed no more frequently than every 96 hours.
- A secondary administration set that has been disconnected from the primary administration set should be changed every 24 hours.
- If disconnected, a new secondary set should be attached and remain connected until the entire system is changed.

Primary intermittent administration set
- Sets used for intermittent infusion should be changed every 24 hours because it is manipulated on both ends with each use.
- When disconnecting either a secondary or primary intermittent administration set, a new, sterile, compatible cover (for example, sterile end cap) is placed on the male luer end of the set. **Do not "loop" or attach the end of the set to a port on the same set. Do not reuse the syringe tip cap on the set.**

Parenteral nutrition and fat emulsions
- Administration set used to deliver parenteral nutrition should be changed every 24 hours.
- Administration sets used to deliver fat emulsions that are infused separately should be changed every 12 hours or with each new container.

Blood and blood components
Administration sets used to deliver blood and blood components should be changed after each unit/component or every 4 hours.

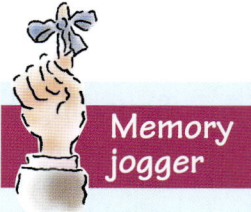

Memory jogger

In selecting the best site for a venipuncture, remember the abbreviation VIP:

Vein

Infusion

Patient

For the vein, consider its location, condition, and physical path along the extremity. For the infusion, consider its purpose and duration. For the patient, consider his ability to cooperate during the procedure; his condition, age, and diagnosis; history of previous I.V. therapy; condition of his vasculature; and his preference.

condition, previous I.V. therapy, and the length and type of therapy to be administered. Select a straight vein that feels soft and bouncy when palpated. When possible, choose a vein in the nondominant arm first. Also for subsequent venipuncture, select a site above a previously used or injured vein."
- Avoid:
  - areas of flexion
  - areas that are painful to palpation

- bruised areas
- red, swollen areas
- veins near a site of an infiltration, phlebitis, thrombosis, or cellulitis
- veins in the same arm with an arteriovenous shunt or fistula
- veins near an area of trauma such as burns or scarring from surgery
- veins in an upper extremity that are on the side of an axillary node dissection from breast surgery
- veins in an upper extremity that have lymphedema, have been affected by a stroke, or have an arteriovenous fistula/graft
- veins on any aspect of the wrist, especially the palm side to prevent pain and possible nerve damage.

> **Best practice**
>
> Risks of cannulating veins in an extremity that has been affected by a stroke, arteriovenous shunt or fistula, axillary node dissection, thrombosis, cellulitis, or trauma could be greater than the benefits. Discuss with the LIP before using.

Commonly used veins

The veins commonly used for placement of venipuncture devices include the metacarpal, cephalic, and basilic veins, along with the branches or accessory branches that merge with them. (See *Comparing peripheral venipuncture sites.*)

Superficial advice: try the hand and forearm

Generally, the superficial veins in forearm offer the best choices. The dorsum of the hand is well supplied with small, superficial veins that may accommodate a small gauge catheter. When using the dorsum of the hand, the length of the I.V. catheter could put the catheter tip in the area of wrist movement and increase the risk of complications. Thorough patient assessment should identify the site most likely to last for the length of the prescribed therapy, decrease pain during insertion, promote self-care, and prevent accidental removal.

Alternatives: upper arms, legs, and feet

Veins of the hand and forearm are suitable for most drugs and solutions. Stay away from the hand, wrist, and antecubital fossa if you are giving vesicant medications. For irritating drugs and solutions, the cephalic and basilic veins in the forearm below the antecubital fossa are more suitable. These veins are larger in diameter and provide better hemodilution for irritating drugs and solutions, and the bones of the forearm provide a natural splint.

Veins in the leg or foot may be used only as a last resort. The saphenous vein of the inner aspect of the ankle and the veins of the dorsal foot network are best for short-term use. Venous access in the

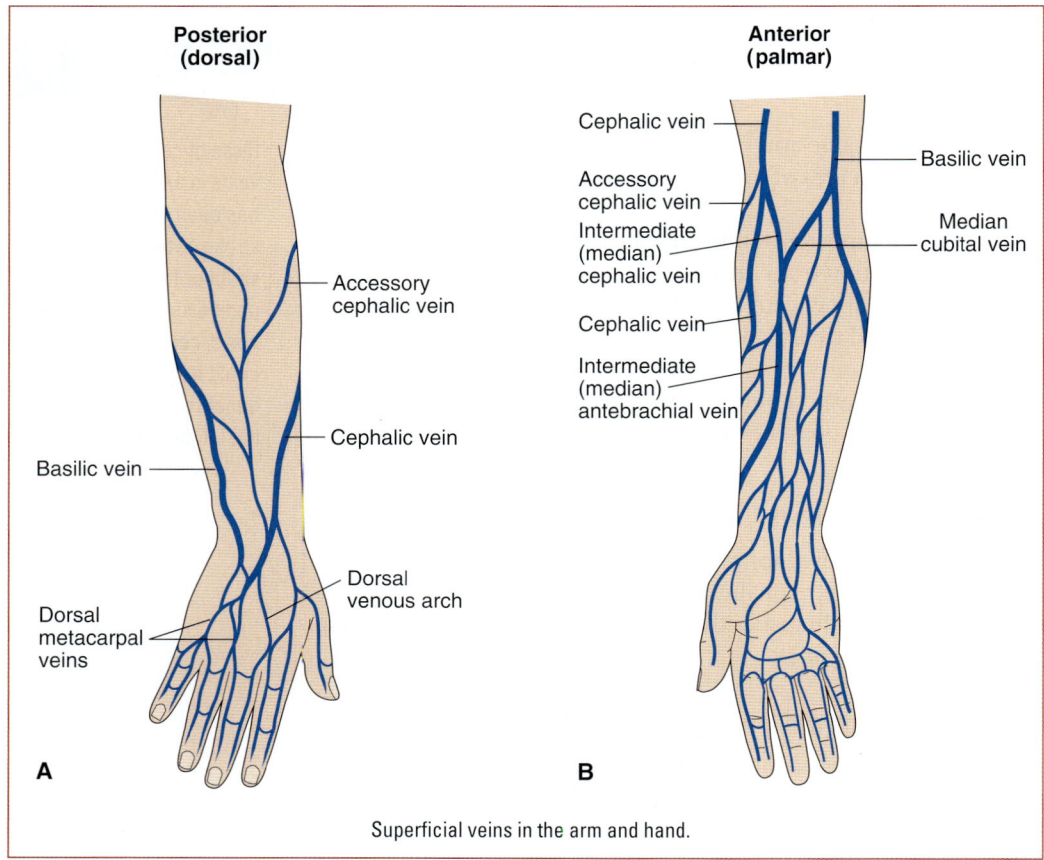

Superficial veins in the arm and hand.

lower extremities can cause thrombophlebitis. Discuss the situation with LIP and make plans to insert a more appropriate venous access device as soon as possible.

The lowdown on the upper arm

An upper arm vein may seem like an excellent site for a venous access device — it's comfortable for the patient and reasonably safe from accidental dislodging. Even so, it has drawbacks. Veins of the upper arm lie deep within the tissue, especially in obese patients. The basilic and brachial veins in the upper arm cannot be palpated and the cephalic vein may be difficult to feel. These veins should be reserved for a catheter inserted with ultrasound guidance such as a Peripherally inserted central catheter (PICC) or midline catheter. It may also be more difficult to identify complications, such as infiltration due to the catheter tip being deeper in the tissue.

(Text continues on page 68)

Comparing peripheral venipuncture sites

Venipuncture sites located in the hand, forearm, foot, and leg offer various advantages and disadvantages. This chart includes some of the major benefits and drawbacks of common venipuncture sites.

Site	Advantages	Disadvantages
Metacarpal veins On dorsum of hand; formed by union of digital veins between knuckles	• Easily accessible • Lie flat on back of hand	• Painful insertion likely because of large number of nerve endings in hands • Greatest risk of all complications at this site • Not acceptable for infusion of vesicant medications
Cephalic vein Along radial side of forearm and upper arm	• Large vein; easy to access • Readily accepts large-gauge catheters	• Joint movement when inserted close to wrist or elbow • Possible difficulty stabilizing vein • Risk of radial nerve injury when inserted close to wrist
Accessory cephalic vein Branches off the cephalic vein along the radial side	• Medium to large vein and easy to stabilize • Readily accepts large-gauge catheters	• May be difficult to palpate in an obese or bariatric surgery patient
Median antebrachial vein Rising from palm and along ulnar side of forearm	• Readily accessible • Acceptable site if located above the wrist	• Many nerves in the wrist area and a high risk of nerve injury
Basilic vein Along ulnar side of forearm and upper arm	• Straight, strong vein suitable for venipuncture • Takes large-gauge catheter easily	• Inconvenient position for patient during insertion • Difficult area to access – extending the patient's arm across their chest and standing on the opposite side of the bed can decrease the difficulty of accessing this vein. • Danger for ulnar nerve injury • Possible difficulty stabilizing vein
Median cephalic In antecubital fossa (on radial side)	• Large vein; facilitates drawing blood • Commonly visible or palpable in children • May be used in an emergency or as a last resort for a short time. Begin to make plans for a more suitable site or catheter type	• Difficult to splint elbow area with armboard, but it should be done if this site is used • Veins may be small and scarred if blood has been drawn frequently from this site • Risk of damage to median and anterior interosseous nerve and the lateral and medial antebrachial nerves
Median basilic In antecubital fossa (on ulnar side)	• Large vein; facilitates drawing blood • May be used in an emergency or as a last resort for a short time; begin to make plans for a more suitable site or catheter type	• Difficult to splint elbow area with armboard, but it should be done if this site is used • Veins may be small and scarred if blood has been drawn frequently from this site • Crosses in front of the ulnar artery • Risk of damage to median and anterior interosseous nerve and the lateral and medial antebrachial nerves

(continued)

Comparing peripheral venipuncture sites *(continued)*

Site	Advantages	Disadvantages
Median cubital In antecubital fossa (rises in front of elbow joint)	• Large vein; facilitates drawing blood • May be used in an emergency or as a last resort for a short time; begin to make plans for a more suitable site or catheter type	• Difficult to splint elbow area with armboard, but it should be done if this site is used • Veins may be small and scarred if blood has been drawn frequently from this site • Crosses in front of the brachial artery • Risk of damage to median and anterior interosseous nerve and the lateral and medial antebrachial nerves
Dorsal venous network On dorsal portion of foot	• Suitable for infants and toddlers who are not walking • Hands are kept free.	• Difficult to see or find vein due to subcutaneous fat • Do not use in patients who are ambulating. • Increased risk of deep vein thrombosis

You aren't an artery, are you?

Before choosing a vein as an I.V. site, make sure that it's actually a vein — not an artery. Palpate for arterial pulsation to identify any nearby arteries prior to performing peripheral venipuncture. Arteries are located deep in soft tissue and muscles; veins are superficial. Arteries contain bright red blood that flows away from the heart; veins contain dark red blood that flows toward the heart. But you cannot always rely on the color of the blood to determine accidental arterial puncture. Sometimes, an artery is located close to the surface in an unusual place. This is an aberrant artery and should not be mistaken for a vein.

A single artery supplies a large area; many veins supply and remove blood from the same area. If you puncture an artery, the blood pulsates from the site; if you puncture a vein, the blood flows slowly. (See *Reviewing skin and vein anatomy*, page 70.)

Avoid valves

All veins have valves, but they're usually apparent only in long, straight forearm veins or in large, healthy veins. Valves may appear as intermittent bulges when a tourniquet is placed on a person with healthy veins. Aging causes loss of valve competency and prevents them from appearing so readily. If the tip of the venous access device terminates near a valve, the flow rate may be affected. Look for a vein that's straight and smooth for about 1" (2.5 cm). Insert the venous access device above the visible bulge. Catheter insertion sites should be proximal to a valve or bifurcation of two veins.

Selection guideline

When selecting an I.V. site, choose distal veins first, unless the solution is very irritating (for example, potassium chloride). Generally, your best choice is a peripheral vein that's full and pliable and appears long enough to accommodate the length of the intended catheter (about 1" to 1.25"). It should be large enough to allow blood flow around the catheter to further dilute the infusing fluid and reduce irritation. If the patient has an area that's bruised, tender, or phlebitic, choose a vein proximal to it. Avoid flexion areas, such as the wrist and antecubital fossa.

How long?

The size and health of the vein help determine how long the venous access device can remain in place before irritation develops. However, the key to determining how long the venous access device will remain functional is the effect of the fluid or drug on the vein, joint and catheter stabilization, catheter size, vein size, site protection, and flushing of the device. Concentrated solutions of drugs and rapid infusion rates can also affect how long the I.V. site remains symptom-free.

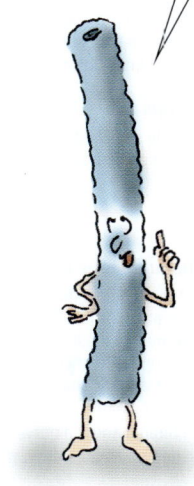

If you inadvertently cannulate an artery, **remove the I.V. catheter immediately.** Apply pressure to the site with a sterile gauze pad until hemostasis is achieved.

Selecting the venous access device

I.V. catheters inserted into peripheral veins have many characteristics designed to improve safety for the nurse and patient. Basically, the chosen vascular access devices should have the shortest length, smallest outer diameter, and fewest number of lumens

(Text continues on page 71)

Reviewing skin and vein anatomy

Understanding the anatomy of skin and veins can help you locate appropriate venipuncture sites and perform venipunctures with minimal patient discomfort.

Layers of the skin
Epidermis
- Top layer that forms a protective covering for the dermis
- Varied thickness in different parts of the body—usually thickest on palms of hands and soles of feet, thinnest on inner surface of limbs
- Varied thickness depending on age; possibly thin in elderly people
- Composed of five layers, with the top layer made up of dead cells and a deeper, living, cellular layer; microorganisms live in all layers

Dermis
- Highly sensitive and vascular because it contains many capillaries
- Location of thousands of nerves, which react to temperature, touch, pressure, and pain

Subcutaneous tissue
- Located below the two layers of skin
- Site of superficial veins
- Varied thickness that loosely covers muscles and tendons
- Potential site of cellulitis if strict aseptic technique isn't observed during venipuncture and care of I.V. site
- Location of nerves which are anatomically very close to veins; direct contact between the needle and the nerve during venipuncture or nerve compression from fluid or blood in the tissue can cause permanent nerve damage

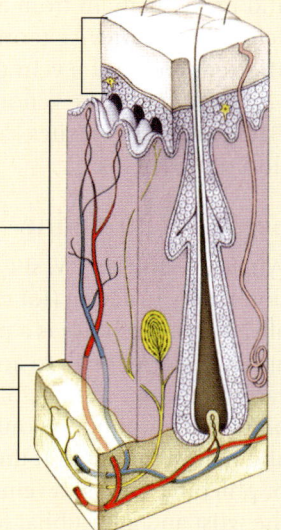

Layers of veins
Tunica adventitia (outer layer)
- Connective tissue that surrounds and supports the vessel and holds it together
- Reduced thickness and amount of connective tissue with age, resulting in fragile veins

Tunica media (middle layer)
- Muscular and elastic tissue
- Location of vasoconstrictor and vasodilator nerve fibers that stimulate the veins to contract and relax (these fibers are responsible for venous spasm that can occur as the result of anxiety or infusion of I.V. fluids that are too cold)
- Use of heat causes this layer to vasodilate (can relieve venous spasm and increase blood flow which can decrease the inflammation and irritation caused by some fluids and medications).

Tunica intima (inner layer)
- Inner elastic endothelial lining made up of layers of smooth, flat cells, which allow blood cells and platelets to flow smoothly through the blood vessels (unnecessary movement of the venous access device may scratch or roughen this inner surface, causing thrombus formation)
- Valves in this layer located in the semilunar folds of the endothelium (valves prevent backflow and ensure that blood flows toward the heart)
- A single layer of smooth, flat endothelial cells lining the internal vein wall;, allows blood to flow smoothly through the blood vessels. Venipuncture and catheter or joint movement disrupts this inner surface, causing thrombus formation. When no longer needed to control bleeding at the puncture site, the body destroys the thrombus

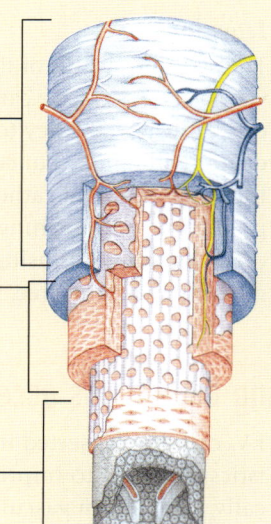

Best practice

- Choose 20-, 22-, or 24-gauge catheters for most infusion therapies based on the size and condition of the palpated vein.
- 20-, 22-, and 24-gauge catheters can be used for blood and blood components.
- Choose 16- or 18-gauge catheters for major surgical procedures, rapid fluid replacement or transfusion, and other life-threatening situations. Veins of the hand or forearm may be too small for these large catheters, leading to early development of complications and the need to change to a different site and a smaller catheter.

and be the least invasive catheter that allows for proper administration of the therapy. Based on this standard, a short peripheral catheter is the most frequent type of catheter used for infusion therapy.

When choosing a short peripheral catheter, assess and confirm the following points:
- The anticipated length of I.V. therapy is less than 1 week.
- The characteristics of the fluids and medications are well tolerated by peripheral veins. Think about the final osmolarity of the solution, the pH of the medications, and the irritant or vesicant nature of each solution.
- Type of procedure or surgery — for an extensive surgical procedure, a larger-gauge catheter may be needed to accommodate the needed flow rate; smaller gauges are useful for other procedures.
- Patient's age — pediatric and elderly patients have veins of smaller diameter.
- Patient's activity level — normal activities of daily living will require use of hands, especially the dominant hand.
- Condition of veins — veins that feel hard or rope-like may be sclerosed and difficult to cannulate.

Venous access devices and safety

Innovations in catheter design provide the clinician with a variety of devices to meet the patient's infusion therapy needs. Catheters range in gauge size, length, and composition. A thin-wall design promotes increased flow rates, allowing for use of smaller gauge catheters. Some catheters are designed with wider wings allowing for ease of stabilization. There are I.V. catheters that have a preattached extension set creating a closed system and reducing the risk for blood exposure. This

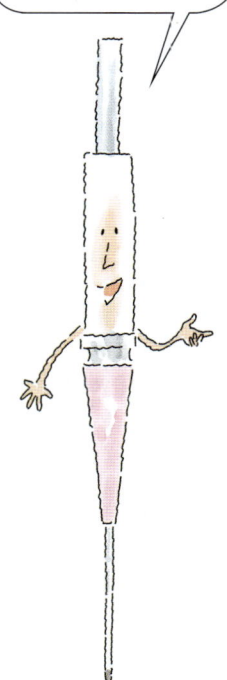

OSHA requires that all peripheral catheters have a safety mechanism to reduce the risk of needlestick injuries

closed system design eliminates the risk of touch contamination during insertion because the extension set does not have to be connected to the open catheter hub.

Your safety

Venipuncture leaves behind a hollow sharp needle filled with blood, which carries the greatest risk of exposure to bloodborne diseases such as hepatitis B and C and HIV if an accidental needlestick occurs. According to the Bloodborne Pathogen Standard from the Occupational Safety and Health Administration (OSHA), a peripheral catheter must have a safety mechanism to house the needle stylet to reduce the risk of accidental needlestick injuries. These mechanisms may be either passive or active in design. Catheters with a passive safety mechanism require no action from the user and are most effective at preventing needlestick injuries. Catheters with an active safety mechanism require some action from the user such as pushing a button or pushing a shield. This means that the safety mechanism may not always completely enclose the sharp needle.

Blood exposure is another safety risk with inserting I.V. catheters. After the needle stylet is removed, blood flows from the round catheter hub while you are connecting the extension set. Also, blood can splash during a peripheral catheter insertion and could reach your mouth, eyes, or areas of skin that are chapped, abraded, or broken. Some peripheral catheters now have a valve inside the hub that automatically closes when the needle stylet is removed, preventing free flow of blood.

To prevent accidental needlesticks and blood exposure:
- Always wear gloves to perform a venipuncture. Learn to palpate the vein with gloves on and don't remove a glove finger.
- Evaluate the patient's ability to cooperate during the procedure. Patients with dementia or other altered mental states may not be able to hold still, increasing the chance of blood splashing into your face. Choose personal protective equipment that will protect your eyes and face, such as a plastic face shield.
- Always use catheters with safety mechanism that houses the needle stylet.
- If using a catheter with an active safety mechanism, always activate the safety device correctly.

Let's go over this needle

An over-the-needle catheter is the most commonly used device for peripheral I.V. therapy. It consists of a plastic catheter attached to a colored hub. The sharp needle, known as a stylet, is inside the catheter and is attached to the safety mechanism on the distal end. The sharp tip of the stylet extends just beyond the catheter tip. The stylet is removed after insertion, leaving the catheter in place.

Over-the-needle catheters are available in varying lengths, from ¾" to 2", with gauges ranging from 14 to 24. Longer-length catheters are needed for insertion into veins lying deeper in the tissue with insertion guided by ultrasound.

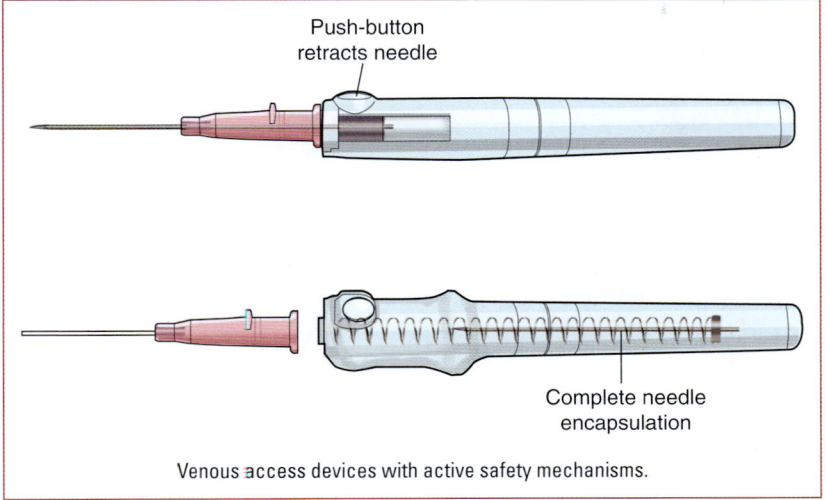

Venous access devices with active safety mechanisms.

Taking wing

Winged infusion needles (sometimes referred to as butterfly needles) have a steel needle and flexible wings you can fold and hold when inserting the device. When the device is in place, the wings lie flat and can be taped to the surrounding skin. Winged needles have a short, small-bore administration set between the needle and hub. They are used for drawing blood and for a very short injection/infusion of medication. They should be removed immediately after the procedure because they are associated with higher rates of complications when left in place. These needles also must have a safety mechanism to house the needle when it is retracted from the vein.

The midline

Midline catheters are considered a peripheral I.V. device that is inserted into veins of the upper arm. The basilic vein is preferred, but cephalic or brachial veins may also be used. Due to the depth of these veins, ultrasound guidance is used. The tip of the midline catheter is located near the axilla, below the shoulder where the vein diameter is larger than in the forearm. They are chosen when 1 to 4 weeks of infusion therapy is planned. Therapies appropriate for placement of a midline device include antibiotics, hydration, and pain control as most of these medications are well tolerated by peripheral veins.

Midlines should not be used for vesicant administration, for parenteral nutrition, or for hypertonic solutions with osmolarity greater than 900 mOsm/L. Insertion of a midline catheter should only be undertaken after competency to place the device has been validated.

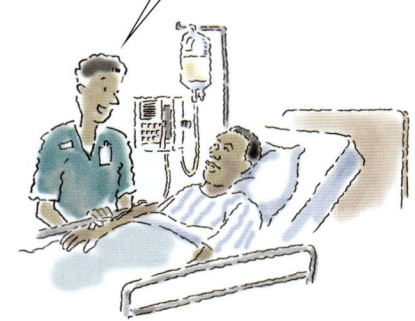

Contact the infusion or vascular access nurse for a complete assessment if you think your patient needs a midline catheter.

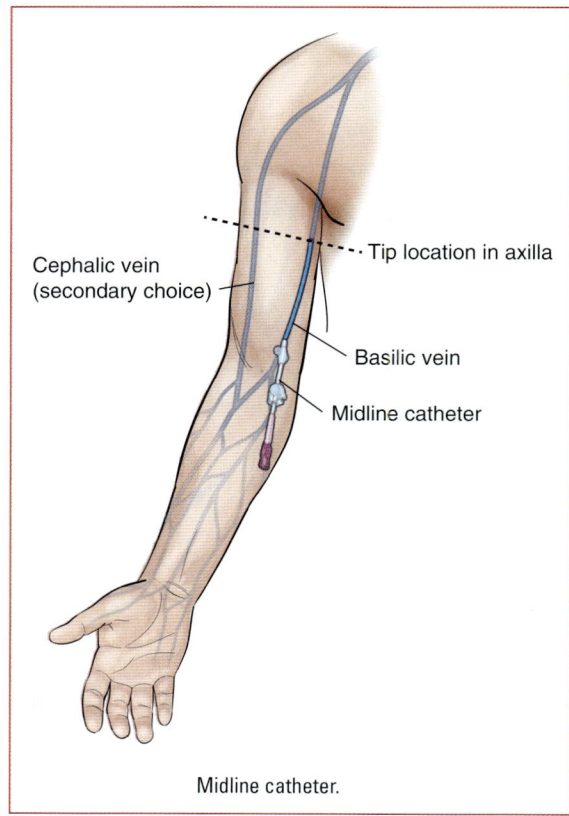

Midline catheter.

Other infusion access options

Peripheral veins may not be readily available for quick insertion in an emergency situation. The condition of veins in patients that have received extensive infusion therapy may not be easily cannulated. There are other options for infusion to meet patient needs but avoid the risk associated with a central venous catheter.

The down low on the IO (intraosseous access device)

During an emergent situation such as a cardiac arrest in either adult or pediatric patients, locating and inserting a catheter into a peripheral vein may be impossible. Intraosseous (IO) access is quickly inserted in these situations and can be used for administration of all fluids and medications. The IO device is limited to a dwell time of 24 hours or less. During this time, an assessment of the needed infusion therapy should lead to insertion of the most appropriate vascular access device for your patient. IO insertion should only be undertaken after your competency with the procedure has been documented.

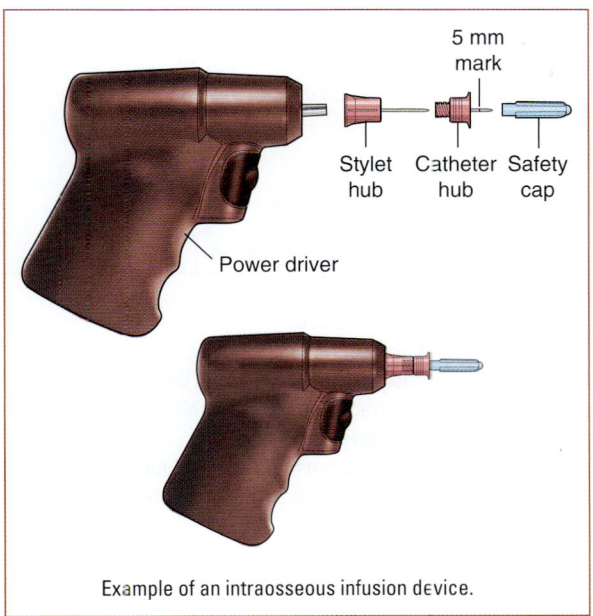

Example of an intraosseous infusion device.

Subcutaneous infusion and access devices

The use of subcutaneous infusions may be the best option in patients with limited vascular access, especially those receiving hospice or palliative care. The subcutaneous route can be used to treat mild to moderate dehydration or provide continuous opioid administration, and medications such as immune globulin. Subcutaneous infusion therapy requires adequate subcutaneous tissue. Assess your patient's needs and their clinical condition and discuss this route with the health care team.

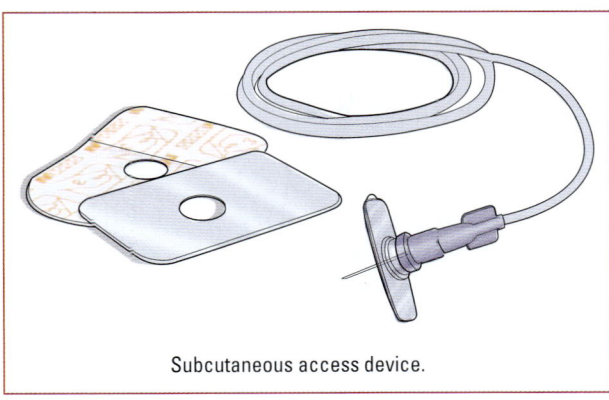

Subcutaneous access device.

When used for hydration, the site should be changed after infusion of 1.5 to 2 L of solution. For medication administration, the site is changed every 7 days or when site assessment reveals clinical signs or symptoms such as redness or swelling. Again, documented competency with placement and monitoring of this device is needed prior to initiating access.

(Text continues on page 78)

Comparing basic venous access devices

Use the chart below to compare the two major types of venous access devices.

Over-the-needle catheter

Advantages
- Easy to insert
- More comfortable for the patient
- Radiopaque
- Safety-engineered mechanism that houses the needle stylet and reduces accidental needlesticks

Disadvantages
- Rounded hub design can be difficult to secure
- Increased risk of phlebitis
- Broken or irritated skin from the round hub if secured tightly or positioned at pressure points
- If sites in the hand, wrist, or antecubital fossa must be used, an armboard is recommended to support the joint and reduce complications

Winged metal needles

Advantages
- Simple device
- Easy insertion
- Easier to use for drawing blood samples in small veins of the hand than straight phlebotomy needles
- Easy insertion
- Easier to use for drawing blood samples in small veins of the hand than straight phlebotomy needles

Disadvantages
- Rigid needle with increased likelihood of infiltration
- Not indicated for infusion or injection of a vesicant medication

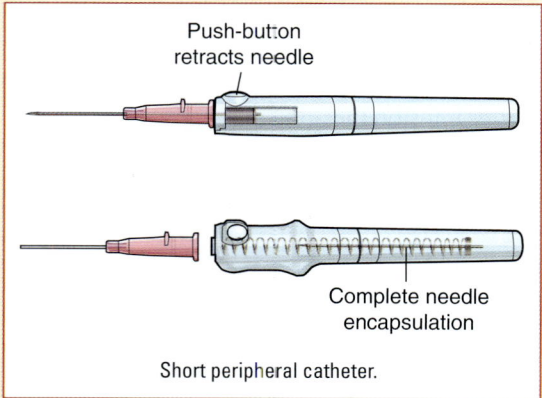

Short peripheral catheter.

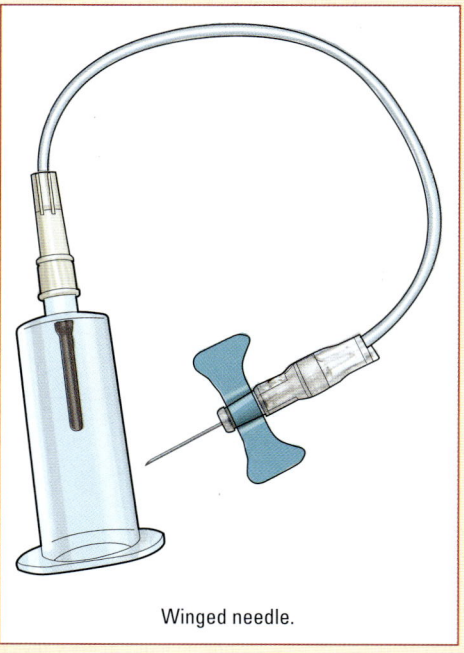

Winged needle.

Guide to needle and catheter gauges

Know your patient's age, primary and secondary medical diagnoses, clinical stability, planned procedures or surgery, and the type of infusion the patient is receiving. This chart lists the uses and nursing considerations for various gauges.

Gauge	Uses	Nursing considerations
16	• Adolescents and adults • Major surgery • Trauma • Whenever large amounts of fluids must be infused rapidly	• Painful insertion • Requires large vein • May require local anesthetic for insertion • Too large for veins of the hand in most patients • Large gauge may lead to early complications; frequent assessment is required
18	• Adolescents and adults • Rapid administration of blood and blood components and other viscous infusions • Routinely used preoperatively if the vein size and condition will accept this large gauge	• Painful insertion • Requires large vein • Large gauge may lead to early complications; frequent assessment is required
20	• Children, adolescents, and adults • Suitable for most I.V. infusions, blood, blood components, and other viscous infusions	• Most commonly used gauge
22	• Toddlers, children, adolescents, and adults of all ages • Suitable for most I.V. infusions, blood, blood components, and other viscous infusions	• Easier to insert into small veins • Commonly used for most infusions
24	• Neonates, infants, toddlers, school-age children, adolescents, and adults of all ages • Suitable for most infusions, but flow rates are slower	• For extremely small veins 　○ Loss of subcutaneous tissue around the vein, such as older adults 　○ Dehydration and decreased blood flow to distend veins • Possible difficulty inserting into tough skin

An intermittent adaption

Adding an extension set to a peripheral catheter has many benefits for both continuous and intermittent infusion or conversion from one to the other. Any venous access device can be made into an intermittent infusion device by attaching an extension set and needleless connector to the catheter hub. An intermittently used catheter is commonly called a "saline lock," as normal saline solution is used to flush and lock them to keep the device patent.

During the insertion of the peripheral catheter, the extension set is added to the catheter hub, allowing for flushing to assess patency before the administration set is attached to the hub of the extension set. If a blood sample during insertion is needed, it should be done from the hub of the extension set, which reduces excess manipulation of the catheter inside the vein. During continuous infusion, it is common practice to leave the extension set attached and change the other components of the administration set as this reduces the manipulation of the catheter hub. For conversion from continuous to intermittent infusion, the administration set is removed and a needleless connector is added to the hub of the extension set. It also provides a slide clamp so that blood exposure from the catheter is reduced.

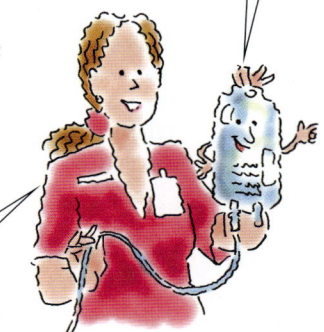

Just attach a needleless connector and extension set to the catheter hub.

Any venous access device that includes a catheter can be made into an intermittent infusion device.

Intermittent venous access devices should be flushed and locked with normal saline solution before and after each use or according to the facility's policy and procedures. Daily flushing and locking are usually not necessary, as the catheter should be removed when it is no longer required for the patient's plan of care.

Performing venipuncture

Performing venipuncture successfully requires assessment, patient preparation, knowledge of the prescribed infusion therapy and venous anatomy and physiology, and clinician competency in placing a vascular access device. The first steps include reviewing the LIPs order for infusion therapy, hand hygiene, gathering and preparing the needed equipment, patient identification, assessment, and education. Next is site and vein selection and vein dilation. Veins must be visible, palpable, or both. When you cannot see or feel the vein, visualization technology such as near-infrared light devices may help to locate superficial veins. Ultrasound may be needed for patients with only deep or difficult venous access.

Patient identification, assessment, and education

Patient identification must be done using two patient identifiers according to your facility policy. Name and date of birth are commonly used. Other verifiable information could be used. Patient assessment begins by gathering the history from the patient's medical record. Look at the primary medical diagnosis along with secondary diagnoses such as diabetes, chronic kidney disease, or other chronic illnesses. What allergies do they have? Has the patient had previous experiences with infusion therapy, and did he or she have any complications? Next, look at current laboratory values such as electrolytes, blood cell counts, and the need for obtaining blood cultures before administering antibiotics.

Next comes your patient assessment. Discuss previous experiences with the patient. Confirm allergies. Ask about any history of fainting during previous venipunctures or from the sight of blood. Explain the reason for the infusion therapy and how the catheter will be inserted. Educate the patient and significant others about activities with the catheter, attached sets, pump, and fluid containers. Patient education about the procedure can help with anxiety and identify the patient's role in the procedure for a successful outcome.

Choosing the actual site for insertion comes next. What is the dominant hand? If possible, begin with the nondominant extremity. Are there reasons for avoiding one side, such as presence of dialysis fistulas or grafts, lymphedema, or paralysis?

Dilating the vein

To dilate or distend a vein effectively, you may need to use a tourniquet, which traps blood in the veins by applying enough pressure to impede venous flow. If you are not able to palpate a radial pulse after applying a tourniquet, the tourniquet is too tight. A tourniquet should be dedicated to a single patient because it could be exposed to blood. A blood pressure cuff may be used as a tourniquet by pumping it up and leaving it at a pressure slightly less than the patient's diastolic pressure. A properly distended vein should appear and feel round, firm, and fully filled with blood as well as rebound when gently compressed. To palpate veins, always use the same finger of your nondominant hand. It may sound odd, but over time, this finger will be able to quickly detect the presence and condition of superficial veins. Also, palpate by gently pressing downward on the site and slowly releasing the pressure. Pay attention to the resilience and elasticity of the vein. Because the amount of trapped blood depends on circulation, a patient who is hypotensive, very cold, or experiencing vasomotor changes (such as septic shock) may have inadequate filling of the peripheral blood vessels. For patients with extra adipose tissue or deep veins, using multiple tourniquets to increase the pressure to fill the veins may be useful, although these patients may need ultrasound guidance for peripheral catheter insertion.

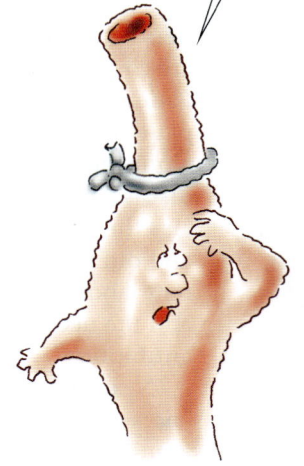

A properly distended vein should appear — as well as feel — round, firm, and full.

Pretourniquet prep

Before applying the tourniquet, place the patient's arm in a dependent position to increase capillary flow to the lower arm and hand. Using dry heat is helpful in getting the vein to fill sufficiently and increase success in accessing the vein. Dry heat is more effective than moist heat. Use caution with heat to prevent burns. Use a method where the temperature can be controlled. Do not heat towels in a microwave oven as you will not know the temperature.

Applying a tourniquet

The ideal tourniquet is one that can be secured easily, doesn't roll into a thin band, stays relatively flat, and releases easily. The most common type is a soft rubber band about 1″ to 2″ (5 cm) wide. (To tie a tourniquet, follow the steps outlined in *Applying a tourniquet*, page 81.)

Intend to distend

After you have applied the tourniquet about 6″ to 8″ (15 to 20 cm) above the intended site, have the patient open and close his fist. Lightly rub the vein downward to help distend the vein. If necessary, gently tap the skin over the vein with one or two short taps of your forefinger. If the vein still feels small, release the tourniquet, reapply it, and reassess the intended access site. If the vein still isn't well distended, remove the tourniquet; apply a warm, dry towel for several minutes; and then reapply the tourniquet. This step is especially helpful if the patient's skin feels cool.

Performing venipuncture 81

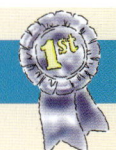
Best practice

Applying a tourniquet

To safely apply a tourniquet, follow these steps:
1. Place the tourniquet under the patient's arm, about 6" to 8" (15 cm) above the venipuncture site. Position the arm on the middle of the tourniquet.
2. Bring the ends of the tourniquet together, placing one on top of the other.
3. Holding one end on top of the other, lift and stretch the tourniquet and tuck the top tail under the bottom tail. Don't allow the tourniquet to loosen. Leave the end of the top tail within easy reach so it can be released by pulling it.
4. Tie the tourniquet smoothly and snugly; be careful not to pinch the patient's skin or pull his arm hair.

Tourniquet: time and tightness
Tourniquets are applied with enough pressure to impede venous blood flow yet maintain arterial blood flow. It should be snug but not uncomfortably tight. If it's too tight, it will impede arterial as well as venous blood flow. Check the patient's radial pulse. If you can't feel it, the tourniquet is too tight and must be loosened. Also, loosen and reapply the tourniquet if the patient complains of severe tightness. Keep it flat against the patient's skin for comfort.

Tourniquets that are left on for extended periods of time can make it more difficult to achieve successful venous access; can lead to circulatory, muscular, neurological, and vascular damage; and can alter certain laboratory results if blood collection is part of the procedure. How long is too long? Recommendations are for no longer than 4 to 6 minutes. If collection of blood is part of the procedure, the tourniquet should be applied for no more than 1 minute. It is recommended to complete the venous device placement and then draw a blood sample to avoid extended tourniquet time and thus potentially altering laboratory results.

Tourniquets should be loosely applied or avoided in patients who have compromised circulation and fragile veins or are at risk for bleeding. For these patients, the hand of a co-worker placed around the patient's arm may be sufficient to distend veins.

Tourniquets are for single patient use. They should not be moved or used between patients.

Use latex-free tourniquets to reduce the chance of a reaction in a latex-allergic or latex-sensitive patient.

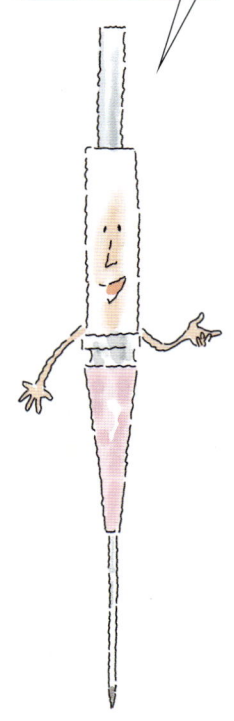

Following these guidelines will ensure safety and promote blood flow, making venipuncture easier.

Top tourniquet technique

A tourniquet that's kept in place too long or is applied too tightly may cause increased bruising, especially in elderly patients whose veins are fragile. Release the tourniquet as soon as you have placed the venous access device in the vein. You'll know the device is in the vein when you see blood in the flashback chamber.

Hidden from sight

Some patient's veins are just not visible and you cannot feel them regardless of how hard you try. The next step may be use of visualization technologies. Visible light devices similar to a flashlight are helpful in infants and adults with very thin arms. Don't use a light that produces heat as burns have been reported. In most adults, the arm diameter is too great for this type of light to be effective, but it could be worth a try.

Near-infrared light devices use a different spectrum of light that works by detecting hemoglobin and reflecting a picture of the veins back to the surface of the skin or a screen. The vein pathway, presence of valves, bifurcations, and tortuosity can be identified. Ultrasound uses sound waves to create a visual image of the vein location and pathway displayed on a screen. However, ultrasound presents a greater challenge to learn because you must look at the screen and not the insertion site during the procedure.

The key to using visualization technologies for I.V. catheter placement is learning the technology, practice with supervision, and documented competency.

Vascular visualization technologies

Use of visualization technologies can improve success rates with peripheral I.V. catheter insertion and decrease the need for central vascular access device placement in patients with difficult venous access.

Before using a visualization technology, the clinician should be knowledgeable in:
- the use of the device (appropriate indications and contraindications, manufacturer's instructions for use)
- vascular anatomy (both arteries and veins), nerves, skin, and pathophysiological changes
- potential complications.

Vascular visualization technologies include:
- visible light devices that provide transillumination of the superficial veins
- near-infrared light technology, which captures and reflects the image of the veins back to the skin surface or onto a screen
- ultrasound that identifies arteries, veins, and nerves and is useful for deep veins, requiring a longer catheter to ensure at least two-thirds of the catheter length resides inside the vein lumen.
- Documented competency is required for the use of these devices.

Preparing the access site

Before performing the venipuncture, you'll need to clean the site and stabilize the vein; you may also need to administer a local anesthetic.

Using a local anesthetic

Use of a local anesthetic is determined by patient assessment and history and the potential for discomfort with the procedure. If the policies and procedures for your organization include the use of a local anesthetic, the patient should be given this option prior to prepping and starting the procedure. Patients should be assessed for allergies to local anesthetic agents. The choice of the local anesthetic agent should be the one that is the least invasive and poses the least risk for potential reactions and patient harm. Local anesthetic agents include injection of intradermal lidocaine, topical transdermal creams, topical vapocoolant sprays, and pressure-accelerated lidocaine. Also, bacteriostatic normal saline solution might be effective due to the preservative agent.

Intradermal lidocaine

Lidocaine works by stopping the initiation and conduction of impulses at the neural membrane, and the result is local anesthetic action. Lidocaine is effective within 20 to 30 seconds, and the patient is able to feel touch and pressure. Due to this fast action, the injection is performed after skin antisepsis and immediately before the actual puncture with the catheter. This added solution within the tissue surrounding the vein could cause difficulty in seeing or feeling the vein. Intradermal lidocaine use requires an order from an LIP if it is not part of an approved protocol within your practice setting. (See *Administering a local anesthetic*, page 84.)

Topical transdermal agents (creams)

Transdermal anesthetic cream may also be used before accessing a peripheral vein and is a good choice for children or anyone who cannot tolerate needlesticks. Like injectable anesthetics, transdermal creams reduce pain, but the patient still feels pressure and touch. To be effective, a transdermal cream usually requires 30 to 60 minutes to be effective. Follow the manufacturer's directions and plan the application in advance of the catheter insertion.

Frozen (not quite)

Topical vapocoolant sprays can produce immediate anesthetic action. The evaporation of the liquid from the surface of the skin causes the temperature of area to decrease and provides a temporary break in pain sensation.

It's electric

Another option is to use pressure-accelerated lidocaine, a technique that delivers dermal analgesia in 7 to 10 minutes with minimal discomfort and without distorting the tissue.

A handheld device with two electrodes uses a mild electric current to deliver charged ions of lidocaine 2% and epinephrine 1:100,000 solution into the skin.

Administering a local anesthetic

A local anesthetic may be prescribed when starting peripheral I.V. therapy. Follow the steps below:

1. Verify patient identity using two patient identifiers.
2. Verify patient allergies.
3. Using a U-100 insulin syringe or 1-mL TB syringe with a 27-G needle, draw 0.1 mL of lidocaine 1% without epinephrine.
4. Don clean gloves.
5. Apply the skin antiseptic agent and allow it to dry thoroughly.
6. Insert the needle, bevel up, at a 15- to 25-degree angle next to the vein. The side approach carries less risk of accidental vein puncture indicated by blood appearing in the syringe. If the vein is deep, however, inject the lidocaine over the top of it. To make sure that you don't inject lidocaine into the vein — thus allowing it to circulate systemically — aspirate to check for a blood return. If this occurs, withdraw the needle and begin the procedure again.
7. Hold your thumb on the plunger of the syringe during insertion to avoid unnecessary movement when the needle is under the skin.
8. Inject the lidocaine until a small wheal appears (as shown). You may not have to administer the entire amount in the syringe.
9. Withdraw the syringe and allow 5 to 10 seconds for the anesthetic to work.
10. Insert the venous access device into the vein.

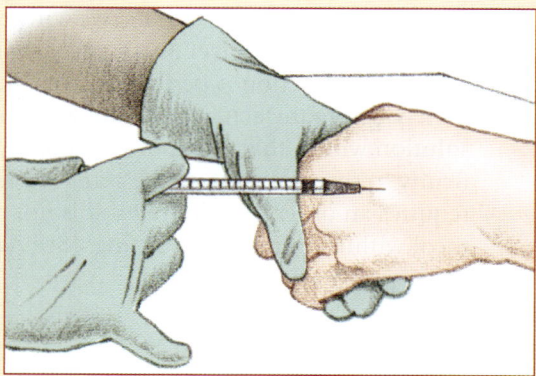

Preparing the venipuncture site

This step focuses on the skin and the infection risks it can present — both the patient's and clinician's skin. While performing the steps for site selection, you have had a good opportunity to notice if the chosen area is dirty or has excessive hair. If necessary, clip the hair over the insertion site to make the veins and the site easier to see and reduce pain when the tape is removed. Do not shave the insertion site as this causes microabrasions and increases the risk for infection. If the site is visibly dirty from sweat, skin oils, blood, or other debris, use soap and water to wash the area.

Perform hand hygiene by handwashing or using alcoholic hand gel. Then, put on clean exam gloves.

Clean the skin surrounding the insertion site with an antiseptic agent. The size of the area to be cleaned should be at least the size of the dressing to be applied, usually about 2" or 3" in all directions from the proposed insertion site.

Alcoholic chlorhexidine solution is the preferred agent. Prep the site for a minimum of 30 seconds using a back and forth mechanical scrub and allow it to dry for 30 seconds. Lightly wiping the skin surface with an antiseptic swab or pad is not adequate because organisms lie within the lower layers of the skin. A scrubbing action does a better job to reach those layers. Use of 70% alcohol alone is acceptable, but it requires the same scrubbing action and multiple pads are needed to thoroughly clean the area. Povidone-iodine may be used for patients when the use of an alcohol or chlorhexidine solution is contraindicated. Do not apply alcohol after applying povidone-iodine, as this will cancel the effects of the povidone-iodine. Povidone-iodine requires 1.5 to 2 minutes to be effective. The site should be allowed to dry completely before insertion of the I.V. catheter.

Never touch the prepared site. If vein palpation is necessary, sterile gloves are required.

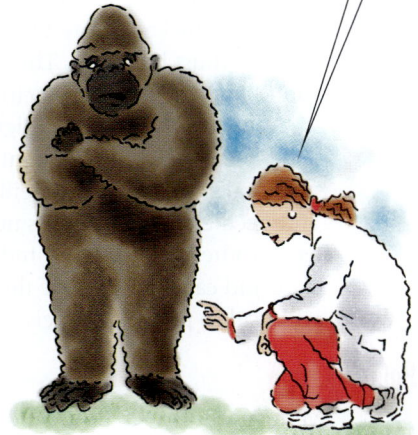

Have a hairy patient? Clip hair at the insertion site. Shaving may increase the risk for infection.

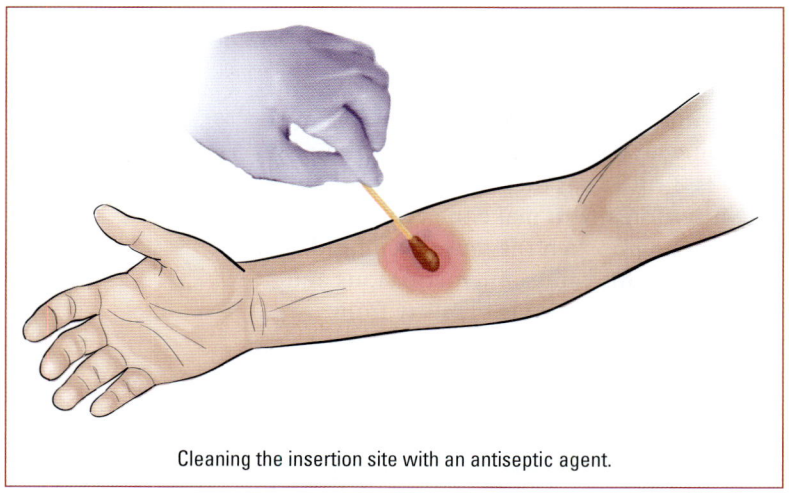

Cleaning the insertion site with an antiseptic agent.

Stabilizing the vein

Stabilizing the vein helps ensure a successful venipuncture the first time and decreases the chance of bruising and infiltration. Subcutaneous probing is not acceptable. Do not make multiple passes into the area to locate the vein. This process increases the chance of vein wall damage leading to bruising and possible hematoma formation. When a vein gets nicked, it can't be reused immediately and a new venipuncture site must be found. Thus, the patient will experience the discomfort of another needle puncture.

Subcutaneous probing significantly increases the risk of damage to superficial nerves. The patient may suddenly complain of feeling an electrical shock moving in either direction on the arm, feeling "pins and needles," or numbness near the site. These complaints are known as paresthesias and are an indication to immediately stop the procedure and carefully remove the catheter. Continuing in the same site will lead to permanent nerve damage.

Hold still, vein

Veins naturally lie in loose superficial connective tissue. As you try to puncture them and advance the catheter into the vein lumen, the force can move the vein. Many patients may say their veins "roll," but that is actually true for everybody. Your technique to stabilize the vein will hold it steady and increase your success. Using your nondominant hand, stretch the skin below the intended insertion site and hold it taut. This traction helps to maintain the stability of the vein and is necessary during the puncture step and the catheter advancement into the vein. (See *How to stabilize veins*, page 87.)

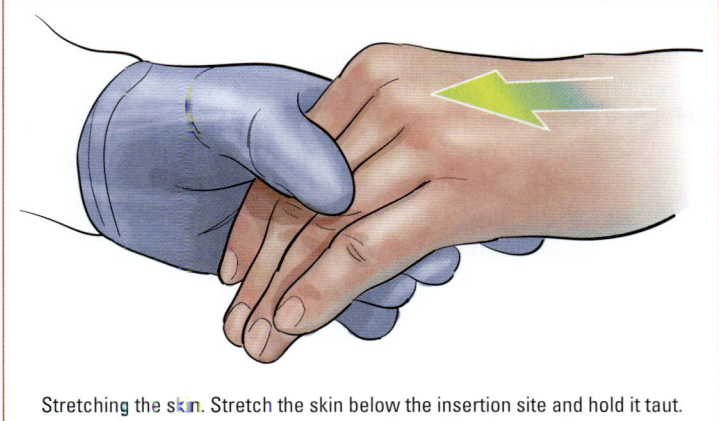

Stretching the skin. Stretch the skin below the insertion site and hold it taut.

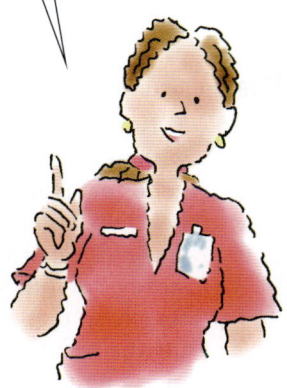

Stabilizing the vein helps ensure a successful venipuncture the first time…
…and also decreases the chance of bruising.

Insertion

Once you've prepared the venipuncture site, you're ready to insert the venous access device. Insertion of a venous access device can be performed using a direct approach or indirect approach. Choice of a direct or indirect approach is based on the patient assessment, device to be inserted, and clinician experience and expertise.

Inserting the venous access device

While still wearing gloves, grasp the plastic hub with your dominant hand. There may be grooves on the side of the hub to indicate the correct place to hold the device; follow the catheter manufacturer's instructions for use. Remove the cover, and visually inspect the device for product integrity. If the device integrity is compromised, remove it from patient use and obtain another device. Report defective devices according to your organizational policy and procedure.

Integrity of an I.V. device includes:
• visual inspection of the catheter before use for torn packaging, expiration date, and signs that the product is contaminated, is not intact, or has been damaged
• not withdrawing and reinserting the needle stylet through the catheter as this could damage the catheter and cause a catheter embolism
• seeing blood in the catheter flashback chamber when the catheter tip is inside the vein lumen
• ensuring that safety mechanisms are functioning per manufacturer's instructions.

You need to know this

Tell the patient that you're about to insert the device. Ask him to remain still and to refrain from pulling away. Explain that the initial needlestick will hurt but should quickly subside. If there is intense shooting pain, tingling, or numbness, this means contact between the needle and a nerve. To prevent permanent nerve damage, immediately stop the procedure and carefully remove the catheter from the site. Choose another site for insertion. There are more nerves in the hand, wrist, and antecubital fossa, so there's a greater chance that this could happen when using these sites.

Steady and direct

This method means the catheter punctures the skin and vein with one motion. It is useful for large prominent veins, but not good for small fragile veins or those not easily seen. Keeping the bevel up, enter the skin directly over the vein at a 10- to 15-degree angle. (Deeper veins require a wider angle.) Make sure to use a steady, smooth motion while keeping the skin taut. Position your fingers so that you are able to visualize blood return upon entering the vein. As soon as the device enters the vein (verified by blood return in the flash chamber), lower the distal portion of the catheter until it's almost parallel with but not touching the skin and advance the catheter slightly to ensure that the tip of the plastic catheter is in the vein. If you pass through the vein lumen completely, blood backflow will occur briefly and then stop as the catheter leaves the vein lumen. You may not see a rapid blood return with a small vein, with low blood pressure or in a dehydrated patient.

If you are unsuccessful in cannulating the vein on the first attempt, remove it and find another location. Continuing to probe the subcutaneous area poses a great risk for nerve damage.

Steady and indirect

With this technique, the catheter enters the skin first, usually slightly below the point where you plan to enter the vein. A second motion pushes the catheter through the vein wall. Using the indirect approach requires the same steady, smooth, motion while stabilizing the vein. Insert the catheter through the skin just distal to but on top of the vein. The vein may appear hidden at this point, but the catheter is very close to the vein. Continue to hold skin traction while you lower the catheter angle to the skin slightly and enter the vein. Confirm the blood in the flashback chamber.

How to stabilize veins

To help ensure successful venipuncture, you need to stabilize the patient's vein by stretching the skin and holding it taut. The stretching technique you'll use varies with the venipuncture site. This chart lists the various venipuncture sites along with a description of the stretching technique used for each.

Vein	Stretching technique
Metacarpal (hand) veins	Stretch the patient's hand and wrist downward, and hold the skin taut with your thumb.
Cephalic vein and wrist	Stretch the patient's fist laterally downward, and immobilize the skin with the thumb of your other hand.
Basilic vein at outer arm	Have the patient flex his elbow. While standing behind the flexed arm, retract the skin away from the site, and anchor the vein with your thumb. As an alternative, rotate the patient's extended lower arm inward and approach the vein from behind the arm. (This position may be difficult for the patient to maintain.) Another method is to place the patient's arm across their chest and stand on the opposite side of the bed. Stretch the skin taut by pulling downward with your nondominant thumb.
Inner arm	Encircle the patient's arm with your nondominant hand and use your thumb or fingers to stabilize the vein and pull the skin taut to stabilize the vein.
Median antebrachial vein	Rising from palm and along ulnar side of forearm.
Antecubital fossa Median cephalic, median basilic, and median cubital.	Have the patient extend his arm completely. Anchor the skin with your thumb, about 2" to 3" (5 to 7.5 cm) below the antecubital fossa.

Don't wing it, follow these steps...

If you're using a winged infusion needle, fold the edges of the wings between your thumb and forefinger, with the bevel facing upward. Remove the protective cover from the needle, being careful not to contaminate the needle. Then, insert the device using either a direct or indirect venipuncture technique. Blood return is seen in the attached extension set.

Advancing the catheter

While stabilizing the vein with one hand by holding skin traction, use the other to advance the catheter up to the hub. For some catheters, there could be a tight seal between the catheter and needle stylet, making separation with one hand difficult. If this happens, temporarily release the skin traction, hold the catheter hub with one hand and the needle stylet hub with the other hand, and pull back slightly on the needle stylet hub. Be very careful to only retract the needle stylet slightly; pulling back on the catheter hub could pull the catheter tip out of the vein. Always re-establish skin traction before advancing the catheter into the vein. Advance the catheter into the vein by holding the sides of the plastic hub or pushing the tab on top of the plastic hub. Do NOT touch the open catheter lumen as this will cause contamination. Be sure to advance only the catheter to avoid puncturing the vein's posterior wall with the needle. At this point, the catheter is inside the skin and vein and the needle stylet extends from the catheter hub and is obstructing the blood from flowing out of the hub. Release the tourniquet.

Reduce your exposure to blood

Next, remove the needle stylet. To minimize blood exposure, if your catheter does not have a valve inside the hub, use one of the following techniques:

- Use a finger of your nondominant hand to apply pressure above the catheter tip. You will also need to hold the catheter hub and the extension set to make this connection, so this method may be difficult if you have small hands.
- Contain blood by placing a dry gauze pad under the catheter hub. This method also prevents blood from escaping onto linens or running down the patient's arm.
- Activate the safety mechanism to shield the needle according to the manufacturer's instructions. A passive safety mechanism does not require activation because the needle is protected as you withdraw it from the catheter lumen. Using aseptic, no-touch technique, attach the extension set to the catheter hub and secure the luer-locking connection. Be very careful to not allow the male luer end of the extension set to touch anything before it enters the catheter hub. Aspirate for a blood return and to make sure all air has been pulled back into the syringe. Flush the catheter with normal saline solution while observing for any swelling and listening for any patient complaints.

"Floating" in

For very small, fragile veins or in dehydrated patients, using the flow of I.V. fluids may help to advance the catheter into the vein. This technique can be tricky because only a very small length of catheter is inside the vein lumen at this point in the procedure and you must prevent the sterile catheter from lying on the skin. Release the tourniquet and remove the needle stylet as described above. Hold the catheter hub off the skin while attaching the primed I.V. administration set and begin the infusion. While stabilizing the vein with one hand, hold the catheter hub to advance the catheter into the vein as the fluid flows. When the catheter is advanced, slow the I.V. flow rate.

Protect the skin

Skin integrity is important for all patients and is a major responsibility for nursing. Medical adhesive–related skin injury includes many types of skin damage. Before using any adhesive device, apply a skin barrier solution to the skin and let it dry thoroughly. This solution not only protects the skin, the dressing remains adherent and intact for longer periods with its use.

Stable and secure

After the venous access device has been successfully inserted, secure the device to the skin using an engineered stabilization device. Stabilization devices are used to reduce catheter dislodgement and risk of complications and should not interfere with monitoring or assessment of the I.V. site.

Although tape is commonly used, it does not adhere well to the plastic hub and is not effective for adequate catheter stabilization. Nonsterile rolls of tape may be contaminated with pathogens and should not be placed near the insertion site. A standard transparent semipermeable membrane (TSM) dressing is not adequate for catheter stabilization; however, a TSM dressing with a cloth border adds greater securement for the catheter. If a stabilization device is not available, use only sterile tape near the puncture site.

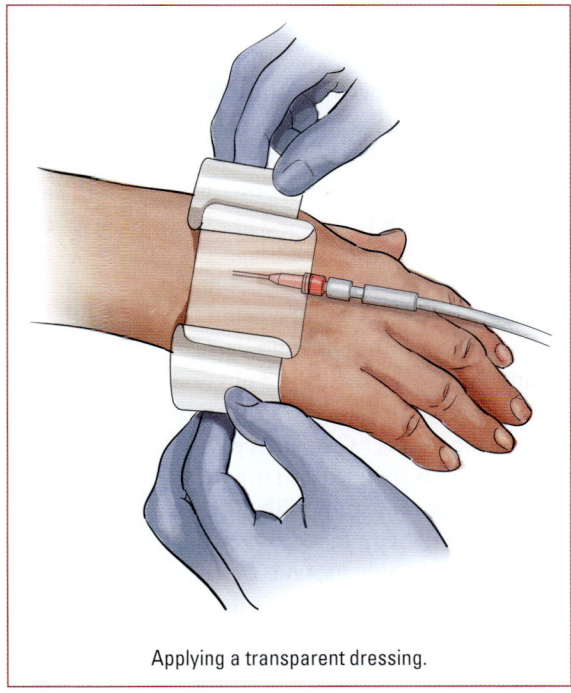

Applying a transparent dressing.

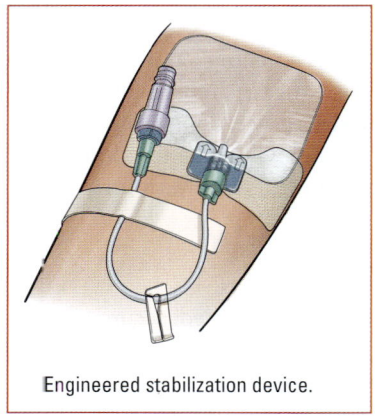

Engineered stabilization device.

Rolled bandages with or without stretchy properties should not be used on the extremity around an I.V. catheter site. They do not provide any securement for the catheter and prevent a complete site assessment. Additionally, they can be wrapped too tightly leading to constriction of venous blood flow and interference with the infusing fluid.

Dressing for success

After stabilizing and securing the catheter, a sterile dressing is applied to the site. Dressings are either a TSM dressing or sterile gauze and tape dressing. A TSM dressing offers the distinct advantage of being able to see the entire site. Dressing changes on short peripheral catheters are done if the dressing becomes damp, loosened, and/or visibly soiled. For a catheter that is allowed to remain indwelling, the TSM dressing should be changed at least every 5 to 7 days and a gauze dressings should be changed at least every 48 hours. TSM dressings should only cover the catheter hub and not the luer connection of the attached extension set or I.V. administration set.

Stabilize the joint

If the catheter insertion site, tip, or dressing is affected by joint motion, add an armboard to support the joint and ensure correct fluid flow rate. Armboards are a single patient device and not considered to be a physical restraint because they protect the patient from harm. Place the armboard on the hand to support the wrist, allowing the fingers to extend beyond the board for movement. The armboard should be padded and not cause any constriction of blood flow. Some armboards now come with attached Velcro strips or you can use a folded gauze or another piece of tape to prevent the tape from adhering to the arm, leaving only the ends of the tape to adhere to the back of the armboard. Do not use a wooden tongue depressor for this purpose as they may increase risk of site contamination.

Remove the armboard periodically according to facility policy so you can check the status of circulation, skin integrity, and range of motion for the joint.

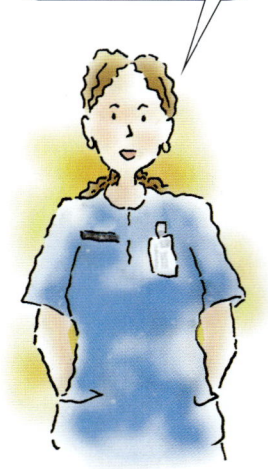

If a vein in the hand, wrist or antecubital fossa is all that is available, use an armboard to stabilize the joint

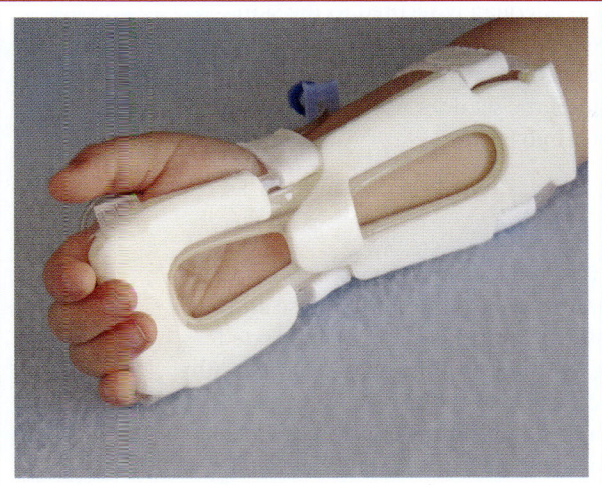
Armboard. Reprinted from I.V. House, Inc., St. Louis, MO, with permission

Finishing touches

Label the insertion site with the date, gauge size of the catheter, and your initials. Return the patient to their preferred position and ensure that the bed is in the lowest level. Make sure that the I.V. pole, fluid container, and/or infusion pump is in the best location for your patient and that no part of the I.V. set is touching the floor. Check all connections to make sure they are securely tightened with their luer-lock device. Check the flow rate for accuracy. Dispose of the needle stylet and safety device in a sharps container. Discard all other supplies and packaging according to organizational policy and procedure. Remove your gloves and perform hand hygiene.

Infection prevention is critical

Infection from a short peripheral catheter includes local site infection and bloodstream infection. Rates of these infections are reported to be very low, but the high number of peripheral catheters used means a large number of infections. Infection prevention is directly in the control of clinicians who insert these catheters. Ensure that you are in compliance with all steps to prevent these infections:

- Adhere to hand hygiene before and after all infusion procedures.
- Use a tourniquet for a single patient only.
- Use gloves for catheter insertion.
- Thoroughly scrub the insertion site with a skin antiseptic agent and allowing it to dry completely.
- After the skin antiseptic is applied, touch the site ONLY with sterile gloves

- Ensure that the catheter hub is adequately secured to the skin.
- Ensure the sterile dressing is totally adherent, clean, and dry.
- Use a new sterile catheter for each insertion attempt.
- Ensure that the male luer end of the set does not touch anything as it is attached to the catheter hub.

Intermittent infusion device

Also called a *saline lock*, an intermittent infusion device may be used when venous access must be maintained for intermittent use and a continuous infusion isn't necessary. Any catheter can be converted from an open catheter allowing continuous infusion to a closed catheter allowing for intermittent access. This is done by adding a needleless connector (NC) to the distal end of a short extension set attached to the catheter hub. The NC can be directly attached to the catheter hub, but the extension set adds many benefits discussed above. All NCs have a luer-lock design to prevent accidental disconnections. NCs function in different ways and it is important to understand what type of device you are using in order to correctly maintain the patency of the venous access device. (See Chapter 1, *Needleless connectors*, page 32.)

Continuous infusion not required

The intermittent peripheral catheter is flushed with preservative-free 0.9% sodium chloride at the completion of an infusion, before and after administration of medications or drawing blood samples, and at a frequency per the organization's policy and procedures. Doing so makes it possible to maintain venous access in patients who must receive regularly scheduled intermittent I.V. medications but don't require continuous infusion. Short peripheral catheters that are no longer needed as part of the patient's plan of care or have not been used for 24 hours or more should be removed. For catheter that is not being used but cannot be removed, flush with 0.9% sodium chloride every 24 hours to assess and maintain patency.

Can't get a blood return from a peripheral catheter?

Try these steps:
- Use a slow and gentle technique to aspirate. Pulling hard and fast on the syringe plunger can prevent the blood return.
- Switch to a smaller syringe; 3- or 5-mL syringes generate LESS force on aspiration than a 10-mL syringe.
- If these fail, place a tourniquet above the site and attempt again. If all of these fail to produce a blood return, the catheter is not functioning correctly and should be removed. If the LIP orders discontinuation of the continous I.V. infusion but I.V. medications are

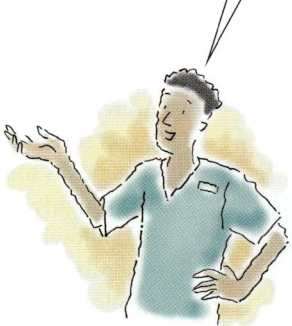

To ensure patency, flush the device before and after infusing the medication...
...aspirating for a blood return is a very important component of assessing the catheter!

From continuous to intermittent

To make the conversion:
1. Assess the site for any signs or symptoms of complications. Proceed with conversion only if the site is free of any problem.
2. Prime the needleless connector with 0.9% sodium chloride solution, leaving the syringe attached.
3. Stop the fluid flow. Clamp the I.V. administration set and detach from the short extension set on the catheter.
4. Attach a needleless connector (see figure) to the extension set.
5. Aspirate for a blood return and flush with the remaining solution.

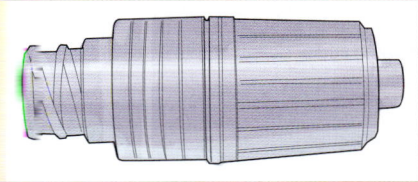

to continue, convert the existing line to an intermittent venous access device or saline lock. (See *From continuous to intermittent,* page 95.)

Don't go blindly

Patients are living longer with chronic diseases that can alter vascular integrity. A history of many venipuncture attempts and peripheral infusion produces vein wasting, leaving very few peripheral sites. Obese patients and patients scheduled for bariatric surgery have veins that cannot easily be seen or palpated. Blindly making venipuncture attempts without a reasonable degree of certainty for success by seeing or feeling the vein is no longer accepted practice. Peripheral veins are damaged or destroyed through multiple failed attempts. These patients may need a central venous catheter based only on the fact that peripheral veins cannot be found, adding unnecessary risk for complications. Vein preservation is now the goal! To meet this goal, it is the national standard of care for one clinician to make no more than two vein puncture attempts. A second clinician can make an additional two attempts, but if those fail, another plan of care is needed. Before making a total of four unsuccessful attempts, use visible light or near-infrared light device if one is available and you are competent to use it. If all of these attempts fail, stop the process. Do not continue sticking!

At this point, a careful assessment of vascular access device needs is required. Notify the infusion or vascular access specialist and ask them to evaluate the patient. Collaborate with the health care team to discuss appropriate options, which include ultrasound guidance for a peripheral catheter insertion, a midline catheter, or, as a last resort, insertion of a central venous catheter.

Take this sample (See also "Applying a Tourniquet")

To smoothly and safely collect a blood sample from a peripheral catheter, follow these step-by-step techniques after assembling your equipment and making the venipuncture:

- Identify the patient using two identifiers according to your facility policy and procedure.
- Perform hand hygiene.
- Place a pad underneath the site to protect the bed linens.
- If fluids are infusing, stop for 2 minutes.
- Close clamp on the extension set.
- Disconnect the administration set from the extension set and cover the male luer end with a sterile end cap.
- Disinfect the needleless connector if used by thorough scrubbing with a new disinfection pad for the time required by facility policy and procedure.
- Use either a syringe or a vacuum tube holder attached to the extension set hub. Syringes require more manipulation of the hub than a vacuum tube holder.
- Draw 1 or 2 mL and label the syringe or vacuum tube as "discard."
- Draw the required amount of blood for the needed lab test. If using a syringe, use a slow gentle technique to aspirate blood. Use a smaller syringe (for example, 3 to 5 mL) instead of a 10 mL size.
- If required, apply a tourniquet on the upper arm to encourage blood aspiration. Ensure that the total tourniquet time is no more than 1 minute.
- Attach a needleless transfer device to the syringe and transfer the blood to the vacuum tubes in the correct sequence according to facility policy and procedure.
- Label all tubes in the presence of the patient.
- Flush the extension set and catheter with normal saline.
- Attach the primary continuous I.V. administration set, if prescribed, and regulate the fluid flow rate.
- Properly dispose of the equipment.
- Place blood specimens in a closed, leakproof bag and deliver to the laboratory immediately.

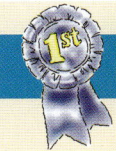
Best practice

How to apply a transparent semipermeable dressing

Here's how to apply a transparent semipermeable dressing, which allows for visual assessment of the catheter insertion site.

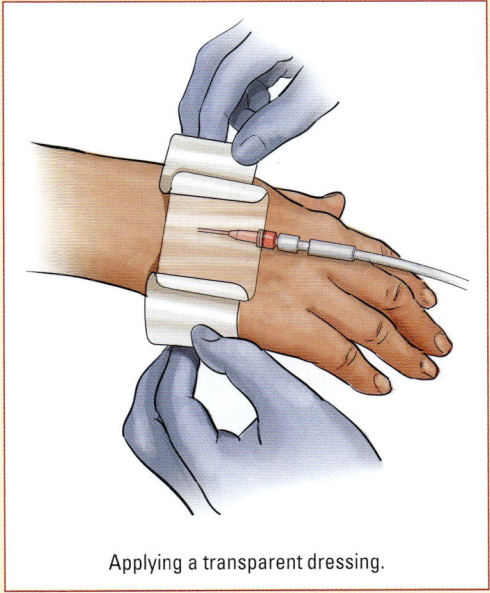

Applying a transparent dressing.

- Make sure the insertion site is clean and dry.
- Remove the dressing from the package and, using aseptic technique, remove the protective seal. Avoid touching the adhesive surface.
- Place the dressing directly over the insertion site and the hub, as shown. Don't cover the administration set or luer connection. Also, don't stretch the dressing; doing so may cause skin irritation and damage, abrasions, or itching.
- Press or mold the dressing around the catheter hub to make the dressing adherent on all sides.

Removing a transparent semipermeable dressing
To remove the dressing, hold the distal portion of the attached set. Begin at the device hub and gently pull the dressing perpendicular to the skin toward the insertion site. Be careful not to accidentally dislodge the catheter, as it may be stuck to the dressing. Use an alcohol pad or other adhesive removal solution if needed to remove the dressing.

Using a stretch net

Patients who are confused and have dementia and those with skin disorders may need some extra help with securing the catheter. Also, patients in home care who are very active can benefit from a little extra securement. Stretch net can help all of these patients. If using the net on the patient's hand, cut a hole in the net sleeve for his thumb. The net reduces the amount of adhesive tape needed and may decrease accidental dislodgment.

Collecting a blood sample

Using a peripheral catheter to collect a blood sample is quite possible, but it should be done after the insertion procedure or during the catheter dwell. Extended tourniquet time may be needed to insert a peripheral catheter, and this can cause changes in lab values. First, gather the necessary equipment: laboratory tubes for the ordered tests, an appropriate-size syringe without a needle, a needleless transfer device, and a protective pad. Then, follow the steps outlined in *Take this sample*, page 96.

Using any venous access device for obtaining a blood sample results in additional manipulation of the system, leading to complications. When the benefit of using the catheter outweighs the risk, it is appropriate to use the catheter. This decision for a short peripheral catheter is simpler than for a central venous catheter. Pediatric patients, adults with difficult venous access, the need for serial blood testing, and those receiving anticoagulants or with a bleeding disorder can benefit from using the short peripheral catheter for this purpose.

If the infusion has already been initiated, stop the fluid flow for at least 2 minutes before obtaining the blood sample. Withdraw 1 to 2 mL of blood and discard before drawing the blood sample for testing.

Documenting the venipuncture

When you insert a peripheral catheter, be sure to document:
- date and time of the venipuncture
- venipuncture site — be specific by using the vein name and its exact location on the extremity and physical description of landmarks or mark the site on a drawing of the arm

- gauge and length of catheter inserted
- number of attempts
- use of local anesthetic
- type of stabilization used
- type of dressing used
- use of visualization technology as appropriate
- presence of blood return
- absence of signs and symptoms of complications (for example, infiltration, nerve damage)
- type and amount of flush solution
- type and amount of fluid infusing including number of the solution container if required by facility policy and procedures
- name and dosage of additives in the solution
- flow rate
- adverse reactions and the actions taken to correct them
- patient teaching and evidence of patient understanding
- name of the person initiating the infusion
- patient response/tolerance to procedure.

Remember to document the information in the appropriate sections of the facility's medical record using the correct forms.

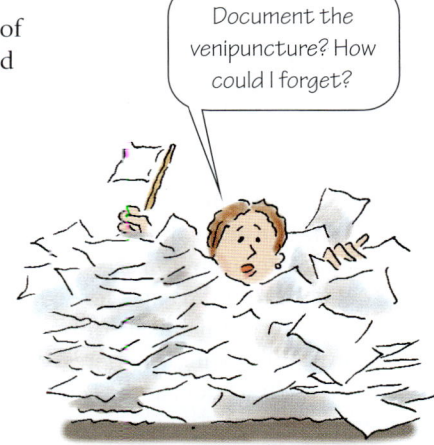

Document the venipuncture? How could I forget?

Best practice

There should be no more than two attempts per clinician and no more than four total attempts. Multiple unsuccessful attempts can delay treatment, increase costs, limit future vascular access sites, cause pain and distress to the patient, and increase the risk for complications.

For the novice clinician: Know your limitations and do not attempt to place a device in a patient with known difficult venous access. Placing a peripheral I.V. device in patients with prominent veins will increase your success, build your confidence, and increase your skill level to move onto those more challenging patients.

Maintaining peripheral I.V. therapy

After the I.V. infusion starts, focus on maintaining therapy and preventing complications. Doing so involves routine and special care measures as well as discontinuing the infusion when therapy is completed. Also, you should be prepared to meet the special needs of pediatric, elderly, and home care patients who require I.V. therapy.

Routine care

Routine care measures help prevent complications. They also give you an opportunity to observe the I.V. site for signs of complications. The infusion system, which is the solution container to the I.V. catheter, is checked on a regular basis for integrity of the system; the correct flow rate and volume infused; expiration dates of solutions, dressings, and administration sets; integrity of the dressing on the site; the site and surrounding area for signs and symptoms of complications; and patient complaints. Perform these measures according to your facility's policy and procedures. Wash your hands and wear gloves whenever you work near the venipuncture site.

Changing the dressing

The insertion site should be inspected for tenderness, drainage, leakage, redness, and other problems. Palpate the site through the intact dressing.

Best practice

Routine assessment of peripheral I.V. infusion therapy

- At least every 4 hours for patients who are alert and oriented
- At least every 1 to 2 hours for patients who are critically ill and sedated and have cognitive defects or impaired sensation.
- At least every 5 to 10 mL for vesicant medications by infusion
- At least once per day for outpatient and home care patients with intermittent infusion; with continuous infusion in these settings, at least every 4 hours. Instruct the patient or family to report any problems immediately to their health care provider.

Maintaining peripheral I.V. therapy

Time to change

All types of dressings must be changed immediately when they are dirty, wet, or loose. Peripheral catheters are changed when there are clinical reasons to change the catheter and not by a specific number of hours or days. This can mean longer dwell times for some catheters, indicating a need for regular dressing changes. Gauze dressings should be changed routinely every 48 hours. A transparent semipermeable dressing should be changed at least every 5 to 7 days.

Getting ready

Before performing a dressing change, gather this equipment:
- skin antiseptic agent — alcoholic chlorhexidine is preferred; povidone-iodine or 70% alcohol are acceptable
- engineered stabilization device, sterile tape, or sterile surgical strips
- transparent semipermeable dressing or sterile gauze pad and tape
- skin barrier solution
- label
- clean gloves.

To change a dressing, follow the steps outlined in *Changing a peripheral I.V. dressing*. Of course, use aseptic technique.

Changing a peripheral I.V. dressing

To change a peripheral I.V. dressing, follow these steps:
1. Gather supplies
2. Perform hand hygiene.
3. Explain the procedure to the patient.
4. Don gloves.
5. Assess the venipuncture site for signs of redness, tenderness, swelling, or drainage. If present, the catheter must be removed.
6. Remove the existing dressing. Begin at the hub of the device and gently pull the dressing perpendicular to the skin toward the insertion site. Be careful not to accidentally dislodge the catheter, as it may be stuck to the dressing. Use an alcohol pad or other adhesive removal solution if needed to remove the dressing.
7. Remove the engineered stabilization device per manufacturer's directions for use.

(continued)

Changing a peripheral I.V. dressing *(continued)*

8. Clean the skin with antiseptic solution; cover the area that will be under the dressing; allow to dry completely.
   - Alcoholic chlorhexidine solution: Use a back and forth scrubbing motion for at least 30 seconds.
   - Povidone-iodine: Should remain on the skin for 1.5 to 2 minutes or longer to completely dry for adequate antisepsis.
   - 70% alcohol: Use enough pads to cover the area.
   - The use of back and forth scrubbing motion will allow penetration to deep skin layers; however, this has not been studied for alcohol or povidone-iodine.
9. Apply skin barrier solution and allow it to dry.
10. Apply engineered stabilization device.
11. Apply TSM (or gauze and tape) dressing to the insertion site.
12. Discard used supplies in appropriate receptacles.
13. Remove gloves, and discard.
14. Perform hand hygiene.
15. Label dressing with date performed.

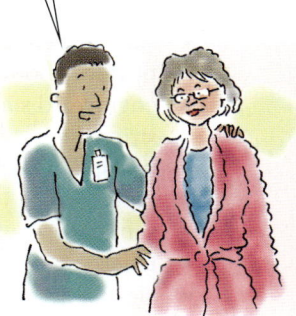

Anticipate the risk for skin injury related to age, presence of edema, joint movement, and medical adhesive–related skin injury (MARSI). Use of a skin barrier solution will reduce the risk of MARSI.

Changing the I.V. solution

A long-standing practice has been to change bags or bottles of I.V. fluids at 24 hours, although this practice is not supported by recent evidence. Change the I.V. fluid container according to facility policies and procedures. Fluids that enhance microbial growth (that is, fat emulsions, parenteral nutrition, blood products) are changed more frequently. Before changing the I.V. container, check the new one for cracks, leaks, and other damage. Also check the solution for discoloration, turbidity, and particulates. Note the date and time the solution was mixed and the beyond-use or expiration date. Plan to change the fluid container and the administration set at the same time to reduce manipulation of the system.

Changing the administration set

Change the administration set according to your facility's policy and whenever you note or suspect contamination. For regular I.V. fluids, changing the administration set more frequently than every 96 hours does not decrease the risk of infection. Administration sets used for parenteral nutrition, I.V. fat emulsion, and blood and blood components require more frequent changes and are discussed in their respective chapters. Inserting a new catheter also requires a change of the administration set.

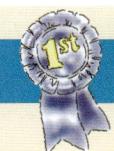

Best practice

A change in administration

- Change the administration set immediately if contamination is suspected or product integrity is compromised.
- Change the administration set when a new peripheral catheter is inserted.
- Administration sets are opened and primed immediately prior to administration.
- Do not leave an unprimed set attached to the fluid container.
- Reduce the number of entries into the system to as few as possible.
- Before disconnecting or reconnecting an administration set, trace the entire length of the set from the patient to the solution container. This should also be done at each transition of care to a new service or setting and as part of the hand-off process to another clinician.
- Choose an administration set with all needed components as an integral part of the set. This reduces the need for add-on devices (for example, filters) as each connection is a potential source of contamination, misuse, and disconnection.
- For intermittent administration sets that are used more than once in a 24-hour period, aseptically attach a new, sterile end cap to the male luer end of the administration set after each intermittent use.
- Do not attach the exposed male luer end of the administration set to a port on the same set. Do not use other objects such as a syringe tip cap to cover the male luer end of the intermittent set.
- Label administration sets with the date of initiation or date of change based on organizational procedures.
- For sets connected to an intraspinal, intraosseous, or subcutaneous device, label administration sets near its connection to the device, indicating the correct administration route and device.

Changing the I.V. catheter: not by a clock or calendar

Previously, a short peripheral catheter was changed on a set schedule, usually every 72 or 96 hours. Research has shown that this practice is less than beneficial. Currently, the condition of the catheter directs when it is removed, and not a clock or calendar. This means that the peripheral catheter is changed at the very first sign or symptom of a problem including:

- any amount of tenderness and/or pain with or without palpation
- redness or blanching at the site
- heat or coolness at the site
- swelling — compare both extremities as this will not always appear as a raised lump near the site

- hardness on palpation
- fluid leakage or purulent drainage from the catheter site
- abnormal functioning such as resistance to flushing and failure to obtain a blood return.

Any of these signs or symptoms represents the development of a variety of complications and requires immediate removal of the catheter. Remember you should be assessing the site at least every 4 hours for an alert and oriented patient and more frequently for other situations.

The clinical need for the peripheral I.V. catheter should be assessed daily. When the peripheral catheter is not needed for the patient's plan of care, it should be removed. Remove the catheter when all I.V. infusion therapy is discontinued. Don't allow it to remain in place just in case it might be needed again.

In situations in which there is an unresolved complication and infusion therapy is still prescribed, assess several factors before automatically restarting the catheter, especially if your patient has difficult peripheral veins. Is the patient eating and drinking? If yes, could the infusion therapy be changed to an oral route? What are the patient's lab values such as electrolytes, blood counts, or culture results? Collaborate with the health care team and discuss the situation for possible changes in the prescribed therapy or the need for an alternative venous access device.

Documentation

Record dressing, administration set, and solution changes, and note the condition of the venipuncture site.

Complications of therapy

Complications of peripheral I.V. therapy can arise from the venous access device, the infusion, or the medication being administered. These complications can be local or near the insertion site or systemic. Even local complications can produce life-altering outcomes, and systemic complications can be life threatening. All clinicians responsible for administering I.V. infusion therapy are also accountable for the outcomes produced. These events add significant costs to patient care in the form of extended treatments and hospital stays. And they are the cause of many lawsuits brought against all clinicians and their employers. The prompt identification of the clinical signs and symptoms and appropriate interventions are critical to decrease the risk of further complications; however, prevention is equally, if not more, important.

Local trouble? It may become system wide...

Local complications include:
- infiltration and extravasation
- phlebitis and thrombophlebitis
- cellulitis and local site infection
- occlusion
- nerve injury.

Systemic complications include air embolism, bloodstream infection, speed shock, circulatory overload, allergic reactions, and numerous adverse reactions to medications. A complication may begin locally and become systemic — as when an infection at the venipuncture site progresses to a bloodstream infection. (For a complete description of local and systemic complications, see *Local complications of peripheral I.V. therapy*, pages 107.)

Infiltration or extravasation!

Perhaps the greatest threat to a patient receiving I.V. therapy is infiltration, which is defined as the unintended infusion of nonvesicant fluid and medication into the surrounding tissues. Extravasation is the unintended infusion of a vesicant fluid or medication into the surrounding tissue. A vesicant is any fluid or medication that can cause tissue damage or necrosis. For this reason, the clinician must know the vesicant or irritant characteristics of all fluids and medications before they are administered. The most severe forms of infiltration and extravasation can lead to the need for surgical debridement and skin grafting due to necrotic ulcers, compartment syndrome requiring immediate surgical fasciotomy to relieve the pressure, and complex regional pain syndrome, which produces lifelong damage to nearby nerves requiring intense pain management.

Phlebitis and thrombophlebitis

Phlebitis is inflammation of the vein wall, while thrombophlebitis is the inflammation plus a clot in the vein. Although the inflammation may start in a very small area, it can progress to involve a very large area of the extremity extending to other superficial veins. This progression can occur after the catheter is removed and is known as postinfusion phlebitis, indicating the need for continued assessment after the catheter has been removed. Mechanical factors associated with the catheter and chemical factors associated with the fluid and medications are probably the most common cause, but microorganisms, especially *Staphylococcus aureus*, can also cause phlebitis.

More information is included in *Local and systemic complications of I.V. therapy*, page 106 and *Systemic Complications of I.V. therapy*, page 111.

The lists of signs and symptoms are comprehensive, but each one may not be present for each complication. For instance, pain may not always be present with phlebitis or infiltration/extravasation. The presence of swelling can be elusive, so compare both upper extremities. Don't always expect to see a raised area of fluid appearing directly at the catheter site. Fluid could be escaping into the compartments, causing the entire extremity to enlarge.

Other Complications

Bloodstream infection (BSI) is caused by all types of vascular access devices; however, more attention has been given to central line–associated bloodstream infection (CLABSI) rather than BSI caused by short peripheral catheters. There are little data about the specific causes related to BSI from peripheral catheters, although attention to aseptic technique should be used for all types of venous access devices. Don't confuse BSI and sepsis. Sepsis is an immune response to a bacterial infection that leads to organ damage and failure. Careful and frequent patient assessment should identify the signs and symptoms of BSI before they have a chance to advance to sepsis or septic shock.

Venous air embolism is another systemic complication that is more common with central venous access devices. This is due to the differences in venous pressure where the catheter tips are located. In the hand, venous pressure is approximately 35 mm Hg. This pressure decreases as veins return blood to the heart, leaving a pressure of 0 in the superior vena cava. Air embolism requires a pressure gradient to allow air to move into the bloodstream. This pressure gradient is not present when a peripheral catheter is open to room air because the venous pressure will cause blood to exit from the catheter instead of allowing air to enter. The opposite is true for a central venous access device, in which the pressure is 0 and an open catheter can easily allow air to move into the lumen and bloodstream.

For air embolism to occur with a peripheral catheter, some force must be pushing the air into the vein such as an unprimed administration set connected to the catheter. A liter bag of I.V. fluids hanging about 3' or 4' above the peripheral I.V. catheter will exert approximately 2 pounds per square inch of pressure, enough to overcome normal venous pressure and force air into the bloodstream. Small air bubbles that are frequently seen in the administration set are not known to cause a sudden catastrophic event for the patient, but they can cause long-term problems. These small air bubbles attract platelets and other blood cells, growing into a larger mass as they move toward the pulmonary circulation. These bubbles pass through the blood vessels in the lungs until they reach a point where the vessel is too small to allow them to go farther. This blocks normal blood flow to that area of the lungs and, over time, could result in pulmonary hypertension in patients that have received many I.V. infusions with these bubbles.

(Text continues on page 113)

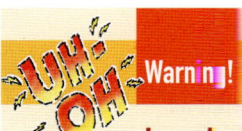

Warning!

Local complications of peripheral I.V. therapy

Definition	Signs and symptoms	Possible causes	Nursing interventions
Phlebitis Inflammation of the vein due to mechanical, chemical, or bacterial causes **Thrombophlebitis** Vein inflammation plus clot formation	• Pain at tip of catheter and above • Redness at tip of catheter and along vein • Edema over vein and extending up or down the extremity • Vein feels hard or cord-like on palpation	• Stiff catheter material • Catheter too large for the vein, obstructing blood flow around the catheter • Excessive movement from inadequate catheter or joint stabilization • Inadequate preparation of medication with correct dilution, if required, or too rapid injection or infusion • Solution with osmolarity greater than 900 mOsm or greater than 10% dextrose concentration • Inexperienced clinician	• Remove the device. • Apply heat. • Administer pain and anti-inflammatory medications as prescribed. • Document the patient's condition using a standardized grading scale. • Document your interventions. • Notify the LIP based on the severity of the condition and the facility policy and procedure. **Prevention:** • Restart the infusion using a larger vein or a smaller-gauge device to ensure adequate blood flow. • Use an engineered stabilization device. • Use an armboard if the catheter must be inserted in or near a joint. • Strictly adhere to all infection prevention methods.
Infiltration Infusion of nonvesicant fluid and medication into the tissue surrounding the vein **Extravasation** Infusion of vesicant fluid or medication into the tissue surrounding the vein	• Swelling at and around I.V. site; may appear as an enlarged arm and not be limited to the catheter site • Discomfort, burning, or pain at site • Feeling of tightness at site, in the distal extremity such as fingers, or above the site • Skin temperature around site may feel cool or warm. • Blanching or redness at site • Absence of blood return • Altered flow rate	• Device dislodged from vein • Perforated vein • Inadequate stabilization of catheter • Inadequate stabilization of joint • Rapid flow rates from power injectors (radiology) and rapid infusers (ED) • Excessive manipulation at the catheter or attached set • Subsequent peripheral catheters after the first insertion • Age-related changes to the vasculature • Disease-related changes to the vasculature • Use of deep veins with insufficient catheter length	• Infiltration: remove the catheter. • Extravasation: disconnect all sets; aspirate all contents from the catheter lumen and tissue if possible and then remove the catheter. • Elevate the arm. • Apply cool or warm compresses depending on the medication in the tissue. • Document using a grading scale. • Notify the LIP based on the severity of the condition and the facility policy and procedure. • Administer the prescribed antidote. • Complete unusual occurrence report. • Periodically assess circulation by checking for pulse, capillary refill, and numbness or tingling. • Restart the infusion, preferably in another limb or above the site. • Document the patient's condition and your interventions.

(continued)

Local complications of peripheral I.V. therapy *(continued)*

Definition	Signs and symptoms	Possible causes	Nursing interventions
		• Patient's inability to communicate/feel pain, tightness, or other discomfort	**Prevention:** • Don't administer vesicant medications through a catheter indwelling for more than 24 hours. • For vesicant medications infusing longer than 60 minutes, advocate for a central venous catheter. • Assess the I.V. site frequently during infusion. • Don't obscure area above site with tape or rolled gauze bandages. • Teach the patient to report discomfort, pain, or swelling. • Stabilize the site with an engineered stabilization device. • Use armboard if the site is in or near a joint.
Local site infection in the vein at the insertion site (suppurative or purulent thrombophlebitis)	• Redness along the line of the vein and/or in the area surrounding the site	• Lack of or inadequate hand hygiene • Inadequate or incorrect aseptic technique for insertion and care of the catheter and the entire infusion system • Inadequate skin antisepsis before venipuncture	• Remove the catheter immediately. • Notify the LIP. • Obtain cultures of drainage and blood, as prescribed. • Administer antibiotics as prescribed. • Suspect an infected thrombus in the superficial veins if the patient does not respond to treatment.
Cellulitis Infection of the subcutaneous tissue surrounding the puncture site	• Swelling • Hardness of the vein • Purulent drainage from the puncture site • An increased body temperature could indicate the progression from a local infection to a BSI.	• Catheters placed during emergent situations that are not changed within 24 to 48 hours • Inadequate catheter and joint stability allowing catheter movement and skin organisms to move into the site	**Prevention:** • If the patient's skin is visibly dirty, wash with soap and water before venipuncture. • Strictly attend to hand hygiene and appropriate use of gloves for all I.V. procedures. • Strictly follow all aseptic techniques for I.V. procedures. • Correctly apply skin antiseptic agents. • Maintain a clean, dry, and intact dressing.

Local complications of peripheral I.V. therapy *(continued)*

Definition	Signs and symptoms	Possible causes	Nursing interventions
Occlusion	• No increase in gravity flow rate when I.V. container is raised • Downstream occlusion alarms from electronic infusion pump • Stagnant blood visible in attached I.V. set • Discomfort at insertion site	• I.V. flow interrupted • Intermittent device not flushed • Reduction of distance between the fluid container and catheter when gravity flow is used • Hypercoagulable patient • Line clamped too long • Venous spasm produced by infusion of cold fluids or a sudden change in infusion pressure • Kinked catheter at insertion site, especially smaller-gauge sizes	• Inspect infusion system for closed clamps or kinked set. • Remove dressing and stabilization device to assess for catheter kinks; never reinsert any external portion of the catheter. • Use 10-mL saline-filled syringe to flush. Don't use force. If resistance is met, stop immediately. If unsuccessful, remove the catheter. • Apply warm compress if venous spasm is suspected. **Prevention:** • Maintain the I.V. flow rate. • Flush promptly after intermittent medications. • Use correct sequence for final syringe disconnection and clamping based on the type of needleless connector being used. • Properly stabilize and secure catheter hub to prevent movement and kinking.
Hematoma Bleeding into the subcutaneous tissue around the vein	• Tenderness and swelling at venipuncture site • Bruising around site	• Vein punctured through opposite wall at time of venipuncture, possibly associated with direct venipuncture technique • Erosion of catheter tip through vein wall due to excessive movement • Subcutaneous probing during venipuncture • Excessively tight or lengthy tourniquet application creating too much pressure inside the vein. Puncture releases this pressure causing blood to enter the tissue. • Inadequate pressure on the site when a catheter is removed, especially in patients receiving anticoagulants	• Remove the venous access device. • Apply pressure and cool compresses to the affected area. • Elevate the arm. • Reassess the site for bleeding. • Document the patient's condition and your interventions. **Prevention:** • Choose a vein that can accommodate the size of the intended device. • Release the tourniquet as soon as successful insertion is achieved. • Use an indirect approach when placing the device. • Use blood pressure cuff for fragile veins.

(continued)

Local complications of peripheral I.V. therapy *(continued)*

Definition	Signs and symptoms	Possible causes	Nursing interventions
Nerve injury	• Extreme pain similar to electric shock when nerve is contacted with needle • Shooting pain up or down the arm • Tingling, feeling "pins and needles" • Numbness • Delayed effects, including paralysis, numbness, and deformity	• Direct contact between needle stylet and nerve; occurs due to close proximity between veins and nerves in normal anatomy • Excessive subcutaneous probing to puncture the vein • Tight taping or improper splinting with armboard • Nerve compression from excessive fluid in the surrounding tissue due to fluid infiltration, hematoma, or edema from severe inflammation	• Stop insertion procedure and carefully remove the catheter to prevent permanent damage. • Do not probe or make multiple passes with the catheter into the area to locate the vein. • Frequently assess the site for infiltration/extravasation, hematoma, and inflammation and remove the catheter at the first appearance of a problem. • Notify the LIP. • Periodically assess neurovascular function for advancing nerve damage. ***Prevention:*** • Make only two venipuncture attempts. • If pain increases or is unrelenting, suspect compartment syndrome. This complication requires an immediate surgical assessment and possible fasciotomy to release pressure. • Don't apply excessive pressure when taping or encircle the limb with tape or rolled bandages. • Pad the armboard and, if possible, pad the tape securing the armboard. It should not cause circulatory impairment. • Remove armboards periodically to assess for circulation, range of motion and function, and skin integrity.

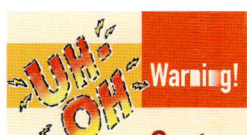

Systemic complications of peripheral I.V. therapy

Definition	Signs and symptoms	Possible causes	Nursing interventions
Bloodstream infection (bacteremia) Invasion of the bloodstream by bacteria	• Fever greater than 101°F (38.3°C) • Chills • Malaise • Nausea and vomiting • Abdominal pain • Shortness of breath • Confusion	• Lack of or inadequate hand hygiene • Failure to maintain aseptic technique during insertion or site care • Phlebitis/thrombophlebitis, which attract organism(s) to the clot • Inadequate stabilization permitting catheter movement and introduction of skin organisms into bloodstream • Prolonged dwell time for catheter • Immunocompromised patient	• Notify the LIP. • Administer medications as prescribed. • Obtain cultures as prescribed; culture of the catheter itself may or may not be ordered. • Monitor the patient's vital signs. **Prevention:** • Perform hand hygiene and use gloves when performing all I.V. procedures. • Reduce disconnection of continuous infusions to as few as clinically necessary. • Always protect the male luer end of any disconnected set when it is to be reconnected to the catheter. • Thoroughly scrub all needleless connectors and injection ports before each entry into the system; use a new disinfectant pad for each entry. • Use scrupulous aseptic technique when handling fluid containers and all components of the infusion system and when inserting and removing the catheter. • Ensure the catheter dressing remains clean, dry, and intact. • Secure all connections with a luer-locking device. • Change fluid containers and administration sets at recommended times.
Vasovagal reaction An involuntary response of the nervous system to certain triggers such a seeing blood or needles	• Feeling light-headed or dizzy • Pale skin • Feeling hot and flushed or cold and clammy • Nausea • Blurred vision • Slow, weak pulse and decreasing blood pressure that progresses to fainting	• Fear of pain or injury • Seeing blood or needles • Being in a sitting position during venipuncture	• Assess for previous fainting episodes and/or the presence of fears. • Assess vital signs. **Prevention:** • Instruct the patient to look in the opposite direction. • Instruct the patient to tighten muscles of the legs during venipuncture. • Position patient in a comfortable supine position for venipuncture procedures to prevent falling if fainting occurs. • For frequent and persistent problems, advise the patient to seek other medical treatment.

(continued)

Systemic complications of peripheral I.V. therapy *(continued)*

Definition	Signs and symptoms	Possible causes	Nursing interventions

Circulatory overload/pulmonary edema	• Discomfort
	• Neck vein engorgement
	• Respiratory distress
	• Increased blood pressure and pulse rate
	• Lung crackles
	• Large positive fluid balance (intake is greater than output)
	• Edema
	• Weight gain
	• Restlessness
	• Cough
		• Uncontrolled rapid fluid flow rate
		  ➢ Roller clamp loosened
		  ➢ Incorrect flow rate on infusion pump
		• Overdose of I.V. fluids
		• History of heart failure or chronic kidney disease
			• Know the patient's history of chronic conditions.
			• Raise the head of the bed.
			• Maintain the infusion rate.
			• Administer oxygen as needed.
			• Notify the LIP.
			• Administer medications, usually diuretics, as ordered.
			Prevention:
			• Use an electronic infusion pump for greatest accuracy of fluid flow control.
			• Recheck calculations of fluid requirements.
			• Monitor the infusion frequently.
			• Monitor intake and output.

Speed shock Sudden physiological reaction when I.V. drugs are given too fast.	• Headache and dizziness • Facial flushing • Chest tightness • Hypotension • Irregular heart rate	• Giving I.V. medications more rapidly than their instructions for use	• Stop the infusion immediately. • Initiate rapid response team as needed. **Prevention:** • Know the correct methods and rate for I.V. medications administration. • Closely monitor all infusions. • Use an electronic infusion pump or syringe pump for adequate rate control.

Venous air embolism
Large amounts of air entering the bloodstream causing a sudden and often catastrophic event
	• Light-headedness
	• Chest pain
	• Respiratory distress
	• Unequal breath sounds
	• Weak pulse
	• Increased central venous pressure
	• Decreased blood pressure
	• Confusion, disorientation, loss of consciousness
		• Existence of a pressure gradient — external pressure is higher than venous pressure, forcing air into the bloodstream.
		  ➢ Unprimed administration set attached to a peripheral catheter
		  ➢ Air in syringe pushed into the vein manually or with a syringe pump
			• Discontinue the infusion.
			• Place the patient in Trendelenburg's position to allow air to remain in the right atrium.
			• Administer oxygen.
			• Notify the LIP.
			• Document the patient's condition and your interventions.
			Prevention:
			• Purge all I.V. sets and syringes of air completely before connection to the catheter.
			• Use an air-detection device on the pump or an air-eliminating filter within the system.
			• Use luer-locking connection and ensure it is securely locked.

Systemic complications of peripheral I.V. therapy (continued)

Definition	Signs and symptoms	Possible causes	Nursing interventions
Allergic reaction	• Itching • Tearing eyes and runny nose • Bronchospasm • Wheezing • Urticarial rash • Edema at I.V. site • Anaphylactic reaction (within minutes or up to 1 hour after exposure), including flushing, chills, anxiety, agitation, generalized itching, palpitations, paresthesia, throbbing in ears, wheezing, coughing, seizures, and cardiac arrest	Allergens such as medications, latex and skin antiseptic agents	• Stop the infusion immediately and infuse normal saline solution. • Maintain a patent airway. • Notify the LIP. • Give aqueous epinephrine subcutaneously for severe reaction. • Administer steroids, anti-inflammatory, and antipyretic drugs, as ordered. **Prevention:** • Obtain the patient's allergy history. Be aware of cross-allergies. • Assist with test dosing. • Monitor the patient carefully during the first 15 minutes of administration of a new drug. • Ensure a latex-free environment for any patient reporting a latex allergy or latex sensitivity.

An ounce of prevention: it's in your hands

Your goal is always prevention of these dangerous conditions. The clinician inserting the I.V. and managing the patient makes many decisions that increase or decrease the risks to patient. The Infusion Therapy Standards of Practice call for each organization to have current policies and procedures to guide the care of patients with these complications. Appropriate treatment requires quick action. There is no time to search for answers, such as the most appropriate antidote to inject around an extravasation injury. Having current information at the ready is essential.

The most important aspects of prevention include the following:
Avoid choosing a site that is at or near a joint.
Check the site for a blood return — it should be the color and consistency of whole blood. A blood return may be present with a complication, and the absence of a blood return may be related to techniques used for aspiration or the catheter or vein size. But this is a significant component of the complete site assessment and cannot be overlooked.

Do not use veins that have previously been used or those near the site of a previous complication. Infusing fluid can escape into the tissue from these damaged sites or worsen the condition of the previous site.

Choose the smallest venous access device to achieve the prescribed therapy.

Stabilize the venous access device with an engineered stabilization device.

Know the fluid and medications you are administering, including the adverse reactions that are associated with each, their characteristics such as irritant or vesicant properties, and the correct dilution and infusion rates.

Proper technique and careful monitoring are a winning team!

Think OPAL

No, not the pretty gemstone, but O-P-A-L:

O = observe the fluid container, infusion system, and insertion site for all signs and symptoms

P = palpate the insertion site for changes in temperature and the presence of hard cord-like vein

A = aspirate for a free-flowing blood return that looks like whole blood

L = listen to the patient's complaints followed by an evaluation of what he is saying. Never simply try to explain away what the patient is telling you about how the site feels.

Always document: thoroughly document!

First, ensure that all actions have been documented in the correct place(s) for the medical record in use. This includes all insertions, removals with the reason for removal, and site assessments before and after medication administration.

When complications do occur, document the signs and symptoms; patient complaints; your immediate interventions such as extremity elevation, etc.; name of the LIP notified; and other treatment(s) prescribed. Use of a grading or ranking scale for phlebitis and infiltration/extravasation is recommended. Signs and symptoms appear gradually and progress to a severe state. The goal is to recognize the complication early in its course as indicated by a low number of the grading scale, as this will reduce the long-term problems for your patient. Photographs are recommended as a more comprehensive way to document exactly what the site looked like. Pictures are better than words but follow your facility policy! Your facility policy may require completion of an unusual occurrence report for certain complications. Documentation allows for better communication among the health care team and provides additional guidance for refining the plan of care. In the event of a lawsuit, your documentation will be a critical component providing the details of medical and nursing interventions.

Discontinuing the infusion

To discontinue the infusion, first clamp the administration set and then remove the venous access device using aseptic technique. Here's how to proceed.

Supplies:
- Gloves, nonsterile
- Gauze, sterile
- Tape

I'm no longer needed

1. Perform hand hygiene.
2. Don gloves.
3. Explain procedure to patient.
4. Discontinue all infusates and/or clamp the extension set.
5. Place patient in a sitting or recumbent position.
6. Remove dressing from insertion site (see *How to apply a transparent semipermeable dressing,* page 97).
7. Remove engineered stabilization device or tape; use appropriate solution as indicated to loosen dressing and securement device adhesive. Be aware of the risk for MARSI.
8. Inspect catheter-skin junction.
9. Hold gauze gently to insertion site with nondominant hand. With your dominant hand, slowly remove catheter using gentle, even pressure and keeping the catheter parallel to the skin.
10. Apply pressure to the site with the gauze until hemostasis is achieved (a minimum of 30 seconds for a short peripheral catheter and longer if anticoagulants are being given).
11. Apply gauze and tape to the site.
12. Inspect catheter to ensure entire catheter was removed (whether it is intact, tip not jagged, and length is appropriate for product).
13. Document in the patient record: date and time of procedure, patient's response to the procedure, and instructions given to the patient.

I need a break. Follow these steps to finish up the infusion.

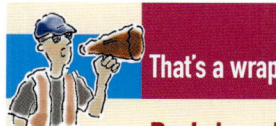

That's a wrap!

Peripheral I.V. therapy review

Basics of peripheral I.V. therapy
Peripheral I.V. therapy involves:
- checking the LIP's orders
- ordering supplies and equipment
- labeling solutions and administration sets
- documenting nursing interventions.

Peripheral I.V. therapy is ordered when venous access is needed for:
- surgery
- transfusions
- emergency care
- maintaining hydration
- restoring fluid and electrolyte balance
- providing fluids for resuscitation
- administering I.V. medications or nutrients.

Preparing for venipuncture and infusion
- Check the patient's medical record for allergies, disease history, and his current diagnosis and care plan.
- Review the LIP's orders and the patient's laboratory studies.
- Describe the procedure to the patient and provide patient teaching.
- Provide privacy.
- Position the patient comfortably.
- Select the appropriate insertion site, venous access device, solution container, and administration set according to the therapy required.
- Use correct flow control devices according to your organizations policy and procedure.
- Assess the fluid container label for complete information about patient's name, flow rate, and contents.
- Attach the administration set as appropriate and label with date and time; label the set if attached to other types of infusion devices such as intraosseous, intraspinal, or subcutaneous devices.

Performing a venipuncture
- Dilate the vein, apply a tourniquet as appropriate, and prepare the access site.
- Stabilize the vein, and then, position the venous access device with the bevel side up.
- Insert the device using a smooth, steady motion.
- Stabilize and dress the venous access device.
- Document the procedure in the appropriate areas according to your facility's policy.

Maintaining peripheral I.V. therapy
- Collect blood samples using appropriate equipment.
- Focus on preventing complications.
- Discontinue the infusion when therapy is completed.
- Discontinue the peripheral catheter when it is no longer part of the patient's plan of care.
- Change a gauze dressing every 48 hours; change a TSM dressing every 5 to 7 days.
- Change the I.V. fluid and medication containers per organizational policy and procedure.
- Change administration sets according to facility policy.
- Change the I.V. site when clinically indicated or according to facility policy.
- Document dressing, set, and fluid container changes and the condition of the venipuncture site.

Patients with special needs
- Intraosseous access is used for fluid resuscitation, medication administration, and blood transfusions until a vein can be accessed and is limited to 24 hours.
- Veins in elderly patients are more fragile and less elastic. Use a blood pressure cuff or light pressure with the tourniquet. Remove the tourniquet promptly to prevent increased vascular pressure.
- Extravasation, phlebitis, thrombophlebitis, local site infection, occlusion, hematoma, venous spasm, vasovagal reaction, and nerve injury
- Bloodstream infection, air embolism, allergic reactions, and circulatory overload.

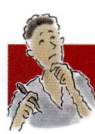

Quick quiz

1. The first step in performing a routine venipuncture is to:
   A. prepare the venipuncture site.
   B. dilate the vein.
   C. use a local anesthetic.
   D. attach the administration set to the device.

   Answer: B. The sequence in performing the venipuncture is to dilate the vein and then prepare the site. An anesthetic may or may not be used.

2. When applying a transparent dressing, it's important to:
   A. stretch the dressing as much as possible.
   B. cover the site and the set connection to the hub.
   C. mold the dressing around and under the hub.
   D. always use a gauze dressing with the transparent dressing.

   Answer: C. Molding the dressing in this manner will make the site more occlusive to microorganisms. Stretching the dressing will cause itching and possible skin injury, and the administration set should never be covered.

3. The preferred skin antiseptic agent is:
   A. 70% alcohol.
   B. tincture of iodine.
   C. povidone-iodine.
   D. alcoholic chlorhexidine.

   Answer: D. Alcoholic chlorhexidine has better results at decreasing the organism on the skin surface and deep in the skin layers.

4. Your patient has swelling at the I.V. site, discomfort, burning, decreased skin temperature, and blanching around the site. These are signs of which of the following I.V. complications?
   A. Phlebitis
   B. Infiltration
   C. Occlusion
   D. Air embolism

   Answer: B. Swelling at the I.V. site, discomfort, burning, decreased skin temperature, and blanching around the site may indicate infiltration.

5. Which location should never be used for insertion of a peripheral catheter?
   A. Dorsum of the hand
   B. Palm side of the wrist
   C. Thumb side of the lower forearm
   D. Upper arm above the antecubital fossa

Answer: B. The palm side of the wrist should always be avoided. The median nerve is very superficial and close to the veins. The site is virtually impossible to stabilize due to joint flexion. Infiltration in this area can produce carpal tunnel syndrome.

6. Short peripheral catheters should be removed:
    A. at 96 hours of dwell time.
    B. when signs and symptoms indicate a problem with the catheter.
    C. when a central venous catheter is inserted.
    D. at 72 hours of dwell time

Answer: B. Immediate removal is required when signs and symptoms create clinical indication for removal. There is no longer a maximum dwell time recommended for removal.

Scoring

☆☆☆ If you answered all six questions correctly, take a bow! At this juncture, fear no venipuncture.

☆☆ If you answered four to five questions correctly, congratulations! For the most part, you delivered the correct solutions.

☆ If you answered fewer than four questions correctly, don't get discouraged! Your quiz score is a peripheral matter. Review the chapter and try again.

Suggested References

Gorski, L., Hadaway, L., Hagle, M., McGoldrick, M., Orr, M., & Doellman, D. (2016). Infusion therapy standards of practice. *Journal of Infusion Nursing, 39*(1S), 159.

Gorski, L., Hadaway, L., Hagle, M., McGoldrick, M., Meyer, B., & Orr, M. (2016). *Policies and procedures for infusion therapy* (5th ed.). Norwood, MA: Infusion Nurses Society.

Gorski, L. A., Hallock, D., Kuehn, S. C., Morris, P., Russell, J. M., & Skala, L. C. (2012). Recommendations for frequency of assessment of the short peripheral catheter site. *Journal of Infusion Nursing, 35*(5), 290–292. doi:10.1097/NAN.0b013e318267f636.

O'Grady, N., Alexander, M., Burns, L., & Dellinger, E. (2011). *Guideline for the prevention of intravascular catheter-related infections.* Retrieved from http://www.cdc.gov/hicpac/BSI/BSIguidelines-2011.html

Polovich, M., Olsen, M., & LeFebvre, K. (Eds.). (2014). *Chemotherapy and biotherapy guidelines and recommendations for practice* (4th ed.). Pittsburgh, PA: Oncology Nursing Society.

Weinstein, S. M., & Hagle, M. (2014). *Plumer's principles and practice of infusion therapy* (9th ed.). Philadelphia, PA: Wolters Kluwer Health.

Chapter 3

Infusion therapy requiring central venous access

Just the facts

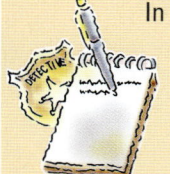

In this chapter, you'll learn:

◀ the purpose of intravenous (I.V.) therapy requiring central venous access
◀ central venous access device (CVAD) insertion equipment
◀ patient preparation for CVAD insertion
◀ the assistant's role in CVAD insertion
◀ maintenance and discontinuation of the CVAD
◀ the proper care of a patient with an implanted port.

Understanding central intravenous (I.V.) therapy

In I.V. therapy given centrally, drugs or fluids are infused directly into the superior vena cava (SVC). I.V. therapy via the central route is used in various situations, including emergencies or when a patient's peripheral veins are inaccessible. It may be ordered when a patient:
- needs infusion of a large volume or rapid infusion of fluid
- requires simultaneous infusion of multiple solutions or medications
- requires infusion therapy for a long period
- needs infusion of irritating medications such as electrolytes, some antibiotics and inotropic agents
- needs infusion of fluids with high osmolarity such as parenteral nutrition (PN).

Bringing it on home

At one time, only patients in intensive care and specialty units received I.V. therapy through a CVAD. Today, patients in any unit or patients in home care and long-term care, as well as infusion clinics, may receive I.V. infusions through a CVAD.

Benefits of a central venous access device

Infusion through a CVAD provides for greater dilution of the infusing fluids and medications because of the larger vessel diameter where the tip is located. Other benefits include:
- rapid infusion of medications or large amounts of fluids
- measurement of central venous pressure and other hemodynamic measures, an important indicator of circulatory function
- obtaining blood samples in some patients with very poor peripheral veins; however, a CVAD is not indicated when there is no infusion therapy and obtaining blood samples is the only need
- preventing multiple failed or very difficult peripheral venipunctures, which increases the patient's anxiety and prevents future use of peripheral veins
- reduced risk of peripheral vein irritation from infusing irritating or caustic substances.

Risks of central venous access devices

Like any other invasive procedure, CVAD insertion for I.V. therapy has its drawbacks. It increases the risk of life-threatening complications, such as:
- pneumothorax
- bloodstream infection
- thrombus formation
- perforation of the vessel at or near its tip location, increasing risk of damage to adjacent organs.
CVADs also have disadvantages such as:
- requiring more time, resources, and skill to insert than a peripheral I.V. catheter.
- a risk of air embolism with insertion, administration set changes, and removal.

Venous circulation

The 5 liters of blood in an average adult body really gets around. After delivering oxygen and nutrients throughout the body, depleted blood flows from the capillaries to ever-widening veins, finally returning to the right side of the heart before collecting a fresh supply of oxygen from the lungs.

Blood enters the right atrium through two major veins: the superior vena cava and the inferior vena cava.

Going down...

Before flowing into the right atrium, venous return from the head, neck, and arms enters the superior vena cava through many other large veins:

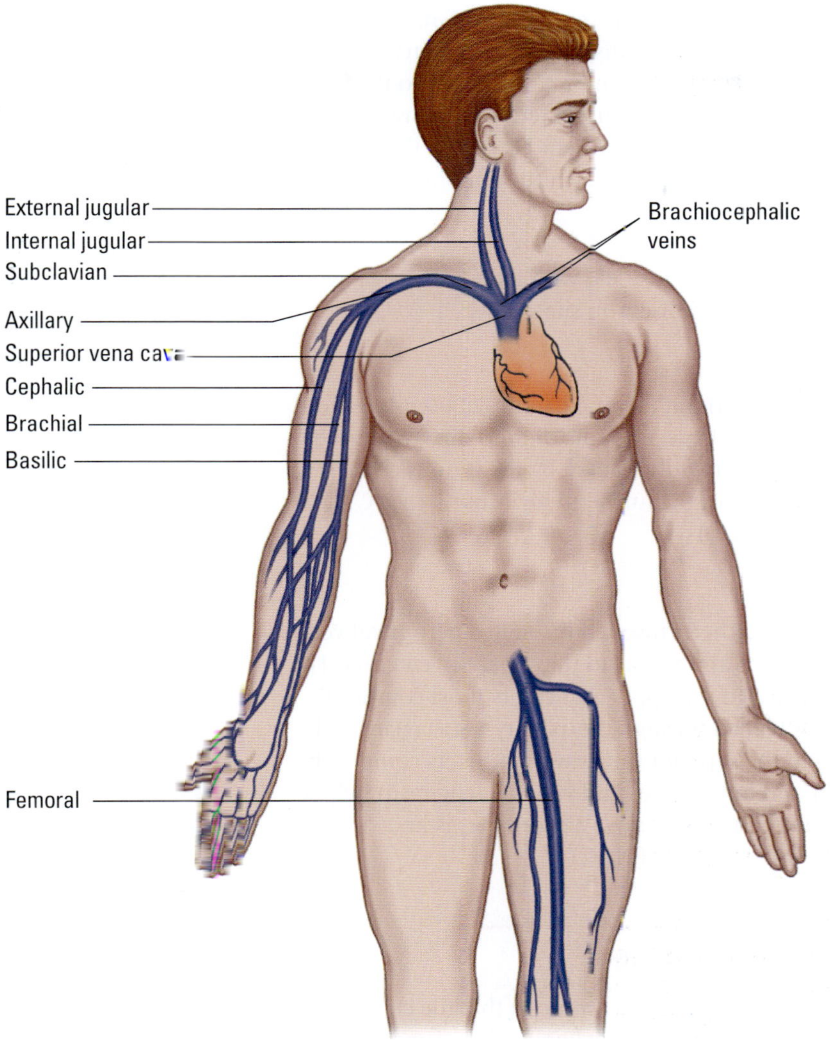

Understanding central intravenous (I.V.) therapy

Venous circulation.

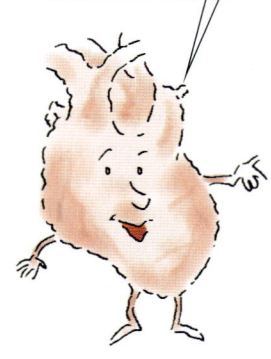

Venous blood enters my right atrium through the superior and inferior venae cavae.

- Internal and external jugular veins in the neck join the subclavian vein.
- Basilic, cephalic, and brachial veins of the upper extremity join the axillary vein and then the subclavian vein.
- The subclavian vein joins the brachiocephalic vein, also known as the innominate vein.
- Finally, the bilateral brachiocephalic veins join to form the superior vena cava.

...and coming up

Venous blood flows from the veins in the legs into the femoral vein on both sides. The femoral vein joins the inguinal veins and then merges into the inferior vena cava and returns blood to the right atrium. Several tributary veins join the inferior vena cava such as the renal, hepatic, and lumbar veins and could be the inadvertent location for a CVAD inserted from the femoral site.

Getting to the point

In central I.V. therapy, a catheter is inserted with its tip in one of two places (depending on the chosen insertion site):
- superior vena cava
- inferior vena cava.

Blood flows unimpeded around the tip at about 2,000 mL/minute, allowing the rapid infusion of large amounts of fluid directly into the circulation. Because fluids are rapidly diluted by the venous circulation, highly concentrated or caustic fluids can be infused. (See *CV access device pathways*, page 123.)

> Because blood flows very quickly and unimpeded around the CVAD's tip, fluids are rapidly diluted by the venous circulation, allowing for the infusion of highly concentrated or caustic solutions.

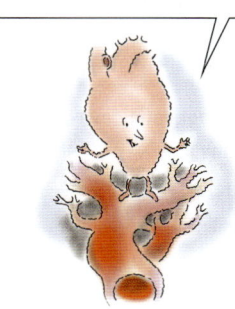

Taking a different route

Another type of CVAD is a catheter inserted through a peripheral vein, and the catheter tip is passed all the way to the superior vena cava. For instance, a catheter inserted in the upper arm enters most commonly the basilic vein and is threaded through the axillary, subclavian, and brachiocephalic veins to the superior vena cava. Catheters come with a variety of introducer and lumen sizes and variable lengths to help tailor the insertion to individual patients. This catheter is known as a peripherally inserted central catheter (PICC).

Central venous access device planning

Patient safety dictates, and guidelines recommend that the clinician placing and using a CVAD should have the knowledge of anatomy, physiology, and therapies for each type of device. Selecting the appropriate CVAD for a patient depends on the type of therapy needed, anticipated duration of therapy, age, number and condition of peripheral veins, comorbidities, infusion therapy history, patient preference for location of CVAD, and resources available to care for the catheter. The process to arrive at the most appropriate device is a collaborative, interprofessional team effort that should also include the patient and the patient's caregivers. Peripheral vein preservation is an important factor in considering which device is most appropriate. It is particularly important to preserve peripheral and subclavian veins for future fistula needs in patients with chronic kidney disease (CKD). Stenosis in these veins can lead to decreased blood flow needed for dialysis.

> CVADs can be used to administer any type of fluid or medication.

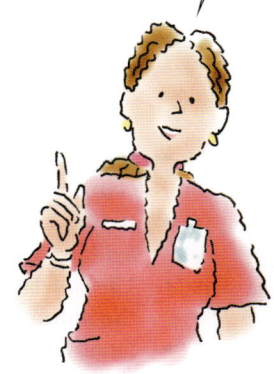

The CVAD should have the smallest outer diameter and the least number of lumens needed for the I.V. therapy ordered.

Types of CVADs include:
- peripherally inserted central catheters (PICCs)
- nontunneled catheters
- tunneled cuffed catheters
- implanted ports.

CVAD pathways

Most commonly a CVAD is inserted into the subclavian vein, internal jugular vein, or veins of the upper arm. All CVADs should terminate in the superior vena cava, at or slightly above the junction of the vena cava and right atrium, known as the cavoatrial junction or CAJ.

The illustrations below show several common pathways of the CVAD.

Inserted into the subclavian vein, this CVAD terminates in the superior vena cava.

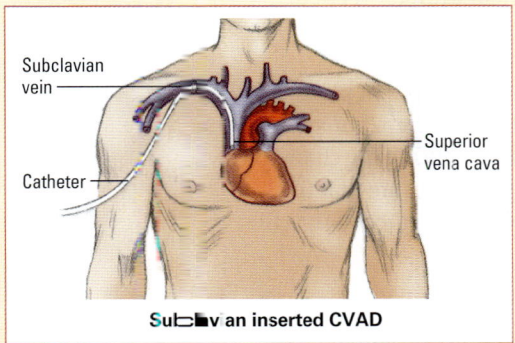

Subclavian inserted CVAD

This CVAD enters the internal jugular vein and terminates in the superior vena cava.

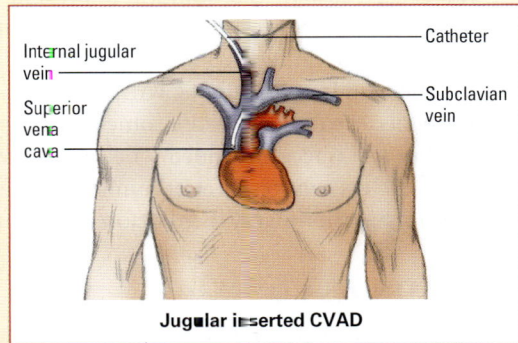

Jugular inserted CVAD

A PICC preferably inserted into the basilic vein of the upper arm terminates in the superior vena cava.

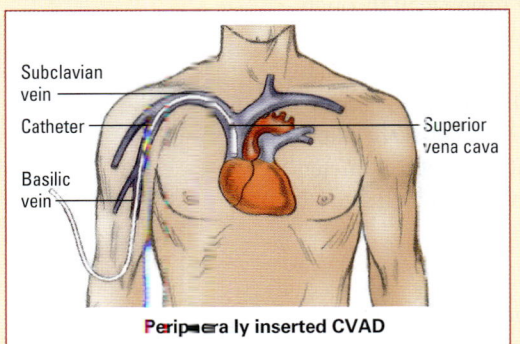

Peripherally inserted CVAD

This CVAD enters the subclavian vein or internal jugular vein and terminates in the superior vena cava. Note the catheter tunnels (shown by broken line) from the insertion site, through the subcutaneous tissue, to an exit site on the skin (usually located by the nipple). Also note how the position of the subcutaneous cuff helps hold the catheter in place.

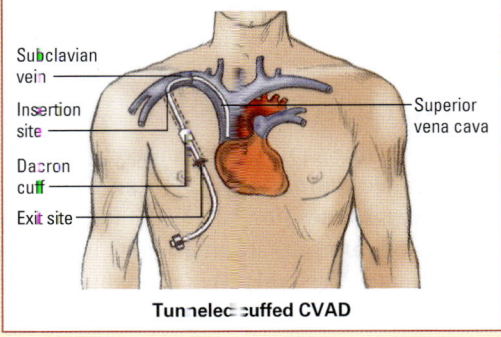

Tunneled cuffed CVAD

CVAD characteristics

CVADs have certain characteristics that apply to all types.

Catheter materials

CVADs are made of either silicone or polyurethane. Silicone is a soft material that requires special insertion techniques. The mechanical strength of silicone is enhanced by making the catheter walls slightly thicker, causing the internal diameter to be smaller or the outer diameter to be larger. Silicone is usually compatible with all types of fluids, medications, and locking solutions.

Polyurethane is a large family of plastic materials that responds to body heat. Once inserted, it becomes softer and more flexible than when it is at room temperature. While polyurethane has greater mechanical strength allowing for thinner catheter walls, there is concern about its ability to tolerate some chemicals. For instance, ethanol is used as a locking solution to prevent or treat catheter-related bloodstream infections; however, this is contraindicated for locking polyurethane catheters.

The rigid female hub of CVADs are made of several types of plastic materials. Alcohol may cause some of these plastics to soften, but an alcohol pad is recommended for cleaning these hubs during the change of needleless connectors or administration sets. Always ensure that the alcohol has thoroughly dried before attaching the new connector or set.

CVAD sizes

CVAD sizes are measured in internal diameter and outer diameter. The internal diameter provides information about the amount of priming volume required to fill the lumen and the maximum flow rate through the catheter. This is measured from one inside wall through the center of the lumen to the opposite internal wall.

The outer diameter is necessary to ensure the catheter is not too large for the vein and is measured from the outside wall through the center of the lumen to the opposite outside wall. Both measurements are taken in millimeters and converted to French size — the number of millimeters multiplied by 3. So a measurement of 2 mm equals a 6-French size.

Power injection

A power injectable CVAD is used for radiology procedures such as a computed tomography (CT) scan. The contrast agents are injected at very fast rates (for example, 3 to 8 mL/second) by using special infusion pumps that can generate infusion pressure up to 325 pounds per square inch (psi). This procedure requires that the CVAD and all add-on devices be able to tolerate this high level of injection pressure.

Integral valves

All types of CVADs can be made with valves built into the catheter; however, many CVADs do not have these valves. These valves may be located near the internal end of the catheter or in the external catheter hub. These valves work by infusion pressure, opening toward the bloodstream during an injection or infusion and opening toward the lumen during aspiration. Slightly more force applied to the syringe plunger may be necessary to open these valves than a CVAD without these valves. The benefit of these valves is to reduce the amount of blood that can move into the catheter lumen, producing a lumen occlusion from a clot formation. Instructions for use with these valved CVADs usually state they can be locked with saline solution and heparin lock solution is not necessary, but follow the policy and procedures for your facility. The presence of these valves may interfere with hemodynamic monitoring, so follow the manufacturer's instructions if this procedure is required.

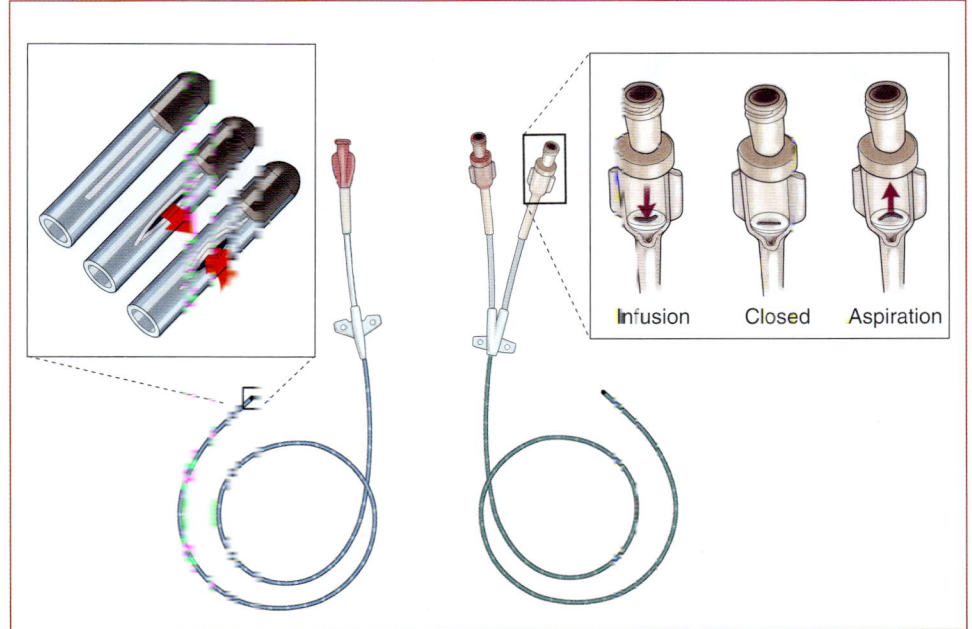

Antimicrobial and antithrombotic properties

CVADs may have antimicrobial and antithrombotic agents added to the catheter material, either as a coating on the internal and external walls or impregnated through the entire catheter wall. Examples of these agents include chlorhexidine, silver, minocycline, and rifampin, used alone or in combination. These CVADs may be chosen when the catheter is required for longer than 5 days or when the patient has risk factors for bloodstream infection such as patients with transplanted organs, burns, or other critical diagnoses. Always assess for patient allergies before insertion of these CVADs.

Multiple lumens, multiple exits

A CVAD can have one lumen or multiple lumens, which are designed as separate channels for the entire length of the catheter. The point where fluid exits on the internal end of the catheter may be staggered or nonstaggered. Nonstaggered exits have fluid from all lumens flowing from the internal tip of the catheter. CVADs with staggered lumen exits have one flowing from the internal catheter tip, with other lumens exiting along the side of the catheter wall, and are usually separated by 0.5 to 2 cm. Those with staggered lumen exits may have different lengths on the external extension legs to indicate the staggering.

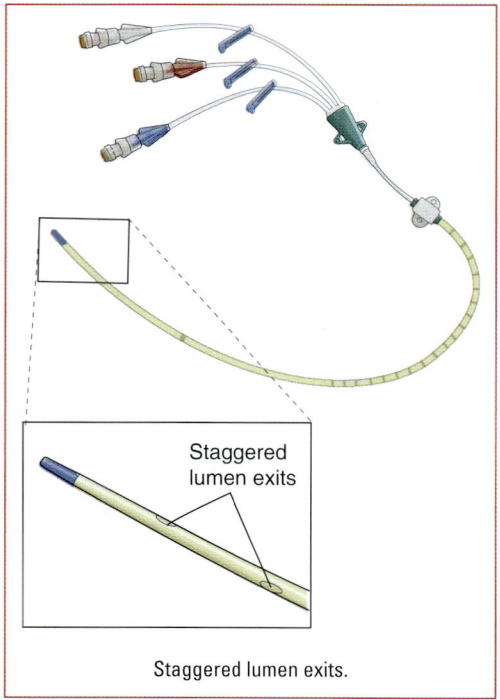

Staggered lumen exits.

Types of CV access devices

Nontunneled CVAD

Nontunneled CVADs enter through a direct venous puncture of the subclavian or internal jugular vein, and the catheter is advanced into the superior vena cava. If the femoral vein is used, the catheter tip should be in the inferior vena cava above the level of the diaphragm. They are usually indicated for short-term use in patients requiring irritant or vesicant medications or fluids and hemodynamic monitoring. They may not be appropriate for a patient requiring long-term I.V. therapy. The nontunneled catheter placed in the subclavian vein may have a lower risk of infection because the dressing is easier to maintain. But the subclavian insertion site can have more mechanical problems. The internal jugular insertion site is more difficult to maintain due to neck motion and growth of beards or long hair.

Nontunneled catheters are radiopaque, so tip location can be checked by a postprocedure chest X-ray. An electrocardiogram (ECG) tip locating system may be used to identify the tip location in relationship to the height of the P wave on the ECG; however, some patients may not have a P wave due to cardiac problems.

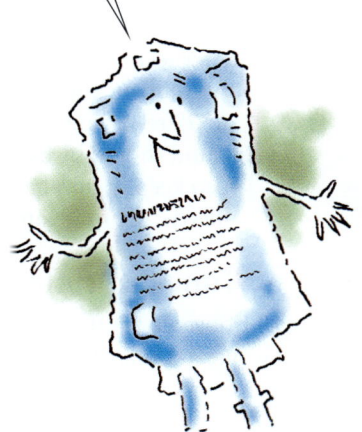

Generally, PICCs are used when patients need infusions of drugs or solutions that are known irritants or vesicants or for more than 14 days of I.V. therapy.

Peripherally inserted central catheter (PICC)

A PICC is a type of CVAD that provides access to the central venous system with its tip located in the lower portion of the SVC at or near the cavoatrial junction. A PICC is inserted into a peripheral vein of the upper arm, usually the basilic or brachial vein, and advanced into the SVC, reducing the risks associated with direct puncture of the internal jugular, subclavian, or femoral vein. A PICC is most appropriate in situations that require venous access greater than 6 days, although a midline may be appropriate depending on the characteristics of the solution and/or medication. (See *Chapter 2, The midline,* page 73.)

PICC specifics

PICCs are available in single-, double-, or triple-lumen configurations, although the triple-lumen sizes can be very large for most upper extremity veins. A stylet wire stiffens the catheter to ease its advancement through the vein, but it can damage the vein if used incorrectly. If an ECG tip location system is used, the guide wire also serves as a lead and assists in confirming tip location, therefore eliminating the need for chest X-ray confirmation in most patients.

The patient receiving I.V. therapy via a PICC must have a peripheral vein large enough to accept the size of catheter being placed. The guidelines recommend the catheter with the smallest outer diameter in the largest vein to reduce the risk of a thrombus from forming around the catheter. For example, a 4-Fr PICC requires the size of the vein to be at least 4 mm in diameter, which is measured by ultrasound. If the catheter has more than one lumen, each lumen has its own gauge size, which is usually written on the external segment of the PICC. For example, a 6-Fr triple-lumen catheter has a total gauge size of 14, but generally, there is one large gauge (18G) and two smaller gauge (21G) lumens. If the patient is to receive blood or blood products through the PICC, you should use at least an 18-G lumen. When caring for a patient with a PICC, make sure that you know where the catheter terminates and what the entire length of the catheter is, both internal and external lengths.

PICC ups

PICCs have a definite upside:
- PICCs provide long-term access to central veins with a single catheter being used for an entire course of therapy.
- PICCs provide a safe, reliable route for infusion therapy.

PICC problems

A PICC may be unsuitable for a patient with bruises, scarring, or sclerosis from earlier multiple venipunctures at the intended PICC insertion site. PICCs are also contraindicated in an extremity on the same side as a mastectomy with lymph node dissection, recent or current deep vein thrombosis, and CKD. It is always best to speak with the nephrologist or LIP regarding vascular access in patients with CKD. Bedside ultrasound should be used to assess whether a vein is suitable for a PICC. Also keep in mind that the best utilization of a PICC is when it is introduced early in treatment; it shouldn't be considered a last resort.

Tunneled cuffed CVAD

Tunneled cuffed CVADs are designed for long-term use, generally greater than 1 to 3 months.

Cuff link

A tunneled cuffed CVAD has a cuff encircling the extraluminal catheter that should be positioned several centimeters away from the skin exit site. The subcutaneous tissue grows into this cuff, acting as an anchor to keep the catheter in place. The cuff also acts as a barrier to reduce migration of microorganisms from the skin into the venous circulation; however, the tunnel can become infected. In most cases, the cuff is made of Dacron.

Tunnel tidbits

Tunneled cuffed catheters are better suited to home care patients than are nontunneled catheters because they're designed for long-term use. They're used in patients who have poor peripheral venous access or who need long-term frequent infusions, such as those with:
- cancer
- acquired immunodeficiency syndrome (AIDS)
- intestinal malabsorption
- transplants
- bone or organ infections
- other chronic diseases.

(Text continues on page 130)

Guide to CVADs

Types of CVADs differ in their design, composition, and indications for use. This chart outlines the advantages, disadvantages, and nursing considerations for several commonly used catheters.

Catheter description and indications	Advantages and disadvantages	Nursing considerations

Peripherally inserted central catheter
Description
• 20"–24" (50–60 cm) long; available in 2–6 French sizes
Indications
• Long-term CVAD need
• Patient with poor peripheral access for proposed therapy ≥6 days
• May be used for 5 days or less for irritating and/or vesicant infusates not well tolerated through peripheral veins
• Patient at high risk for complications from insertion at subclavian or jugular insertion sites (i.e., infection, pneumothorax)
• Patient with medical or surgical conditions preventing use of subclavian or jugular sites such as:
  ○ respiratory diseases
  ○ increased intracranial pressure
  ○ spinal curvatures
	Advantages
	• Peripheral insertion site is not near the lungs or large arteries.
	• It can be inserted at bedside with minimal complications and does not require LIP to be present.
	• It may be inserted by a clinician (i.e., RN, radiological technologist, respiratory therapist) with documented competency. Inserters must follow the rules and regulations for their profession in their states.
	Disadvantages
	Catheter outer diameter may occlude smaller peripheral vessels; evaluation of vein's internal diameter using ultrasound is required to choose an appropriately sized catheter.
		• Patency assessment includes the ability to aspirate a blood return from the catheter, the absence of resistance when flushed with a saline-filled syringe, and the absence of all signs and symptoms of complications.
		• Check frequently for signs of phlebitis, thrombosis, and infection.
		• Insertion site should be above the antecubital fossa.
		• Know the gauge and purpose of each lumen.
		• Use the same lumen for the same task (e.g., to administer total parenteral nutrition or to collect a blood sample).

Nontunneled central venous catheter ***Description*** • Double, triple, or quadruple lumen • Variety of lumen gauges ***Indications*** • Short-term CVAD for several days to weeks in hospitalized patients • May be used for 5 days or less for irritating and/or vesicant infusates not well tolerated through peripheral veins • Patient with limited insertion sites who requires multiple infusions	***Advantages*** • Insertion and removal at bedside • It allows infusion of multiple solutions through the same catheter (e.g., incompatible solutions). • Preferred for critical care patients instead of PICC • Nonphysician clinicians are placing these catheters in many states. ***Disadvantages*** • Increased risk for complications on insertion if real-time ultrasound guidance is not used • Requires Trendelenburg position for insertion; may be contraindicated or not well tolerated by patients with increased intracranial pressure, respiratory diseases, and spinal curvatures	• Know the gauge and purpose of each lumen. • Use the same lumen for the same task (e.g., to administer total parenteral nutrition or to collect a blood sample). • Patency assessment includes the ability to aspirate a blood return from the catheter, the absence of resistance when flushing with a saline-filled syringe, and the absence of signs and symptoms of complications.

(continued)

Guide to CVADs (continued)

Catheter description and indications	Advantages and disadvantages	Nursing considerations
Tunneled cuffed catheters *Description* • Presence of subcutaneous cuff placed in subcutaneous tunnel several centimeters away from the skin exit site • Subcutaneous tunnel separates skin exit site from vein entrance site. *Indications* Continuous or intermittent infusion therapy needed for ≥30 days	*Advantages* Subcutaneous cuff anchors catheter and reduces bacterial ingress. *Disadvantages* • Requires surgical insertion • Removal requires complete removal of the subcutaneous cuff, sometimes by a minor surgical procedure. • Fluoroscopy or ultrasound may be needed to ensure the complete removal of the cuff. • Retained cuff components could produce a subcutaneous abscess.	• Two surgical sites (i.e., skin exit and venipuncture site) require dressing after insertion. After healing, the LIP may allow for no dressing on the skin exit site. • Check the external portion frequently for kinks or leaks. (Repair may be possible but a brand-specific repair kit should be used.) • Patency assessment includes the ability to aspirate a blood return from the catheter, the absence of resistance when flushing with a saline-filled syringe, and the absence of signs and symptoms of complications.

Implanted ports

Patients with long-term chronic diseases often require long-term but intermittent I.V. therapy. An implanted port may be better suited for these patients as it has no external components requiring care. (See *Comparing implanted ports and long-term CVAD*.)

A surgical pocket is created in the subcutaneous tissue, most commonly in the area under the clavicle. The catheter is inserted into the internal jugular or subclavian vein and advanced into the superior vena cava at or near the cavoatrial junction. A short subcutaneous tunnel extends from the venipuncture site to the port body. The catheter is attached to the stem extending from the base of the port body, the body is sutured into place, and the incision is sutured closed. The port body is made of titanium, stainless steel, or plastic. It contains a thick septum covering an open chamber and the outflow track through the stem on its side.

An implanted port is also used for epidural, intra-arterial, or intra-peritoneal placement, so make certain of the actual location before any infusion.

The implanted port is accessed with a special, noncoring needle. The bevel of the needle is angled to allow it to slice easily through the dense septum, and the angled tip resides in the open chamber or reservoir. A regular needle is never used to access an

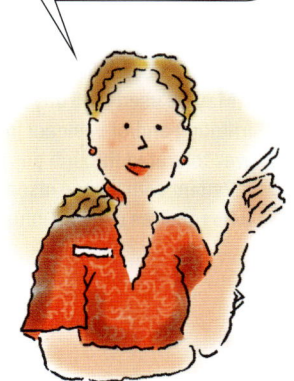

An implanted port functions much like a long-term CV access device except that it's implanted in a pocket under the skin.

implanted port as it can easily cause a small piece of the septum to be cut and embolize to the lungs. Also, a small hole can be left in the septum producing leaking of infusion fluids into the subcutaneous tissue. The port access procedure requires a needle-stick and may be painful for some patients. Use of an ice pack over the port body immediately before accessing may help reduce the discomfort, or other local anesthetics may be required. The access procedure should be performed with aseptic technique using sterile gloves and mask.

Comparing implanted ports and long-term CVADs

An implanted port offers the patient many of the advantages of a long-term CVAD, along with an unobtrusive design that many patients find easier to accept. Both devices are indicated when poor venous access and certain medications and solutions prohibit peripheral I.V. therapy. Deciding which device to use depends on the type and duration of treatment, the frequency of access, and the patient's condition. This chart shows how these devices compare.

Type of treatment	Implanted port	Long-term CVAD (tunneled cuffed or PICC)
Continuous infusion of drugs or fluids	Yes, especially when infusions will last less than a week. Maintaining constant needle access longer than a week eliminates the benefits of implanted ports.	Yes
Self-administration of drugs or fluids	Yes, but inserting the needle may be more difficult for the patient or caregiver. Some may be agreeable to learn, and it should be the patient's choice.	Yes
Injection or infusion of vesicant or irritant drugs	Yes	Yes
Duration of treatment		
<1 month	No, because of the high cost of surgical insertion and removal	Yes
More than 1 month	Yes, if infusion therapy is prescribed for long-term intermittent needs (e.g., 1–3 days of infusion every 3 or 4 weeks)	Yes
Patient concerns		
Negative effect on body image	No	Possibly
Negative reaction to needle punctures	Possibly	No
Ability to care for external catheter	Not needed when not accessed	Needed
Cost of dressing changes, flushing, and locking	Minimal	Considerable

Implanted port: out of sight

Implanted ports are easier to maintain than an external CVAD for patients who can tolerate needlesticks. They require flushing and locking periodically (for example, usually once per month, but it may be extended) to maintain patency when not being used for infusions. Implanted ports are reported to have lower rates of bloodstream infection; however, the port pocket may become infected.

Implanted ports offer several other advantages for patients, including:
- minimal activity restrictions
- few self-care measures to learn and perform
- dressing over the port needle site only when accessed for continuous or intermittent infusions.

Finally, because implanted ports create only a slight protrusion under the skin, many patients find them easier to accept than CVADs with an external component. A patient with an implanted port may shower, swim, and exercise without worrying about the device, as long as the device isn't accessed. The LIP decides how soon after insertion the patient may undertake these activities.

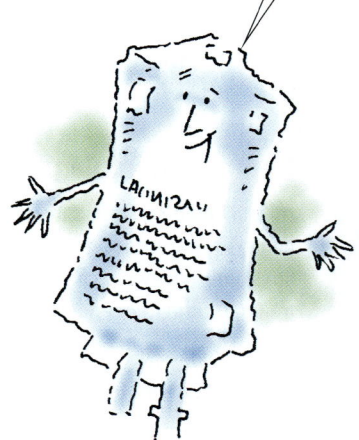

For more information about implanted port insertion and infusions, turn to page

CVAD use — what can go through them?

CVADs are indicated for the infusion of all types of fluids and medications including irritant or vesicant medications. This includes antineoplastic agents, parenteral nutrition, vasopressors, and high concentration of electrolytes such as potassium and calcium. CVADs may also be used for hemodynamic monitoring. A CVAD should only be inserted when:
- the rapid blood flow of the SVC is needed to provide greater dilution of the fluid or medication
- the patient is not clinically stable and multiple infusion therapies are required
- hemodynamic monitoring is needed, for example, central venous pressure reading
- long-term infusion therapy is needed
- the patient has very difficult peripheral veins and the use of ultrasound guidance for peripheral catheter insertion has failed.

Blood sampling from a CVAD

Prior to using any CVAD for obtaining a blood sample, assess the patient for the risk associated with this use. Blood sampling from a CVAD increases manipulation of the catheter hub and subsequent contamination that leads to bloodstream infection. Blood samples from a CVAD may produce erroneous lab values such as test for coagulation factors in a CVAD locked with heparin or errors in therapeutic drug monitoring when that drug is being infused through the CVAD (for example, vancomycin trough levels). Frequent blood samples taken from a CVAD contributes to hospital-acquired anemia. Alternatively, using the CVAD may be the most appropriate option when the patient has extremely difficult peripheral veins, has a history of vasovagal reactions due to needlesticks, or is anticoagulated with a risk of venipuncture-associated hematomas.

Syringe sizes and CVADs

Prior to infusion through a CVAD, assess for the patency of the catheter. The insertion site, surrounding area, and chest, extremity, and neck should be free of any signs or symptoms of complications. When flushed, the saline should flow easily into the catheter lumen without feeling any resistance. When aspirated, the CVAD should produce a blood return that looks like whole blood. If resistance is felt or there is no blood return, do not use the catheter until the cause has been evaluated and corrected.

Follow these key points when giving medications:
- Assess the patency of the CVAD using a 10-mL syringe or a syringe designed to generate lower pressure (that is, the barrel size equals the barrel size of the 10-mL syringe but may hold smaller amounts of fluid).
- Do not use force to flush any vascular access device. If resistance is met and/or blood cannot be aspirated, look for the cause, either external (clamped, kinked sets) or internal (kinked catheter, catheter occlusion). This may require chest X-ray to confirm tip location, check for pinch-off syndrome or color duplex US or fluoroscopy to determine intravascular causes.
- If patency is confirmed by aspiration of blood and no resistance when flushed, give the medication in syringes appropriately sized for the medication such as a 3- or 5-mL syringe. Do not transfer the medication to a larger syringe.

So a 10-mL syringe (or 10-mL barrel-size syringe) is only required to assess for patency.

CVAD removal

The optimal time interval for removing CVADs is unknown; therefore, the length of the dwell time should not be a factor for removal. Current standards do not recommend removal of a CVAD on the presence of fever alone before diagnostic studies such as blood cultures indicate that the CVAD is the source of an infection. The catheter should only be removed when there is evidence of local or systemic complications caused by the catheter, after collaboration with the LIP. Ongoing and frequent monitoring of the patient and insertion site should be performed. If signs or symptoms of any complication are detected, notify the LIP immediately. Following a daily assessment for hospitalized patients, all CVADs should be removed immediately when the therapy is completed and no longer needed for the plan of care.

Removing the tunneled cuffed CVAD and implanted ports requires a short surgical procedure. Consult with the LIP about removal for patients with chronic illness such as cancer, sickle cell disease, or cystic fibrosis as there may be a future need for infusion through the CVAD.

Preparing for central venous therapy

The first step in preparing for CVAD insertion is selecting a site for the catheter. Although the clinician trained to place the catheter will determine the insertion site, you will be assisting with the procedure. You also need to prepare the patient physically and mentally and then gather and prepare the appropriate equipment. An insertion checklist is required for every CVAD insertion to monitor best practices for prevention of complications. It may be your responsibility to observe the insertion and fill in a checklist. It is everybody's responsibility to stop the procedure if the sterility has been compromised. (See *Central Line Insertion Practice Adherence Monitoring in appendix.*)

Selecting the insertion site

Although traditionally a CVAD is inserted by an LIP, many states allow registered nurses to insert centrally inserted central catheters. Additionally, this procedure is also performed by respiratory therapist and radiologic technologists in some states. If inserting a central line is an elective rather than an emergency procedure, you may collaborate with the patient and other members of the patient's care team in selecting a site.

The insertion site varies for CVADs, depending on:
- type of catheter
- patient's anatomy and age
- duration of therapy
- vessel integrity and accessibility
- history of previous neck or chest surgery
- history of mastectomy with lymph node removal
- coagulopathies
- vein size
- presence of chest trauma
- recent history or current DVT
- presence of a pacemaker or automatic implantable cardioverter-defibrillator (AICD)
- possible complications
- some diagnoses such as CKD.

Commonly used insertion sites include the basilic vein in the upper arm, axillosubclavian vein, and internal and external jugular veins. The femoral vein may also be used.

Comparing CVAD insertion sites

The chart below lists the most common insertion sites for a CVAD and the advantages and disadvantages of each.

Site	Advantages	Disadvantages
Subclavian vein	• Easy and fast access • Easier to keep dressing in place • High flow rate	• Proximity to subclavian artery. (If artery is punctured during catheter insertion, hemorrhage can occur.) • Difficulty controlling bleeding • Difficulty assessing vein with US due to presence of the clavicle • Increased risk of pneumothorax • Deeper vein • Risk of pinch-off syndrome
Internal jugular vein	• Straighter, direct route to superior vena cava from the right side • Decreased risk of pneumothorax • Site of choice for renal patients • Easy access using ultrasound	• Proximity to the common carotid artery. (If artery is punctured during catheter insertion, uncontrolled hemorrhage, emboli, or impedance to flow can result.) • Difficulty keeping the dressing in place due to neck motion • Proximity to the trachea
External jugular vein	• Easy access, especially in children • Decreased risk of pneumothorax or arterial puncture	• Less direct route • Difficulty keeping the dressing in place • Tortuous vein, especially in elderly patients
Veins in the upper extremity: • Cephalic vein • Basilic vein • Brachial vein • Median cubital vein	• The basilic vein is generally the vein of choice due to its large diameter and straight pathway. • The cephalic vein in the upper arm may be easily palpated especially in patients with weight loss. • The brachial vein is a deep vein but may be used when basilic or cephalic veins are not available. • The median cubital vein located in the antecubital fossa may be only choice for obese patients. • Easy to keep the dressing in place	• Use of basilic or brachial veins requires ultrasound guidance due to their depth in the tissue. • Cephalic vein narrows and has a high risk of malposition on insertion due to tortuous route through shoulder area. • Brachial vein has increased risk for cannulating artery and damage to nerve bundle. • Median cubital vein in the antecubital fossa is an area of joint flexion, with a higher risk of complications due to catheter movement.

Subclavian vein

The subclavian vein is one of the most common insertion sites for central I.V. therapy. It affords easy access and a short, direct route to the superior vena cava and central circulation. It is preferred over IJ or femoral vein sites for infection prevention purposes. The subclavian site also allows for greater patient mobility after insertion. It is difficult to safely access when using only anatomical landmark techniques. Several guidelines recommend dynamic or real-time US guidance, but this is difficult because the clavicle obscures the subclavian vein. For this reason, some clinicians are moving out from the center of the body and accessing the axillary vein in the deltopectoral groove.

Axillary vein

The axillary vein may be preferred over the subclavian vein due to its distance from the pleura and ultrasound can be used with insertion. The insertion site will be at the deltopectoral groove, further away from the center of the body. Otherwise, the insertion and care and maintenance are identical to a CVAD inserted in the subclavian vein.

Internal jugular vein

The internal jugular vein provides easy access and is actually preferred for some patients such as those with CKD. This insertion site is commonly used in adults and children, but not infants.

Careful! It's close to the common carotid

The right internal jugular vein provides a more direct route to the superior vena cava than the left internal jugular vein. However, its proximity to the common carotid artery can produce accidental puncture of this large artery. Possible outcomes include uncontrolled hemorrhage, emboli, or impeded blood flow to the brain. The risk of carotid artery puncture is greatly reduced using ultrasound guidance.

Using the internal jugular vein has other drawbacks. The puncture site is in the neck, an area of high movement. It is difficult to adequately stabilize and secure the catheter, which can mean lack of dressing integrity and an increased risk for infection. The site could limit the patient's movement and may be a poor choice for home infusion therapy. However, if the insertion site is low on the neck and the catheter is situated close to the chest, the dressing will remain intact. This also helps with movement, as the catheter is no longer affected when moving the head.

Femoral veins

Femoral veins may be used if other sites aren't suitable, especially in emergent situations. Although the femoral veins are large vessels, the moist skin around this insertion may increase risk of bloodstream infection. Insertion may be difficult, especially in obese patients, and carries the risk of puncturing the local lymph nodes. As with other insertion sites, ultrasound use reduces these risks. The catheter used should be long enough for the tip to be correctly positioned in the inferior vena cava above the level of the diaphragm. Confirmation of tip location with either ECG or postprocedure chest X-ray is needed. Additionally, patient ambulation may be more difficult with a femorally inserted CVAD. Many hospitals have policies that require femorally inserted catheters to be replaced with another type of CVAD as soon as possible due to higher risk of infection and thrombosis at this site.

Dress code

Dressing adherence is a big concern when selecting an insertion site. The femoral site inherently carries a greater risk of local infection because of the difficulty of keeping a dressing clean and intact in the groin area.

Straighten it out

When a femoral vein is used, the patient's leg needs to be kept straight and movement limited. Doing so prevents bleeding and keeps the catheter from becoming kinked internally or dislodged. Infection can also occur at the insertion site from catheter movement into and out of the incision.

Peripheral veins

The peripheral veins most commonly used as insertion sites for PICCs include:
- basilic
- brachial
- cephalic
- external jugular.

Veins located directly in the antecubital fossa are no longer recommended for PICC insertion. Moving the insertion site to the upper arm and out of the bend of the arm reduces mechanical irritation and subsequent thrombophlebitis. Insertion sites in the upper arm require the use of ultrasound because the basilic and brachial veins are deep in the tissue and cannot be palpated.

Far from internal organs

Because they're located far from major internal organs and vessels, peripheral veins cause fewer traumatic complications on insertion. However, accessing peripheral veins may cause phlebitis and increased risk for thrombus formation. Therefore, it is critical to measure the vein's internal diameter with ultrasound guidance and place the smallest size catheter in the largest vein to prevent complications. Catheter movement may irritate the inner lumen of the vein or block it due to the vein to catheter ratio, causing blood pooling (stasis) and thrombus formation.

Vein pursuits

The brachial vein is situated near the artery and median nerve bundle. The cephalic vein is generally large in the forearm, is generally smaller in diameter than the basilic vein, and narrows as it joins the axillary vein. These factors increase the risk of thrombus formation. Therefore, the larger, straighter basilic vein is usually the preferred insertion site. Bedside ultrasound should be used to locate these veins and determine which vein is appropriate for catheter insertion.

The external jugular vein may provide a CVAD insertion site. Using the external jugular vein this way presents few complications. However, threading a catheter into the superior vena cava may be difficult because of the sharp angle encountered on entering the axillary-subclavian vein and it is generally smaller than the internal jugular vein. For this reason, it is not first choice for a CVAD but may be used in acute situations when other veins cannot be accessed.

Accessing peripheral sites in the antecubital space limits the patient's mobility because the device exits the skin at the bend of the elbow, increasing the risk for infection and thrombophlebitis. Inserting the catheter above the antecubital space increases patient mobility and prevents kinking. The use of US is necessary to locate and access the veins of the upper arm. However, in obese patients, the antecubital fossa may be the only site that is accessible, even with US.

Dilution dilemma

A CVAD is only considered centrally located when the tip is in the superior (SVC) or inferior vena cava (IVC), close to the cavoatrial junction, where the SVC or IVC and atrium meet. This tip location provides high blood flow rates and turbulence of the blood flow to reduce chemical damage to the intima of the vein. If the tip is higher in the SVC, or lower in the IVC, the risk for complications increases. Tip migration to smaller vessels or erosion of the catheter tip through the vessel wall leading to extravasation is more common when the tip is located more distal to the cavoatrial junction.

Insertion site concerns

There are notable concerns in choosing an insertion site for a CVAD. Examples of these include:
- presence of scar tissue
- interference with the surgical site or other therapy (for example, radiation, physical therapy)

- configuration of the lung apices
- implanted intracardiac devices such as pacemakers
- patient's lifestyle or daily activities
- whether the patient's arms can abduct (for a PICC).

Scar wars

In some patients, scar tissue from previous surgery or trauma may prohibit access to major blood vessels or make catheter insertion difficult. Alternatively, if the patient is facing surgery in the area of a central vein, another site is chosen. A peripheral site, such as the basilic vein, and a central site on the side of the body unaffected by surgery are likely alternatives.

Tracheostomy treachery

An alternative site may be necessary if the patient is receiving other therapy that interferes with the insertion site. For example, if the patient has a tracheostomy, the internal or external jugular site should be avoided because the tracheostomy tapes come too close to these insertion sites. This proximity predisposes the patient to infection and may cause the catheter to dislodge.

Look out for the lungs

Another site consideration is the location of the lung apices. In patients on mechanical ventilation — especially those receiving positive end-expiratory pressure therapy — intrathoracic pressures increase, which may elevate the lung apices and increase the chance of lung puncture and pneumothorax. Patients with COPD also have displaced lung apices, so consideration should be given to venous access sites outside the thorax in these patients.

Be practical and alert

Practical considerations play a role in site selection. For example, patients on home infusion therapy will be managing their own infusions and flushing. A PICC in one arm may mean only one hand with which to work. A woman with a long-term tunneled catheter or implanted port that exits near her bra straps would have a limited choice of clothing.

Be aware of the catheter's insertion site and the location of the catheter tip. That way, you can be alert for potential problems, such as thrombosis, catheter displacement, and infection.

Preparing the patient

Accurate and thorough patient teaching increases the success of I.V. therapy. Before therapy begins, make sure that the patient understands the procedure and its benefits. Be sure to let the patient know what to expect during and after catheter insertion. Also, cover all self-care measures.

Informed consent may be required by the policy in your facility. This is an educational process that usually ends with the patient's signature on a consent form. The patient must understand the procedure, the reason for its recommendation, the risk and benefits, alternative treatment options, common complications, and any serious risk. The primary responsibility for explaining this information rests with the inserter; however, regulations in some states put this responsibility exclusively on the physician. Your role may include allaying the patient's fears and answering questions about:
- movement restrictions
- cosmetic concerns
- management regimens
- and confirming the patient's comprehension of the information provided.

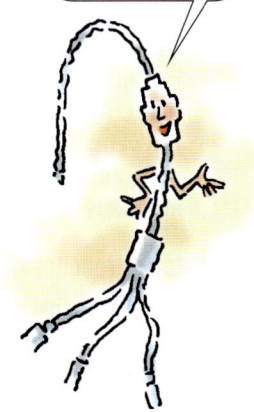

Be aware of the insertion site and where my tip is located.

Explaining the procedure

Ask the patient if he or she has ever received I.V. therapy before, particularly central I.V. therapy. Evaluate the patient's learning capabilities and adjust your teaching technique accordingly. Age- and culturally appropriate methods are needed. For example, use age-appropriate language when describing the procedure to a child. Also, ask the parents to help you phrase the procedure in terms their child understands. If time and resources permit, use pictures and physical models to enhance your teaching.

Getting all dressed up

Explain that sterile procedures require the staff to wear gowns, masks, and gloves and that the patient be completely covered with a full-body drape. Tell your patient that he or she may need to wear a mask as well. If time allows, let your patient, especially a child, try on the mask.

An important position

To minimize the patient's anxiety, explain how he or she will be positioned during the procedure. If the subclavian or jugular vein will be used, the patient will be in Trendelenburg position for at least a short period, and a towel may be placed under the back between the scapulae. (In Trendelenburg position, the head is low and the body and legs are on an inclined plane.)

Reassure the patient that he or she won't be in this position longer than necessary. Stress the importance of this position for dilating the veins, which aids insertion and helps prevent air embolus during insertion.

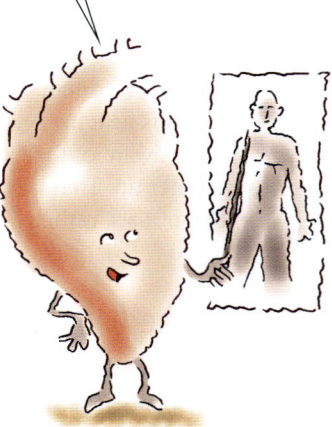

The use of pictures and physical models can enhance your patient teaching. Remember to tailor your teaching to the patient's age, primary language, and learning capabilities.

This may sting

Warn the patient to expect a stinging sensation from the local anesthetic and a feeling of pressure during catheter insertion.

Testing, testing

Explain any other tests that may be done. For example, the inserter may obtain a venogram before the catheter insertion to check the status of the vessels, especially if the catheter is intended for long-term use. Prior to surgical catheter insertion, blood samples are commonly drawn to establish baseline coagulation profiles, and a chest X-ray is always done to confirm catheter placement if the catheter is not inserted using fluoroscopy or a tip locating system. When an ECG or ECG/Doppler system or fluoroscopy is used for tip location, no chest X-ray is needed; however, there should be some form of permanent documentation for the original tip location.

Explaining self-care measures

In explaining self-care measures to your patient, make sure that you cover the following topics:
- Instruct the patient to keep the dressing clean, dry, and intact and how to protect during showering or bathing.
- If the catheter will be managed at home, thoroughly explain all care procedures, such as hand hygiene before touching the catheter, disinfecting the needleless connector, connecting the flush syringes and medication administration sets, and clamping the catheter after each use.
- Ask the patient to demonstrate the various techniques and procedures, and include other family members, as appropriate.

The home care nurse should coordinate teaching and follow-up assessments until the patient is capable of independently managing infusions. Assessing patency by aspirating for a blood return and dressing changes are most commonly performed by the home care nurse on weekly visits. Ensure that the patient knows when and whom to call for help.

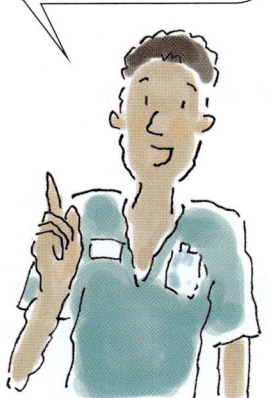

Make sure the patient thoroughly understands self-care measures, infusion techniques, and methods to prevent infection.

Preparing the equipment for CVAD insertion

Besides the I.V. solution, infusion equipment typically includes an administration set appropriate for the solution to be infuse (for example, set with an in-line 0.2-micron filter if parenteral nutrition is being infused). An electronic infusion pump should also be used when solutions are administered through a CVAD.

Getting equipped

When you're assisting with an insertion at the patient's bedside, first collect the necessary equipment. Preassembled disposable trays or kits that include the CVAD and all supplies are used by many facilities, although others will use a dedicated cart stocked with all supplies. Although most trays include the necessary equipment, be sure to check. If you don't have a preassembled tray, gather the following items, which should be bundled and on a CVAD insertion cart:
- linen-saver pad
- clippers for hair removal
- sterile gauze pads
- alcoholic chlorhexidine skin antiseptic
- local anesthetic
- 3-mL syringe with 25-G needle for local injection of anesthetic
- sterile syringe for blood samples, if needed
- sterile towels
- large full-body sterile drape
- sterile gloves
- sterile gown
- an engineered stabilization device (ESD) (recommended instead of sutures)
- sterile dressing
- CVAD.

You also need to obtain extra syringes and blood sample containers if venous blood samples are to be drawn during the procedure.

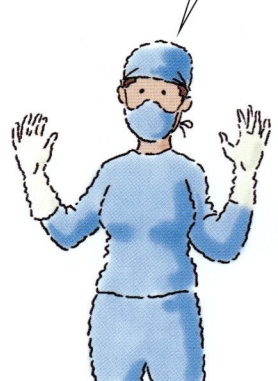

Gowns, masks, caps, and gloves are standard issue for a bedside CVAD insertion.

Mask, gown, and gloves required

Make sure that everyone participating in the insertion of a CVAD has a cap, mask, gown, and gloves. You may also need facial protection for the patient, especially if there's a risk of site contamination from oral secretions or if the patient is unable to cooperate.

Some assembly required

To set up the equipment, follow these steps:
- Attach the administration set to the solution container.
- Prime the set with the solution.
- Prime and calibrate any pressure monitoring setups.

Aseptic, air-free, secure, and sealed

In addition, take the following precautions:
- Priming the administration set must be done immediately before insertion using aseptic no-touch technique.
- All sets must be free from air.
- After you have primed the set, recheck all the connections to make sure that they are luer-locked securely.

- Make sure that all open ends are covered with sealed caps. Some administration sets will allow fluid to flow without removing the cap on the male luer end.

Performing CVAD insertion

Although specific steps may vary, the same basic procedure is used whether catheter insertion is done at the bedside or in the operating room. Before the CVAD insertion, you need to:
- position the patient
- prepare the insertion site.

Gonna be sedated?

Some patients may require sedation for the catheter to be placed. Such patients must be carefully monitored by staff trained in this procedure.

Positioning the patient

After you have assembled the administration set and infusion pump, position the patient to make him or her as comfortable as possible.

Visible and accessible

Position the patient in Trendelenburg position for insertion in the subclavian, internal, or external jugular veins. This position distends neck and thoracic veins, making them more visible and accessible. Filling the veins also lessens the chance of air emboli because of the distended veins at the insertion site.

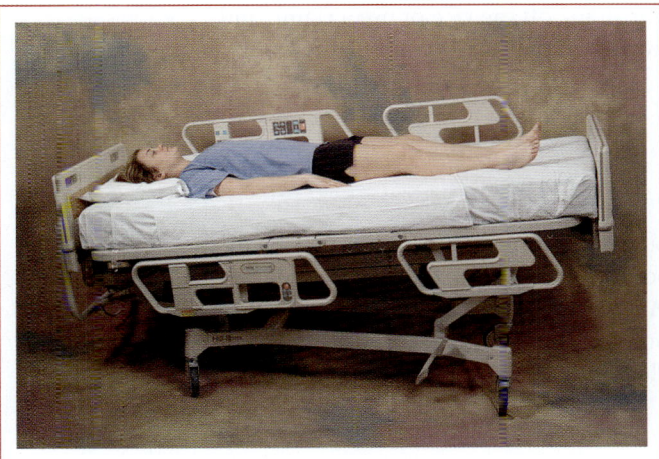

Trendelenburg position.

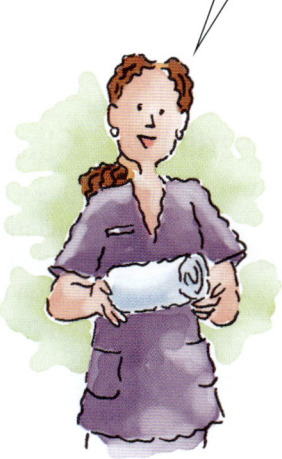

A rolled towel or blanket may be helpful when positioning the patient, to promote visibility of anatomic landmarks and reduce puncture of the lung apex and adjacent vessels.

On a roll

If the subclavian vein is to be used, you may need to place a rolled towel or blanket between the patient's scapulae. Doing so allows for more direct access, reducing the risk of puncturing the lung apex or adjacent vessels.

If a jugular vein is to be used, place a rolled blanket under the opposite shoulder to extend the neck.

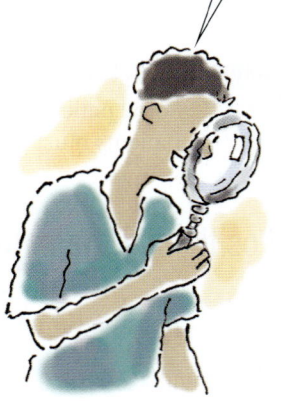

Always prep clean skin. If the skin is visibly soiled, wash first.

Preparing the insertion site

If the planned insertion site is visibly dirty (for example, sweat, skin oils, blood), wash with soap and water. Make sure that the skin is free from hair because the follicles can harbor microorganisms. (See *Removing hair from a CV insertion site.*) Place a linen-saver pad under the site to prevent soiling the bed.

To prepare for insertion, the inserter will do the following:
- Prepare the catheter by trimming to a patient-specific length as needed and flushing the catheter with normal saline.
- Perform skin antisepsis, preferably with alcoholic chlorhexidine gluconate (CHG) solution using a back-and-forth scrubbing motion. The solution must dry completely before proceeding with vascular access device insertion.

Sterile drape style

After the site is prepared, the inserter uses maximal sterile barriers by placing sterile drapes around it and using a full-body drape, covering the patient's entire body. (This makes the patient's mask unnecessary.) The patient may become anxious with the drape directly over his face. You can simply lift the drape off the face or use a clamp and I.V. pole to hold the drape away from the face but still maintaining a barrier.

Inserting the catheter

During catheter insertion, you may be responsible for monitoring the patient's tolerance of the procedure and providing emotional support. The inserter prepares the CVAD for insertion, which requires aseptic technique. Don't forget to complete the insertion checklist as you observe the procedure. And don't hesitate to inform the inserter to stop the procedure if a step was not performed or there was a breach of technique.

In some cases, radiologic techniques, such as fluoroscopy or an injectable contrast agent, may be used to assist with catheter placement. Current recommendations to use US guidance for visualization requires the US probe to be covered with a sterile sheath and the use of sterile coupling gel. You may be asked to assist with this part of the setup.

Blood samples

You may obtain venous blood samples after the catheter is inserted. If the sample is drawn while the sterile field is still in place, you'll need a sterile syringe that's large enough to hold all of the needed blood such as a 10-mL syringe. Another option is to draw the blood sample after the sterile field has been removed so that the vacuum tube holder can be attached directly to the catheter hub. This allows for the sample to be drawn directly into the vacuum tubes and eliminates the need to manually transfer the sample to the appropriate tubes. If blood transfer is needed, a needleless transfer set must be used. Do not remove the cap on the vacuum tubes to facilitate this blood transfer.

Patient participation

Each time the catheter hub is open to air — such as when the needleless connector or administration set is changed — tell the patient to perform Valsalva's maneuver or clamp the catheter's extension leg to decrease the risk of air embolism.

Catheter inserted. Now what?

After the catheter is inserted, your primary responsibilities are monitoring the patient and administering therapy. You'll also need to document your interventions and all information related to the catheter insertion.

Monitoring the patient

After the catheter has been inserted, monitor the patient for complications. Make sure that you tailor your assessment and interventions to the particular catheter insertion site. For example, if the site is close to major thoracic organs, as with a subclavian or internal

Best practice

Removing hair from a CVAD insertion site

Infection prevention practitioners and the Infusion Nurses Society recommend clipping the hair close to the skin rather than shaving.

Irritation, open wounds, infection
Shaving may cause skin irritation and create multiple, small, open wounds, increasing the risk of infection. To avoid irritation, clip the patient's hair with single-patient–use clipper blades.

Rinse, wash, and remove
After you remove the hair, rinse the skin with water to remove hair clippings. You may also need to wash the skin with soap and water to remove surface dirt and body oils before application of the skin antiseptic agent.

jugular vein site, you should closely monitor the patient's respiratory status, watching for dyspnea, shortness of breath, and sudden chest pain.

Arrhythmia alert

Inserting the catheter can cause arrhythmias if the catheter enters the right atrium (irritating the node) or right ventricle (irritating the cardiac muscle). For this reason, make sure that you monitor the patient's cardiac status. (Arrhythmias usually abate as the catheter is withdrawn.) If the patient isn't attached to a cardiac monitor, palpate the radial pulse to detect rhythm irregularities.

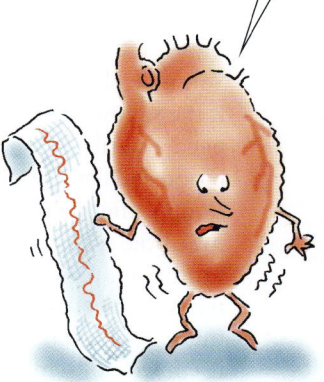

Be aware that catheter insertion can cause arrhythmias if the device inadvertently enters my right atrium or right ventricle.

No suture in his future

Most nontunneled CVADs are designed to accommodate an adhesive engineered stabilization device. Standards and guidelines recommend against suturing due to increased risk of sharps injury, local infection, and subsequent catheter-related bloodstream infection. A subcutaneous stabilization device is now available for CVADs. This is not visible, so check the insertion documentation for its use.

Where is the tip?

Final tip location is confirmed by using an electrocardiogram (ECG) tip locating system during the procedure or a postprocedure chest X-ray. An X-ray is ordered to confirm the location of the catheter tip before starting infusions when an ECG system cannot be used. Use of the ECG system is contraindicated in patients with atrial fibrillation, atrial pacemaker, or atrial flutter because the P wave on the ECG tracing is not easily found. While waiting on results of the chest X-ray, each lumen of the CVAD must have a luer-locking needleless connector on the hub and be locked with normal saline solution until confirmation of tip location is obtained. After confirmation, begin the infusion by connecting a new I.V. administration set to the catheter hub.

Poor catheter positioning poses problems

The external portion of the catheter may be positioned poorly, causing several problems. It can:
- make dressing changes difficult
- make maintaining a totally adherent dressing impossible
- cause the catheter to kink.

Documenting access device insertion

The inserter will document the procedure; however, your involvement should also be documented. Record all pertinent information in the appropriate section of the medical record (for example, nurses' notes, the I.V. flow sheet). Make sure that your documentation includes:
- type of CVAD used
- location of insertion site
- catheter tip position as confirmed by ECG tip locating system or X-ray
- patient's tolerance of the procedure
- blood samples taken, if any
- type of stabilization and dressing applied.

A measure of dislodgment

The length of catheter remaining outside the body should be documented so other nurses can compare the measurements, checking for catheter dislodgment.

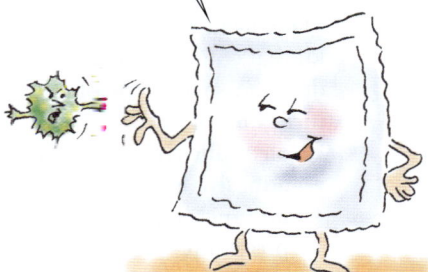

Prevent infection: Keep the insertion site clean and dry and the dressing adherent on all sides.

Maintaining central venous infusions

One of your primary responsibilities is maintaining infusions. Doing so includes meticulous care of the CVAD insertion site as well as the catheter and entire administration system.

Routine care

Expect to perform the following care measures according to your institution policy:
- Change the transparent semipermeable dressing, adhesive stabilization device, and dressing weekly or whenever it becomes moist, loose, or soiled.
- Assess catheter patency before each use by observing for any resistance during flushing and aspirating for the presence of blood return that is the color and consistency of whole blood.
- Flush and lock the catheter when used for intermittent medication.
- Change the needleless connector, I.V. administration set, and fluid containers according to facility policy and procedure.
- Administer I.V. medications.
- Obtain blood samples, if needed and peripheral venipuncture sites are not available.
- Record your assessment findings and interventions.

Changing dressings

To reduce the risk of infection, always wear sterile gloves and a mask when changing the dressing. The patient should also wear a mask. If the patient can't tolerate a facial mask, have the patient turn the head away from the catheter during the dressing change.

> *Wear sterile gloves and a mask when you change a dressing.*

Getting equipped

Many facilities use a preassembled dressing-change tray or kit that contains all the necessary equipment. If your facility doesn't use this type of tray, gather the necessary equipment, including:
- alcoholic chlorhexidine skin antiseptic
- adhesive ESD, if the subcutaneous ESD is not in use
- antimicrobial dressing per your facility's policy and procedure
- skin barrier solution
- transparent semipermeable dressing
- sterile drape
- sterile gloves and masks
- sterile paper tape measure
- clean gloves
- bag to dispose of old dressing.

A different brand of dressing

Expect to change your patient's CVAD dressing every 48 hours if it's a gauze dressing and at least every 5 to 7 days if it's a transparent membrane. Dressings should be changed immediately if they become soiled, moist, or loose or if the integrity of the dressing is compromised. (See *Changing a CVAD dressing*, page 149.)

Changing fluid containers and administration sets

Change the I.V. solution according to what is infusing. For example, parenteral nutrition requires a new bag and administration set every 24 hours. Continuous primary and secondary sets are changed every 96 hours or as directed by your facility's policy, maintaining strict aseptic technique. You don't need to wear a mask unless there's a contamination risk, for example, if you have an upper respiratory tract infection. (See *Chapter 1* for more information about administration sets and fluid containers.)

Plan to change the solution container and the administration set at the same time if possible to minimize the number of times the system is opened. You may not be able to do this if, for example, the set is damaged or the solution runs out before it's time to change the set.

(Text continues on page 150.)

Changing a CVAD dressing

After you assemble all needed equipment, follow the step-by-step technique below to safely change a CVAD dressing.

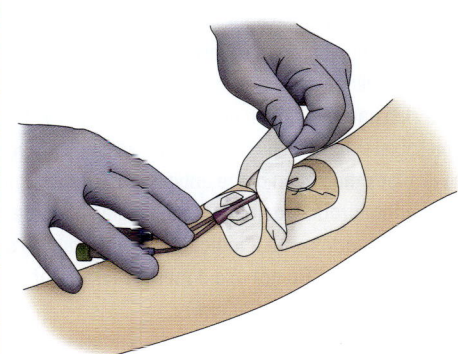

Step 1: Remove the old dressing, stabilization device and antiseptic dressing.

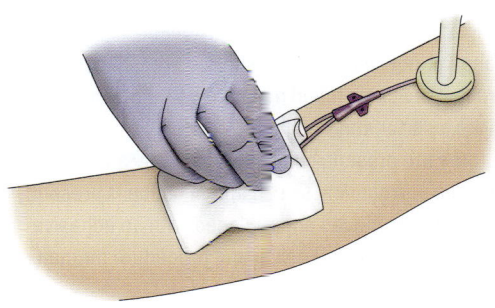

Step 2: Application of the skin antiseptic in a back and forth motion

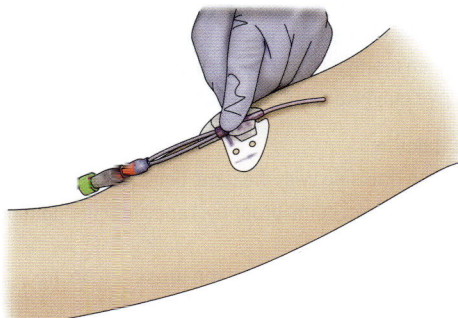

Step 3: Application of the new stabilization device.

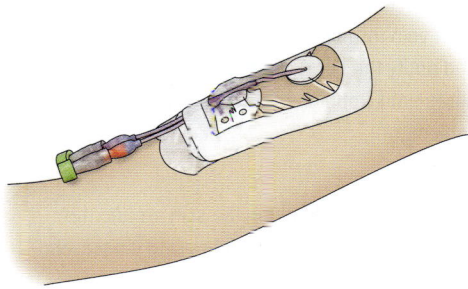

Step 4: Apply the new antiseptic and transparent membrane dressing

Getting ready
- Perform hand hygiene by washing or using antiseptic hand gel. Then place the patient in a comfortable supine position.
- Prepare a sterile field. Open the bag, placing it away from the sterile field but still within reach.

Out with the old
- Put on clean gloves and remove the old dressing and adhesive ESD.

- Inspect the old dressing for signs of drainage. If purulent drainage is present, assess the insertion site for other signs of infection; apply a sterile temporary dressing. Discard the dressing and gloves in the bag. Immediately notify the LIP of the site condition and follow the orders for obtaining drainage cultures, blood cultures, or both. Document your actions in the medical record. If the site is without complications, proceed with the dressing change.

(continued)

Changing a CVAD dressing (continued)

- Check the position of the catheter, measuring the external catheter length to assess for dislodgment by comparing to external length on insertion. Never readvance a CVAD into a vein once it has been dislodged. A catheter exchange or new insertion may be required. Simply secure the device as found once the site is cleaned and notify the inserter and/or LIP.
- If sutures are present, check their integrity and the condition of the surrounding skin. If inflammation is present, they should be removed and replaced with an adhesive ESD. Know your facility's policy and procedure for managing this problem.
- For a PICC, measure upper arm circumference in the presence of arm edema or patient complaints of tightness or discomfort in the extremity, shoulder, or neck. Measure 10 cm above the antecubital fossa. Compare to baseline measurement. A significant increase in arm circumference could be related to the presence of vein thrombosis. Document in medical record and notify the LIP. Anticipate an order for a color duplex ultrasound Doppler study to facilitate a diagnosis of the problem.

In with the new

- Put on sterile gloves and clean the skin around the catheter with alcoholic chlorhexidine using a back-and-forth or side-to-side motion.
- Apply a skin barrier solution to the skin where all adhesive products will be applied, and allow to dry. This will decrease the risk of medical adhesive-related skin injury (MARSI). If using an antimicrobial dressing such as a foam disc or gel pad built onto the transparent dressing, avoid placing the skin barrier solution under the small area where the antimicrobial dressing will be located. The skin barrier solution will block the action of the antimicrobial dressing.
- Apply the antimicrobial foam disc dressing around the catheter at the insertion site if indicated by your facility's policy and procedure. (Do not use if there is history of reactions to the antimicrobial agent.)
- Apply the ESD, the preferred method for securing an access device; it should be changed whenever you change the dressing. Sterile tape or surgical wound closure strips are not adequate to ensure catheter stabilization and securement.
- Apply a sterile transparent semipermeable dressing to the site, ensuring it is adherent on all sides.
- Remove gloves and perform hand hygiene.

Write it down

- Label the dressing with the date, time, and your initials.
- Discard all used items properly; reposition the patient comfortably.
- Document site condition and the procedure in the patient's medical record.

Open air prevention

To prevent air embolism, clamp the catheter or attached extension set before the catheter hub is open to air, such as with a change of needleless connector or administration set.

Switching solutions

To change the solution, follow these steps:
1. Assess the LIP order for fluids prescribed.
2. Obtain a solution container, checking the label for the correct fluids as prescribed.
3. Perform hand hygiene.
4. Identify the patient using two identifiers according to facility policy and procedure.

5. Stop or pause the electronic infusion device.
6. Remove the seal from the solution container.
7. Remove the spike from the empty solution container, and reinsert it into the new container, being careful not to allow the spike to touch anything.
8. Hang the new container and restart the electronic infusion device, ensuring the correct flow rate.
9. Apply the appropriate time strip labels according to facility policy and procedure.

Turning over the administration set

Gather an I.V. administration set, an extension set, an alcohol wipe, and gloves.

Changing the CVAD administration set

Administration sets are changed any time a new CVAD is inserted, when changing from a peripheral infusion to a CVAD infusion, and at scheduled intervals based on the type of therapy being given. The administration sets are changed based on solution, frequency (continuous or intermittent), and suspected contamination or the integrity of the system has been compromised. The administration set and the fluid container should be changed at the same time. Changing only the administration set and keeping the existing fluid container is not the preferred method because it easily allows unfiltered room air to enter the container and, for a plastic bag, the appearance of the fluid level is altered. But there might be times when it is necessary.

Follow these guidelines to safely change the administration set:
- Obtain the necessary set.
- Verify the patient identity using two identifiers according to facility policy and procedure.
- Perform hand hygiene.
- Stop the electronic infusion pump.
- Remove the covering from the port intended to receive the spike end of the administration set. Open the administration set package, close the set clamp, and remove the cover from the spike. Do NOT allow the spike to touch anything. Insert the spike into the fluid container.
- Squeeze the drip chamber to fill it halfway.
- Open the clamp and purge all air from the administration set, inverting injection ports and filters to allow all air bubbles to be flushed out. Do NOT remove the tip cap from the male luer end of the set as most will allow fluid to flow through with the tip cap intact. Alternatively, the set can be inserted into the electronic infusion pump and air purged according to the pump instructions.
- Put on clean gloves.
- Close the clamp on the catheter extension leg.
- Disconnect the used set and clean the hub with the alcohol pad. Allow the hub

(*continued*)

Changing the CVAD administration set (continued)

to dry thoroughly. If the old set is difficult to remove, wrap a tourniquet around the set to enhance your grip. Use of hemostats on the catheter hub can easily cause the hub to crack.
- Remove the tip cap from the male luer end of the new set, and connect directly to the hub.

Your facility may use a needleless connector on the CVAD hub for all continuous infusions. If present, assess the date for it to be changed and change it with the addition of the new set as needed. If the current needleless connector will not require changing before the next administration set change is due, disconnect the used set from the connector. Disinfect the connector surface with 70% alcohol solution, povidone-iodine, or alcoholic chlorhexidine solution. Perform a vigorous mechanical scrub according to your policy, and connect to the new set to the needleless connector.
- Unclamp the CVAD and restart the electronic infusion pump at the correct flow rate.
- Label all sets appropriately with date of change according to your institution's policy.
- Label the set near its connection to the CVAD hub with the type of solution being infused.

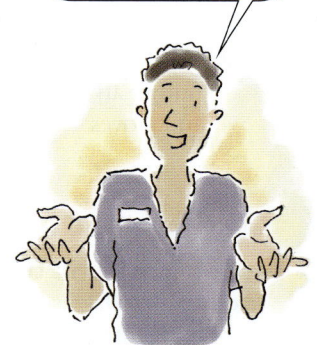

The administration set is changed when a new CVAD is placed. Hmm, that's new.

Changing the administration set without changing the infusing fluid container is not preferred but could be necessary in some situations. To do this safely:
- Remove the administration set from the package.
- Stop the electronic infusion pump and close the catheter clamp.
- Remove the fluid container from the pole. For a plastic bag, pinch the outlet to prevent air from entering the bag if possible. Withdraw the spike from the used administration set and drape it over the I.V. pole.
- Remove the cover from the spike on the new administration set and insert into the existing fluid container.
- Suspend the container from the pole and purge all air from the set manually or with the electronic infusion pump.
- Detach the used set from the CVAD hub. Scrub the female catheter hub or needleless connector with an antiseptic solution according to facility policy and procedure.
- Attach the new administration set.
- Restart the electronic infusion pump and regulate the flow rate as prescribed.

Flushing and locking the CVAD

Flush the CVAD with saline solution routinely, according to your facility's policy, to maintain patency, remove the previous locking solution from the CVAD lumen, and prevent contact between incompatible solutions. Flushing may be needed with continuous infusion if the electronic infusion pump has an occlusion alarm or if the flow rate is slow or interrupted. Flushing is necessary before and after intermittent infusions.

Locking the CVAD lumen involves putting a solution into the CVAD lumen to maintain patency between intermittent infusions. Low-dose heparin (that is, 10 units/mL) or normal saline are common locking solutions, and studies now show there is no difference in patency outcomes between these two lock solutions. A variety of antimicrobial locking solutions are used to prevent or treat catheter-related bloodstream infection. The antimicrobial lock solutions often contain high concentrations of antibiotics, causing concern about developing resistance to those antibiotics. This concern requires that all antimicrobial lock solutions be aspirated from the lumen rather than being flushed into the bloodstream.

When the system is maintained as an intermittent infusion device, the flushing procedure varies, depending on:
- facility policy
- type of catheter used
- medication administration schedule.

How often? How much?

All lumens of a CVAD must be assessed for patency prior to each use. According to the Infusion Therapy Standards of Practice from the Infusion Nurses Society (INS) and guidelines from the Institute for Safe Medication Practices (ISMP), a minimum 10-mL diameter-sized syringe filled with preservative-free 0.9% sodium chloride should be used for assessment of central line patency. Using bacteriostatic normal saline may result in administration of too much preservative. Laboratory studies have shown that using a pulsatile flushing technique of short, 1-mL boluses interrupted by brief pauses may remove a greater amount of solid deposits like fibrin.

The recommended frequency for flushing CVADs varies. For a continuous infusion with a slowed flow rate or an electronic infusion pump with an occlusion alarm, flushing is done to assess the lumen and encourage patency on an as-needed basis. When the CVAD is only used for intermittent infusion, flushing is done before and after the medication administration.

The recommended amount of normal saline for flushing varies due to different internal volumes for the catheter lumen plus any add-on devices such as extension sets. The INS recommends a volume of at least twice the internal volume of the entire catheter system (that is, catheter plus add-ons). Five, ten, and even twenty mL of saline may be needed. The smaller amount is often used for small-sized CVADs, but 20 mL is used following blood draws, blood administration, parenteral nutrition, contrast media, and other viscous solutions.

Mismatched medications

A normal saline solution flush should also be performed before and after the administration of incompatible medications.

Flushing made simple

Solutions for flushing and locking should come from a single-dose system such as a single-dose vial or prefilled syringe. Use of a bag of normal saline for multiple patients is never recommended as this practice has caused several infectious outbreaks among patients. If you only have access to multiple-dose vials, one vial should be dedicated to a single patient and not shared between patients to prevent spreading infection.

When flushing a CVAD, use a 10-mL syringe with the appropriate flush solution. Follow these steps:
1. Perform hand hygiene.
2. Put on clean gloves.
3. Disinfect the needleless connector using a 70% alcohol solution, povidone-iodine, or alcoholic chlorhexidine solution by applying a vigorous mechanical scrub. The length of scrubbing time may vary from 5 to 15 seconds or more, so follow your facility's policy. Discard the disinfectant pad after each use.
4. Allow the needleless connector to dry completely.
5. Attach the syringe and inject a small amount of flush solution, observing for any resistance. Aspirate by pulling back on the syringe plunger to obtain a blood return that is the color and consistency of whole blood. Absence of resistance and presence of a blood return confirm patency. Do not apply excessive force to overcome resistance and do not continue without a blood return. Stop and investigate the possible causes.
6. Follow instructions for use from the manufacturer of the specific type of needleless connector in use. The sequence for clamping and disconnecting the syringe depends on the type of needleless connector being used. (See *Chapter 1, Needleless connectors,* pages 31–33 for more discussion of needleless connectors)
7. The process for disinfection is needed before each entry into the system. Giving an intermittent medication usually requires multiple entries for flushing, administering the medication, flushing again, and instilling the lock solution.

Changing needleless connectors

CVADs used for intermittent infusions have needleless connectors attached to the catheter hub. These connectors must be luer-locked to prevent inadvertent disconnection and air embolism.

The frequency of connector changes varies according to facility policy and how often the connector is used. If used with a continuous infusion, the needleless connector should be changed when the administration set is changed every 96 hours. For intermittent use, the administration set is changed every 24 hours and the needleless connector should be changed at least every 7 days.

Integrity check

The integrity of a connector should be checked before and after each use. If at any time the integrity is compromised, or blood is seen in the connector, it should be changed. Remember, always use strict aseptic technique when changing these connectors.

Exception to the rule!

The needleless connector should be removed, discarded, and replaced with a new one:
- if the connector is removed for any reason
- when residual blood or debris is noted in the connector
- prior to drawing a sample for blood cultures
- on contamination
- per institutional policies, procedures, and guidelines
- per manufacturer's instruction for use.

To change the connector, follow these steps:
1. Close the clamping mechanism on the catheter.
2. Disconnect the used connector, clean the catheter hub with alcohol swab, allow to dry, and place the new connector, using aseptic technique.

Under cover

Passive disinfectant caps containing isopropyl alcohol are placed on needleless connectors if the CVAD is used intermittently. These caps have been found to reduce contamination of the internal lumen of the CVAD and, consequently, rates of catheter-related bloodstream infection (CRBSI). These caps are removed prior to using the CVAD and are discarded; they are single-use items. Use the caps according to your policy and the manufacturer's instructions for use.

After the disinfecting cap is removed, and the CVAD will be accessed multiple times (for example, giving several I.V. medications) use a 5- to 15-second scrub to clean the connector between connections.

Secondary piggyback sets

Administration sets used for primary continuous infusion and secondary *piggyback* medications should remain connected together and be changed no more frequently than 96 hours. If a secondary piggyback administration set is used with an *intermittent* medication and disconnected from the primary set, the secondary set must be changed every 24 hours. When only intermittent medication is prescribed, the administration set must be changed every 24 hours also. Each connection and disconnection potentially increases the risk for CRBSI.

To infuse a piggybacked medication, make sure that solutions running in the same line are compatible and connections are luer-locked. Secondary I.V. lines may be piggybacked into a side port or Y-port of a primary infusion line.

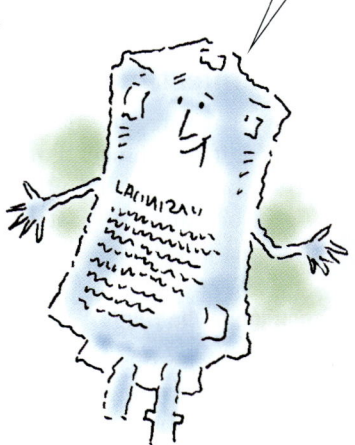

Make sure that solutions running in the same line are compatible and the connections are secure.

Documentation

Record your assessment findings and interventions according to your facility's policy. Include such information as:
- type, amount, and rate of infusion
- dressing changes, including the type, appearance, and location of the catheter and site
- how the patient tolerated the procedure
- administration set and solution changes
- connector changes
- flushing and locking procedures, including any problems encountered, and the amount and type of solution used
- the blood samples collected, including the type and amount.

Blood samples from a CVAD

Keep in mind that a CVAD should only be used to draw blood when no other venipuncture options are available. Consider using a CVAD phlebotomy checklist and direct observation periodically for adherence to the checklist. Risk factors for using a CVAD for obtaining blood samples include hub manipulation, intraluminal contamination, erroneous lab values, and hospital-acquired anemia. Dedicate a lumen to blood sampling if possible, and if not, direct venipuncture may be necessary. If a CVAD is used, pay close attention to any lab values that require a dose change based on the lab value, as test results may be inaccurate.

(Text continues on page 158)

Drawing blood from a CVAD

- Assemble your equipment.
- Perform hand hygiene and put on gloves.
- Clamp the catheter lumen, and disinfect the needleless connector per institution policy.
- Stop all infusions and flush with preservative-free 0.9% sodium chloride (USP). No length of time for stopping infusions or the amount of saline flush has been established by research, although using 10 to 20 mL of flush may provide more accurate results for coagulation values and other therapeutic drug monitoring.
- Using the empty flush syringe, aspirate and discard 6 mL from PICCs and non-tunneled catheters and 9 mL from tunneled catheters and implanted ports.
- Clamp the catheter and remove the syringe for discard. Label this syringe to prevent confusion with the syringes containing the sample to be sent to the lab.
- Disinfect the injection surface, and connect an empty syringe.
- Release the clamp, and withdraw the blood sample.
- Clamp the catheter and remove the syringe.
- Disinfect the needleless connector and connect the syringe with normal saline solution.
- Open the clamp and flush with solution. Close the clamp.
- For an intermittent CVAD, instill the appropriate locking solution according to facility policy. The sequence for final clamping and disconnection depends upon the type of needleless connector in use. For a negative displacement needleless connector, flush, clamp, and then disconnect. For a positive displacement needleless connector, flush, disconnect, and then clamp. For a neutral needleless connector, the sequence of clamping and disconnection can be done in any order.
- For continuous infusion, restart the appropriate infusion rate.
- Attach a needleless transfer device to the syringe with the blood sample and inject the blood into the appropriate blood collection tube after cleaning it with appropriate solution per policy. Use the appropriate sequence for filling the vacuum tubes based on the color of the tube top and the manufacturer's instructions.

Using a vacuum tube system

- Wash your hands and put on gloves.
- Clamp the catheter lumen, and clean the connector per institution policy.
- Stop all infusions and flush with preservative-free 0.9% sodium chloride (USP). No length of time for stopping infusions or the amount of saline flush has been established by research, although using 10 to 20 mL of flush may provide more accurate results for coagulation levels and other therapeutic drug monitoring.
- Attach the vacuum tube holder to the needleless connector or directly to the catheter hub. Insert the first tube and draw the volume to be discarded. Label this tube for discard to prevent confusion with the other tubes.
- Insert the vacuum tubes in the appropriate colored sequence, filling to the desired level. Label each tube with the patient information in the presence of the patient.
- Close the catheter clamp and detach the tube holder and discard in a sharps container.
- Disinfect the connection surface and connect the saline-filled syringe. Flush to clear the lumen of all visible blood.
- For an intermittent CVAD, instill the appropriate locking solution according to facility policy. For continuous infusion, restart the appropriate infusion rate.

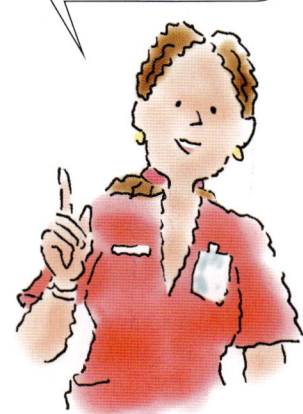

Remember, when drawing blood cultures to determine CRBSI, remove the connector, and draw from the hub.

The mixing method is another acceptable technique for obtaining a blood sample. Hospital-acquired anemia is associated with excessive blood sampling and discarding the initial sample. The mixing method eliminates the need for discarding any blood. To perform this method:
- Perform handing hygiene and don clean gloves.
- Stop all infusions if present.
- Disinfect the connection surface.
- Attach a saline-filled syringe and flush the lumen.
- Leave the syringe attached and aspirate 5 mL of blood into the empty syringe. Inject this blood back into the catheter lumen.
- Repeat this aspiration and injection process for a total of five times.
- Disconnect the empty syringe. Attach a new empty syringe or a vacuum tube holder and draw the blood sample. Do not draw a sample to be discarded.
- Attach a saline-filled syringe and flush the lumen. Lock the lumen with the appropriate locking solution or restart continuous infusions as appropriate.
- If using a syringe, transfer to the vacuum tubes using a needleless transfer device. Label all filled tubes in the presence of the patient and send to the lab.

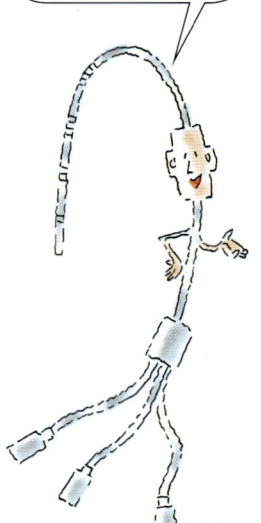

Protect me from tears by using a nonserrated clamp.

Special care

Besides performing routine care measures during infusions, be prepared to:
- prevent or handle common problems that may arise during infusion, such as a damaged or kinked catheter, fluid leaks, and clot formation at the catheter's tip
- tailor your interventions to meet the special infusion requirements of pediatric, elderly, and home therapy patients
- manage potential traumatic complications, such as pneumothorax, and systemic complications such as bloodstream infection. (See *Managing common problems in central I.V. therapy*, page 161.)

Common infusion problems

During infusions, problems arising from the catheter may call for special care measures.

Catheter breakdown

A serrated hemostat will eventually break down the catheter producing a tear, causing blood to back up and fluid to leak from the device. If air enters the catheter through the tear, an air embolism could result. Prevent catheter tears by using nonserrated clamps. If the catheter or part of the catheter breaks, cracks, or becomes nonfunctional, contact the LIP to discuss the patient needs, which could include changing to another route for completion of the therapy, replacing the entire catheter with a new one, or repairing the existing catheter if a brand-specific repair kit is available.

Working out the kinks

The catheter can become kinked or pinched either internally or externally. Internal kinks are detected by X-ray and are usually located between the clavicle and the first rib, known as pinch-off syndrome. This problem only occurs with subclavian insertion sites and indicates the need for catheter replacement. For a PICC, aberrant venous anatomy may cause kinking in the veins of the arm, requiring an extremity X-ray to locate it.

You may be able to prevent external catheter kinks by positioning and securing the catheter properly with an ESD. Additional securement may be needed for the attached extension set. Loop this set to the side and secure with a piece of tape or a secondary type of securement device. If the catheter is pulled, this secured set would receive the force rather than the catheter at the insertion site.

Occlusions

If you have difficulty withdrawing blood or infusing fluid, there are several causes of lumen occlusion including intraluminal fibrin/thrombus, a fibrin sheath or thrombosis at the tip of the catheter, intraluminal drug precipitate, or other mechanical causes. To evaluate the cause, assess the recent history of how the catheter has performed. Was there a gradual loss of blood return or slowed flow rate over an extended period? Did the signs appear quickly? What fluids and medications have recently been infused through the catheter? Was the correct flushing procedures performed before and after each infusion?

Thrombotic occlusion is one of the most common causes of lack of blood return and/or difficulty infusing fluid. Fibrin can accumulate as the body's natural defense against the foreign object — the catheter. It may appear inside the lumen, or as a sheath around the exterior wall of the catheter, or directly surrounding the catheter tip. This type of sheath impedes the flow of blood and provides a protein-rich environment for bacterial growth. Occasionally, this sheath forms so that fluids infuse easily, but acts as a one-way valve, making blood aspiration difficult or impossible.

Instilling a thrombolytic agent will remove the intraluminal fibrin and the portion of the extraluminal fibrin sheath or thrombosis located at the tip. The agent may be instilled by a clinician who has documented competency in the procedure. This procedure can be performed on all CVADs but is more common on long-term CVADs in patients with difficult venous access or when the CVAD is costly to replace.

Changes in drug pH due to contact between incompatible medications may lead to precipitate formation that causes lumen occlusion. When the precipitated drug is acidic, hydrochloric acid is instilled to reverse the precipitate; for precipitate from alkaline drugs, sodium bicarbonate or sodium hydroxide is used.

Attempting to salvage a CVAD isn't always appropriate or possible. Collaborate with the LIP and infusion/vascular access specialist in your facility about the best action to take.

Managing a CVAD occlusion

If clotting threatens to occlude a CVAD, making flushing and infusions sluggish, a thrombolytic agent is used to clear the catheter. Gather the necessary equipment, including:
- clean gloves
- 20-G or 22-G noncoring needle with an extension set for an implanted port
- syringe filled with a thrombolytic agent
- empty 10-mL syringe
- two 10-mL syringes filled with saline solution
- syringe filled with appropriate locking solution as prescribed.

Clear the way

Follow these steps to clear the catheter:
1. Perform hand hygiene. Don clean gloves.
2. Assess CVAD patency by attempting a gentle flushing technique and aspiration for a blood return. For an implanted port, the existing noncoring port needle may need to be removed and a new one inserted to rule out the needle position as the cause. (See *Access the implanted port* on page 179.)
3. While pulling backward on the syringe plunger, close the clamp on the extension tubing. This removes as much intraluminal fluid as possible and creates a vacuum inside the lumen.
4. Detach the empty syringe. Attach the syringe containing the thrombolytic agent and unclamp the extension tubing.
5. The thrombolytic agent will be pulled into the lumen when the clamp is released. To fully instill the entire quantity of the agent, use a gentle pull-push motion on the syringe plunger to allow the agent to reach the thrombus inside the CVAD lumen.
6. Clamp the extension set, and leave the solution in place for 30 minutes or according to your policy.
7. Then, attach an empty 10-mL syringe, unclamp the extension set, and aspirate the thrombolytic and other lumen contents with the 10-mL syringe. Discard this syringe.
8. If a blood return can't be aspirated, a second instillation may be required with a wait time of 120 minutes. Follow your facility policy and procedure.
9. After the occlusion is cleared and blood can be aspirated, flush the catheter with 10 to 20 mL of saline solution. Follow with the prescribed locking solution or restart prescribed fluids for continuous infusion.

(Text continues on page 162.)

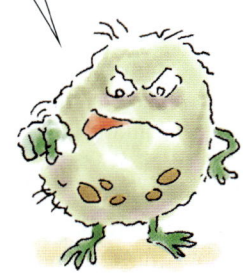

A sheath at the catheter tip provides a protein-rich environment for bacterial growth.

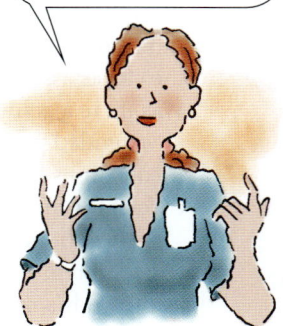

If clotting threatens to occlude a CVAD, a thrombolytic agent may be used to clear the catheter.

Maintaining central venous infusions 161

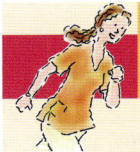

Running smoothly

Managing common problems with CVADs

Maintaining a CVAD requires being prepared to handle potential problems. This chart tells you how to recognize and manage some common problems.

Problem	Possible causes	Nursing interventions
Fluid won't infuse.	• Closed clamp • Displaced or kinked catheter • Vein thrombus/fibrin sheath • Catheter lumen occlusion	• Check the infusion system and clamps. • Change the patient's position. • Have the patient cough or breathe deeply. • Remove the dressing and examine the external portion of the catheter. • Try to aspirate blood. • Try a gentle flush with saline solution. • If an internal occlusion is apparent, notify the LIP. A catheter clearance procedure with a thrombolytic agent and/or a chest X-ray may be ordered, depending on the recent history of the CVAD performance.
Unable to obtain a blood return *Patency must be assessed prior to each use of CVAD.*	• Closed clamp • Displaced or kinked catheter • Thrombus or fibrin sheath • Catheter movement against vessel wall • Catheter tip has eroded through the vein wall. • Catheter tip has migrated into a smaller vein.	• Check the infusion system and clamps. • Change the patient's position • Have the patient cough or breathe deeply • Remove the dressing and examine the external portion of the catheter. • If an internal occlusion is apparent, notify the LIP. A catheter clearance procedure with a thrombolytic agent and/or a chest X-ray may be ordered.
Fluid leaking at the site	• Displaced or malpositioned catheter • Tear in catheter • Complete fibrin sheath • Thrombus	• Check the patient for signs of distress (e.g., respiratory, chest discomfort). • Change the dressing and observe the condition of the insertion site. • Notify the LIP. • Obtain an X-ray order to check catheter tip placement. Contrast agent injection under fluoroscopy may be indicated.
Administration set or needleless connector disconnected from catheter	Lack of secure luer-locked connection	• Immediately close catheter clamp, if available, or tightly fold and tape the catheter to temporarily occlude the lumen. • Place a sterile syringe on the catheter hub. • Don't reconnect the contaminated set or needleless connector. Obtain a new needleless connector, extension set, or complete administration set, as needed.

(continued)

Managing common problems with CVADs *(continued)*

Problem	Possible causes	Nursing interventions
		• Disinfect the catheter hub using a swab pad with 70% alcohol or alcoholic chlorhexidine. Don't soak the hub. Allow the solution to dry completely before connecting a new set. • Connect new administration or needleless connector to the hub. • Restart the infusion at the prescribed rate. • Notify the LIP of the incident to determine if CVAD removal is required.

Patients with special needs

There are a few additional considerations involved in caring for pediatric, elderly, and home therapy patients.

Across the generation gap

Essentially the same access devices are used in both pediatric and elderly patients. However, four possible differences include:
- catheter length
- lumen size
- insertion sites
- amount of fluid infused.

For more information about infants and children, see *Chapter 9, Pediatric I.V. Therapy*. For more information about elderly patients, see *Chapter 10, Geriatric I.V. Therapy*.

Homework

Long-term CVADs allow patients to receive fluids, medications, and blood infusions at home. These catheters are designed to have a longer life. They are less prone to infection due to organisms from the skin but require careful attention to hub maintenance to prevent organisms from entering through the lumen.

The care procedures used in the home are the same as those used in the hospital, including aseptic technique. A candidate for home I.V. therapy must have:
- a family member or friend who can assist in safe and competent administration of I.V. fluids
- a suitable home environment
- a telephone
- transportation
- the ability to prepare, handle, store, and dispose of medication and equipment.

Patient teaching may begin before the patient's discharged from the hospital, but that is not always possible. Sometimes, a patient may

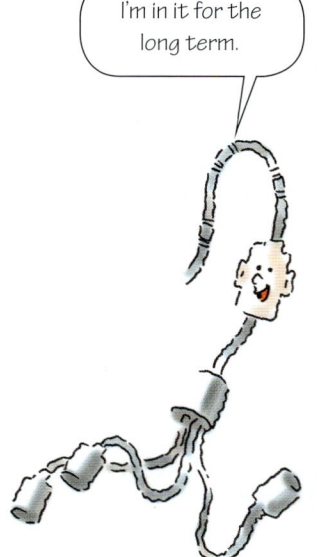

I'm in it for the long term.

start home infusion without being hospitalized first. Nurses from the home care company provide educational materials, demonstration, and return demonstration until the patient or family caregiver is able to perform infusion independently. CVAD dressing changes may be done by the patient, caregiver, or the home care nurse. This decision is based on the location of the insertion site, the patient/caregiver's ability to learn, and their manual dexterity to perform the procedure.

Traumatic and systemic complications

Complications can occur at any time during dwell time of a CVAD. Traumatic complications, such as pneumothorax, occurs on insertion but may not be noticed until after the procedure is completed. Systemic complications such as bloodstream infection typically occur later in therapy. (See *Complications of IV therapy via the central venous system*, pages 164–167)

Traumatic topic: pneumothorax

Pneumothorax, or air entering the space between the lungs and chest wall when the lung collapses, is the most common traumatic complication of catheter insertion. It is associated with the insertion of a CVAD into the subclavian or internal jugular vein. A bedside ultrasound of the chest is an excellent way to diagnose this problem but is not performed routinely after all subclavian or jugular CVAD insertions. It may or may not be discovered on the postprocedure chest X-ray; therefore, the patient must be closely monitored for signs and symptoms for several hours after the procedure.

Pneumothorax may be minimal and may not require intervention (unless the patient is on positive-pressure ventilation). For a small pneumothorax, close observation may be the chosen management. For larger pneumothoraces or those producing acute distress, a thoracotomy is performed and a chest tube inserted. Signs and symptoms include:
- chest pain
- dyspnea
- cyanosis
- decreased or absent breath sounds on the affected side.

Sneaky signs and symptoms

Initially, the patient may be asymptomatic; signs of distress gradually show up as pneumothorax gets larger. For this reason, you need to monitor the patient closely and auscultate for breath sounds for at least 3 hours after catheter insertion.

If unchecked, pneumothorax may progress to tension pneumothorax, a medical emergency. The patient exhibits such signs as:
- acute respiratory distress
- asymmetrical chest wall movement
- possibly, a tracheal shift away from the affected side.

(Text continues on page 167)

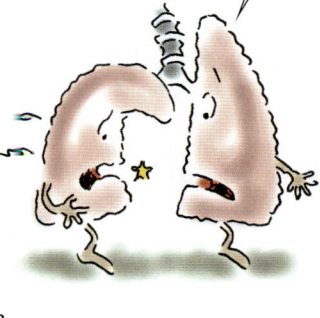

Yikes! Insertion of a catheter into subclavian or internal jugular veins may cause pneumothorax.

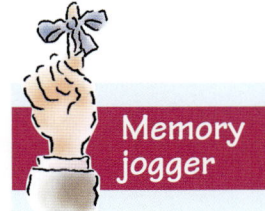

Memory jogger

Use the mnemonic

ACT to remember the signs and symptoms of tension pneumothorax so that you can "act" fast to protect your patient:

Acute respiratory distress

Chest wall motion that's asymmetrical

Tracheal shifting.

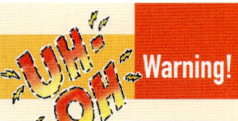

Warning!

Complications of IV therapy via the central venous system

As with any invasive procedure, CVAD insertion and I.V. therapy poses risks, including pneumothorax, air embolism, thrombosis, and infection. This chart outlines how to recognize, manage, and prevent these complications. The Infusion Therapy Standards of Practice calls for each organization to have established policies and procedures for prevention and management of CVAD complications.

Signs and symptoms	Possible causes	Nursing interventions	Prevention
Pneumothorax, hemothorax, chylothorax, or hydrothorax			
• Chest pain • Dyspnea • Cyanosis • Decreased breath sounds on affected side • Decreased hemoglobin because of blood pooling (occurs with hemothorax) • Abnormal chest X-ray	• Lung puncture by catheter during insertion or exchange over a guide wire • Large blood vessel puncture with bleeding inside or outside lung • Lymph node puncture with lymph fluid leakage • Infusion of solution into the chest area through a catheter that has perforated the vein wall	• Stop the infusion and notify the LIP. • Remove the catheter or assist with its removal. • Administer oxygen as ordered. • Set up and assist with chest tube insertion. • Document interventions.	• Position the patient's head down with a towel roll between scapulae to distend and expose the internal jugular or subclavian vein as much as possible during catheter insertion. • Assess for early signs of fluid infiltration, such as swelling in the shoulder, neck, chest, and arm area. • Ensure immobilization with adequate patient preparation and restraint during the procedure; patients unable to cooperate may need to be sedated or taken to the operating room for catheter insertion. • Confirm CVAD position by ECG tip locating device or X-ray.
Air embolism			
• Respiratory distress, tachypnea, coughing • Chest pain • Tachyarrhythmias • Altered speech • Decreased blood pressure • Change in or loss of consciousness	• Intake of air into central venous system that may move through the heart into the lungs. Air may bypass lungs by passing through a patent atrial septal defect and into the arterial circulation or move retrograde into the brain	• Immediately clamp or tightly fold and tape the catheter to prevent more air from entering. • Cover the catheter exit site with an air-occlusive dressing if catheter has been inadvertently removed.	• During insertion and removal, teach the patient to perform Valsalva's maneuver at the appropriate time (bear down or strain and hold breath to increase CVP) unless contraindicated (cardiac dysfunction, recent MI, glaucoma).

Complications of IV therapy via the central venous system *(continued)*

Signs and symptoms	Possible causes	Nursing interventions	Prevention
	• Occurs during subclavian and jugular CVAD insertion and removal • For all CVAD insertion sites, can occur during changes of administration set or needleless connector; inadvertent opening, removal, cutting, or breaking of catheter	• Turn the patient on his left side, Trendelenburg, so that air remains in the right atrium, preventing it from entering the pulmonary artery. • Don't have the patient perform Valsalva's maneuver. (Large intake of air worsens the situation.) • Administer 100% oxygen. • Notify the code team in hospital or EMS if at home or other facility and LIP. • Document interventions.	• Purge all air from the administration set before connection. • Instruct the patient/family not to disconnect or reconnect any I.V. sets without proper instruction for managing their CVAD in the home. • Use ONLY luer-locking connections on all junctions of the CVAD and administration system. • Clamp CVAD prior to changing the set/connector. • Do not leave unprimed administration sets connected to solution container. • Apply sterile dressing with petroleum-based ointment for 24 hours after removal of all CVADs. • Patient should lie flat or at least reclining for 30 minutes postremoval
Thrombosis			
• Edema in the ipsilateral extremity, shoulder, neck, or chest • Pain in the extremity, shoulder, neck, or chest • Erythema in the extremity • Engorged peripheral veins on the extremity, shoulder, neck, or chest	• Sluggish blood flow rate related to a large catheter placed in a small vein • Suboptimal CVAD tip location • Known genetic coagulopathies (factor V Leiden) • Chronic diseases associated with hypercoagulable state such as cancer, diabetes, or end-stage renal failure • Pregnancy or oral contraceptives • Surgical and trauma patients	• Notify the LIP and anticipate order for diagnostic studies and for anticoagulant therapy if diagnosis confirmed. • Measure arm circumference prior to PICC insertion and when clinically indicated (presence of edema). • Do not remove a CVAD with confirmed thrombosis if the catheter tip is in the appropriate position, functioning with blood return, and no evidence of infection.	• Assist with measuring the internal diameter of vein using ultrasound before insertion. (The catheter should occupy no more than 45% of the vein.) • PICCs are associated with higher rates of DVT than other CVADs; carefully consider PICC in patients at high risk of DVT. • Verify that the catheter tip is in lower segment of superior vena cava near the cavoatrial junction before using the catheter.

(continued)

Complications of IV therapy via the central venous system (continued)

Signs and symptoms	Possible causes	Nursing interventions	Prevention
	• History of multiple CVADs especially with a difficult or traumatic insertion and other devices such as pacemakers • Age extremes • Critical care patients	• Be aware that pulmonary emboli and postthrombotic syndrome are associated with upper extremity vein thrombosis. • Anticipate anticoagulant therapy while CVAD remains in place and for at least 3 months after CVAD is removed. • Document interventions.	• Encourage patient to mobilize ipsilateral extremity early, normal activities of daily living, adequate hydration, and gentle range of motion.
Local infection			
• Redness, warmth, tenderness, and swelling at insertion or exit site, subcutaneous tunnel, or port pocket • Possible exudate of purulent material • Local rash or pustules • Fever, chills, malaise	• Lack of adequate hand hygiene before insertion or maintenance procedures • Lack of appropriate skin antiseptic use • Failure to maintain aseptic technique during catheter insertion or dressing changes • Failure to comply with dressing change protocol • Wet or soiled dressing remaining on site • Immunosuppression • Irritated suture sites	• Adequate hand hygiene before all procedures involving a CVAD • Monitor vital signs as needed. • Assess CVAD site through intact dressing at least once daily by visual inspection and gentle palpation. • Perform appropriate stabilization and dressing change procedures. • Treat systemically with antibiotics or antifungal drugs, depending on the culture results and LIP orders. • Anticipate and assist with catheter removal, if necessary. • Document interventions.	• Select the site for CVAD best suited to prevent local infection (subclavian, PICC). • Maintain strict aseptic technique. Use gloves, masks, and gowns when appropriate. • Adhere to dressing change protocols. • Teach the patient about restrictions (bathing, swimming), if applicable. • Use appropriate site protection devices to keep the dressing dry during bathing, etc. • Change a wet or soiled dressing immediately.
Systemic bloodstream infection			
• Fever, chills without other apparent reason • Leukocytosis • Nausea, vomiting • Malaise • Hypotension if infection is severe	• Contaminated catheter or infusate • Failure to maintain aseptic technique during set change or upon accessing the catheter • Frequent opening of catheter • Immunosuppression	• Draw central and peripheral blood cultures as ordered. • Anticipate leaving a long-term CVAD in place with an uncomplicated CRBSI, and certain types of microorganisms. Administer systemic antibiotics and/or antibiotic lock solutions as prescribed.	• Examine infusate for cloudiness and turbidity before infusing. • Check the fluid container for leaks. • Do not disconnect a continuous administration set from the catheter hub unless it is time to change the set.

Complications of IV therapy via the central venous system *(continued)*

Signs and symptoms	Possible causes	Nursing interventions	Prevention
	• CVAD site (femoral and IJ sites pose a greater risk than subclavian site)	• Culture the tip of the catheter upon removal only if CRBSI is suspected and ordered by the LIP. • Expect CVAD removal when CRBSI is present and associated with severe sepsis, suppurative thrombophlebitis, and endocarditis and CRBSI continues after 72 hours of antimicrobial treatment. • Assess for other sources of infection. • Monitor vital signs closely. • Document interventions.	• Thoroughly disinfect all connection surfaces by vigorous scrubbing before each entry into the system. • Only use a sterile device to enter the CVAD; maintain all administration sets with adequate sterile covers when not in use. • Use strict aseptic technique for connection and disconnection of fluid containers and administration sets. • Teach the patient infection prevention techniques for home care.

Let's talk puncture at this juncture

The second most common life-threatening complication is arterial puncture. Arterial puncture may lead to hemothorax and internal bleeding, which may not be detected immediately. A hemothorax is treated like pneumothorax, except that the chest tube is inserted lower in the chest to help evacuate the blood.

Left untreated, internal bleeding caused by arterial puncture leads to hypovolemic shock. Signs and symptoms include:
- increased heart rate
- decreased blood pressure
- cool, clammy skin
- obvious swelling in the neck or chest
- mental confusion (especially if the common carotid arteries are involved)
- formation of a hematoma (a large, blood-filled sac), which causes pressure on the trachea and adjacent vessels.

Arterial bleeding may be prevented by the tamponade action of the presence of the CVAD. Before CVAD removal, diagnostic tests are needed to determine the safest method for removal.

Rare but risky

There are a few additional, but rare, complications of CVADs:
- Tracheal puncture is associated with insertion of a catheter into the subclavian vein.
- Development of a fistula between the brachiocephalic vein and the subclavian artery may result from perforation by the guide wire on insertion into the vessel.
- Chylothorax results when a thoracic duct is punctured and lymph fluid leaks into the pleural cavity.
- Hydrothorax (or infusion of solution into the chest), thrombosis, and local infection are also potential complications of CV therapy.

Sepsis is systemic and serious

Sepsis is severe organ dysfunction caused by the inability of the patient's immune system to respond to infection. Without early recognition and treatment, it may progress to septic shock and death. CVADs can be the source of microorganisms leading to sepsis. It might be possible to treat a patient with a bloodstream infection from a tunneled cuffed catheter or implanted port, however the presence of sepsis means that the CVAD should be removed immediately after a new vascular access device has been inserted. Aggressive treatment will require rapid fluid infusion and many types of IV medication including antibiotics, coritcosteroids, and vasopressors and a new CVAD may be necessary.

The most common organisms causing septic shock are gram-negative and gram positive bacteria along with Candida species. When sepsis occurs in a hospitalized patient, the most common organism is methicillin-resistant Staphylococcus aureus (MRSA) and vancomycin-resistant Enterococci. Be prepared to draw blood cultures from a peripheral vein and the infected CVAD as prescribed. Strict attention to aseptic technique when performing all care and maintenance of any VAD is necessary, but patients with a compromised immune system from other diseases such as cancer are at the greatest risk.

PICC-specific complications

PICCs have a risk for catheter-related bloodstream infection (CRBSI) and venous thrombosis, especially in critical care patients. Phlebitis of the veins in the arm may also develop with PICC insertion.

Phlebitis — mechanical, bacterial, or chemical?

Phlebitis is painful inflammation of a vein and possibly erythema, warmth, swelling, induration, purulence, or palpable venous cord. It may occur after PICC insertion and can be mechanical, bacterial, or chemical in nature.

Mechanical phlebitis occurs when the vein wall is irritated. This can happen if the PICC is too large for the vein, with rapid or forceful insertion techniques, and with excessive movement of the PICC due to inadequate stabilization. If the patient develops mechanical phlebitis, apply warm, moist compresses to the upper arm, elevate the extremity, and restrict activity to mild exercise. If the phlebitis continues or worsens within 24 hours of starting treatment, remove the catheter, as ordered. Avoid this type of phlebitis by using the smallest catheter possible for therapy, securing with an ESD, and avoiding insertion at the antecubital fossa.

Bacterial phlebitis can occur with CVADs; however, it is more common with peripheral I.V. devices. If drainage occurs at the insertion site and the patient's temperature increases, notify the practitioner. The catheter may need to be removed.

Chemical phlebitis is associated with vein wall irritation from the prescribed medication. It is usually associated with the dilution and/or infusion techniques especially in peripheral veins. Since the tip location for a PICC is in the SVC, this type of phlebitis is unlikely; however, it could occur if the skin antiseptic solution is not allowed to dry completely before catheter insertion and is pulled into the vein. Allow skin to dry completely.

Deeds for those who bleed

Bleeding from the PICC insertion site may occur. Bleeding that persists needs additional evaluation. If pressure or other methods do not stop bleeding, a hemostatic agent should be considered. If there is no further bleeding, the dressing can be changed and a new transparent dressing applied.

Tame the pain

Some patients complain of pain at the PICC insertion site, usually because the insertion was traumatic. Unresolved pain after sufficient treatment should be removed. Pain may be treated by:
- applying warm compresses
- elevating the limb
- giving analgesics
- giving nonsteroidal anti-inflammatory medications.

Be sure to document treatment and phlebitis score using your facility's phlebitis scale.

Spared of air (embolisms)?

Air embolism with PICCs is less common than in traditional CVADs because the line is inserted below the level of the heart, but it can happen, especially upon removal, if the catheter has been in place for a long period. A skin tract can develop, from the skin through the subcutaneous tissue into the vein. The patient should be lying flat for removal, and the site covered with an occlusive dressing, created by adding a petroleum-based ointment to a gauze dressing and covering with tape or a transparent membrane dressing.

Malposition disposition

Intravascular malposition or tip migration of any CVAD can occur at any time, especially with coughing, vomiting, heavy lifting (home care patients), increased intrathoracic pressure, and the presence of congestive heart failure. If the patient complains of hearing a flushing sound in the ear when the CVAD is used, notify the LIP and expect an order for a chest X-ray to check position of CVAD and tip location. A PICC is particularly prone to malposition; due to its smaller size, it is usually more pliable than other CVADs.

Discontinuing central venous therapy

You or the LIP may remove the catheter, depending on your state's nurse practice act, your facility's policy, your documented competency, and the type of catheter. Tunneled cuffed catheters and implanted devices are removed by the LIP. However, PICCs and nontunneled CVAD may be removed by a nurse with documented competency.

Discontinue continuous, implement intermittent

You may receive an order to discontinue continuous infusion therapy and begin intermittent infusion therapy. If so, follow the same procedure used for peripheral I.V. therapy. (See Chapter 2, *Peripheral I.V. therapy*.)

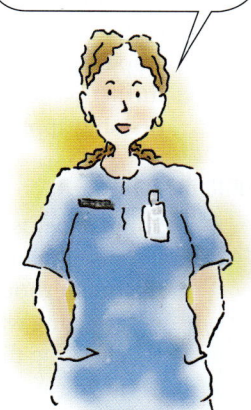

Remember: VADs, central or peripheral, are not removed based exclusively on the length of dwell time. There is no known optimum dwell time for any type of VAD.

Is the CVAD still needed?

The INS, CDC, and others recommend having a standardized procedure for determining if a CVAD is still needed, and if it is not, it should be removed for infection prevention purposes. Some institutions have a daily assessment form that is used in daily rounding to determine if a CVAD is still necessary. There are several questions that should be asked to determine whether a CVAD should be removed or retained, such as an unresolved complication, plan of care change where CVAD is deemed no longer necessary, or therapy is complete.

Removing the catheter

Begin catheter removal with a couple of precautions:
- First, check the patient's record or other documentation (such as the nurses' notes, LIP notes, or the written X-ray report) as directed by facility policy. An order must be written by the LIP for removal of a CVAD.

- Then, make sure that backup assistance is available if a complication, such as uncontrolled bleeding or venous air embolism, occurs during catheter removal.

Patient preparation

Before you remove the catheter, explain the procedure to the patient. Inform that the patient will need to turn the face away from the site and perform Valsalva's maneuver when the catheter is withdrawn, unless contraindicated, such as with cardiac dysfunction. If necessary, review the maneuver with him. Alternatively, remove catheter on exhalation or instruct patient to not breathe during removal of the last portion of CVAD removal.

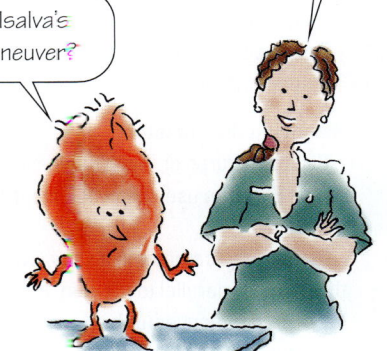

Remember…bearing down or straining while holding your breath? It's done to increase central venous pressure during catheter changes and withdrawal, whenever the catheter is open to air, to prevent air emboli.

Valsalva's maneuver?

Getting equipped

Before removing the catheter, gather the necessary equipment, including:
- sterile gauze
- clean gloves
- sterile gloves if catheter culture is to be obtained
- sterile scissors if catheter culture is to be obtained
- antimicrobial swab
- petroleum-based ointment
- alcohol swabs
- sterile transparent semipermeable dressing
- tape.

If you're sending the catheter tip for culture, you also need a sterile specimen container. Routine culture of catheter tip on removal is no longer indicated. If the CVAD is being removed due to a suspected bloodstream infection, culture of the extraluminal side of the catheter will not culture what is on the intraluminal side. Special techniques could be possible in the lab, but they must be informed of this need. (See *Removing a CV catheter*, page 172.)

Note this

After removing the catheter, be sure to document:
- patient tolerance
- condition of the catheter, including the length
- time of discontinuation of therapy
- cultures ordered and sent
- dressings applied
- other pertinent information.

Removing a CVAD

After assembling your equipment, follow the step-by-step guidelines listed below to safely remove a CVAD.

Getting ready
- Place the patient in a Trendelenburg position if possible to prevent emboli. If this is not possible, the patient should be lying flat in bed for removal of a CVAD inserted through the jugular or subclavian veins. For a PICC removal, the exit site should be at or below the level of the heart.
- Perform hand hygiene and put on clean gloves.
- Turn off all infusions.
- Remove the old dressing.
- Inspect the site for signs of drainage or inflammation.

Removing the catheter
- Clip the sutures or remove adhesive ESD. If a subcutaneous ESD is in use, follow the manufacturer directions for removal.
- Remove the catheter in a slow, even motion, keeping the catheter parallel to the skin. Have the patient perform Valsalva's maneuver (unless contraindicated) as the catheter is withdrawn to prevent air emboli.
- Apply pressure with a sterile gauze pad immediately after removing the catheter. Hold pressure until bleeding has stopped.
- Apply petroleum-based ointment to the insertion site to seal it.
- Place a transparent semipermeable dressing over the site. Label the dressing with the date and time of the removal and your initials.
- Inspect the catheter and measure the length to see if any pieces broke off during the removal. If so, notify the LIP immediately and monitor the patient closely for signs of distress.
- If a catheter tip culture is to be obtained, use sterile scissors to clip approximately 1" (2.5 cm) off the distal end of the catheter, letting it drop into the sterile specimen container. This may require an assistant, one to hold site pressure and one to prevent the catheter from coming into contact with anything until the tip is cut and dropped into the sterile container.
- Properly dispose of the I.V. set and equipment used.

Monitoring the patient
Bleeding may develop after removing the catheter but the greatest risk is air embolism. Remember that some vessels, such as the subclavian vein, aren't easily compressed. The occlusive dressing should remain in place for at least 24 hours. If the site is not healed, continue to change the dressing every 24 hours until it has healed.

Make a notation on the nursing care plan to recheck the patient and insertion site frequently for the next few hours. Check for signs of respiratory decompensation, possibly indicating air emboli, and for signs of bleeding, such as blood on the dressing, decreased blood pressure, increased heart rate, paleness, or diaphoresis.

Noteworthy
- Document the time and date of the catheter removal and any complications that occurred, such as catheter fracture, bleeding, or respiratory distress. Also, record the length of the catheter and signs of blood, drainage, redness, or swelling at the site.

Implanted port insertion and infusion

Positioned securely under the skin, an implanted port consists of a catheter attached to a titanium, stainless steel, or plastic reservoir covered by a self-sealing silicone rubber septum. Inserting an implanted port requires a minor surgical procedure. The device may be placed in the arm, chest, abdomen, or thigh. An unusual site could mean that the catheter goes to a site other than a vein, such as the epidural space or intraperitoneal space. Confirm venous location before using the implanted port.

When to tap a port

Usually, you'll use an implanted port to deliver intermittent infusions. For example, you may use one to deliver:
- antineoplastic medication
- antibiotics and all other I.V. medications
- I.V. fluids
- blood products.

On punctures and patients

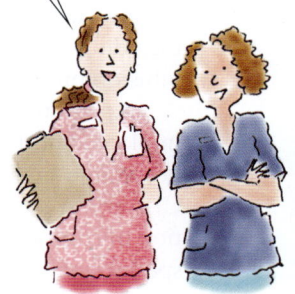

Do you know what an implanted port is? Sure do. It's a catheter attached to a reservoir covered by a self-sealing silicone rubber septum.

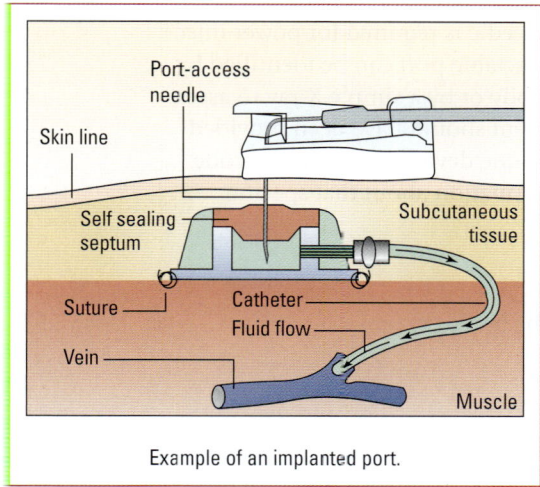

Example of an implanted port.

A regular-sized implanted port placed in the upper chest can typically tolerate approximately 2,000 punctures. A small port body, commonly used in the upper extremity, can tolerate approximately 750 punctures. The benefit of an implanted port is an easy central venous access only when required. Most implanted ports are accessed for a few hours or 3 to 5 days to receive a course of continuous I.V. medication. Implanted ports may also be used for intermittent infusion by flushing and locking after each infusion just like other CVADs. An implanted port may be preferred for some patients receiving cyclic parenteral nutrition for a few hours at night. The patient accesses their port, infuses, and removes the access needle daily allowing freedom from an external catheter during the daytime. Typically, the port access needle is changed every 7 days. Continuous or intermittent infusions over extended periods would mean that the implanted port is constantly accessed. This could increase the risk of needle dislodgment and bloodstream infection. When the infusion need is long-term and constant, an implanted port may not be the best choice.

Selecting the equipment

The selection of infusion equipment will depend partly on the type of implanted port selected and the insertion site. Generally, you'll use the same infusion equipment as with other central I.V. therapy, including an infusion solution, administration set, and an electronic infusion pump.

Depending on the patient's size and the type of therapy, an implanted port catheter with one or two lumens may be chosen. A power injectable port should be considered if the patient will need CT scans. A power injectable port needle is required for power injection of contrast agents. A power injectable port can be identified by special surface design of the port body or by a simple X-ray to assess for markings. Additionally, the patient should have been provided with a special card containing a unique device identification code. Use of this code can lead to all information about that specific implanted port.

Material matters

The implanted port reservoir may be made of:
- titanium
- stainless steel
- molded plastic.

The type of reservoir used depends on the patient's therapeutic needs. For example, a patient undergoing magnetic resonance imaging should have a device made of titanium or plastic, instead of stainless steel, to avoid distorting test results.

A close look at an implanted port

An implanted port is typically used to deliver intermittent infusions of medication, antineoplastic agents, and blood products. It offers several advantages over a CVAD with an external component. Because the device is completely covered by the patient's skin, the risk of extrinsic contamination is reduced. In addition, patients may prefer this type of CVAD because it doesn't alter the body image and requires less routine catheter care.

The implanted port consists of a catheter connected to a small reservoir. A septum designed to withstand multiple punctures seals the reservoir. To access the port, a special noncoring needle is inserted perpendicular to the reservoir.

Noncoring needles needed

To avoid damaging the port's silicone rubber septum, use only noncoring needles with an engineered safety mechanism. A noncoring needle has an angled or deflected point that slices the septum on entry rather than coring it as a conventional needle does. When the noncoring needle is removed, the septum reseals itself. (See *A close look at noncoring needles*, page 175.)

Noncoring needles have multiple designs. The needle has a right-angle configuration attached to wings or a round disc with a safety mechanism to house the needle upon removal. An extension set is preattached and may or may not have an additional injection port. Each configuration comes in various needle lengths (depending on the depth of septum implantation) and gauges (depending on the rate of infusion). (See *Choosing the right implanted port needle*.)

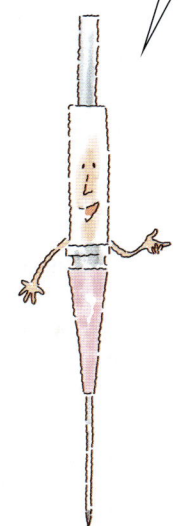

Implanted ports require special noncoring needles to access the device. Also, ensure that it has a safety mechanism to prevent accidental needlesticks on removal.

A close look at noncoring needles

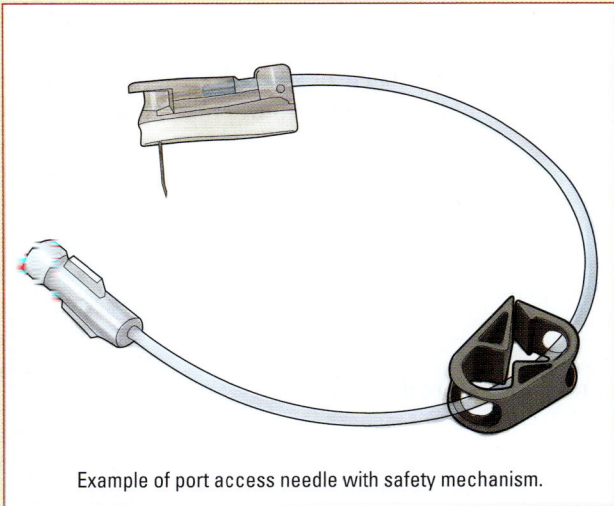

Example of port access needle with safety mechanism.

Unlike a conventional hypodermic needle, a noncoring needle has a deflected point, which slices the port's septum instead of coring it. Noncoring needles must contain a mechanism to safely trap the needle as it is removed from the port body.

Implanted port insertion

An LIP inserts the implanted port, usually using local anesthesia with conscious sedation. Occasionally, general anesthesia may be used.

It begins with an incision

Inserting the implanted port involves the following steps:
1. After vein identification with ultrasound, a small incision is made and the catheter is introduced and advanced into the superior vena cava through the subclavian or internal jugular vein. Fluoroscopy is used to verify placement of the catheter tip.
2. A subcutaneous pocket is surgically created over a bony prominence on the chest wall and the catheter is tunneled to the pocket.
3. The catheter is connected to the reservoir. A noncoring needle is inserted into the port, flushed, and aspirated to confirm patency.
4. The reservoir is sutured to the underlying fascia and the incision is closed with sutures. A dressing is applied.

The patient may return from the procedure with or without the port needle in place. The port may be used immediately or when the insertion site is healed, depending on the LIP instructions and when infusion therapy must begin.

Preparing the patient

Because implanted port insertion is a surgical procedure, teaching should cover preoperative and postoperative considerations.

Pre-op pointers

Use these pointers to guide your teaching before implanted port insertion:
- Make sure that the patient understands the procedure, its benefits, and what's expected of him or her after the insertion. Be prepared to supplement information provided by the LIP. You'll also need to allay the patient's fears and answer questions about movement restrictions, cosmetic concerns, and maintenance regimens. Clear explanations help ensure the patient's cooperation.
- Describe how the patient will be positioned during the procedure.

Obtaining consent

Most facilities require a signed informed consent form before an invasive procedure. Tell the patient he or she will be asked to sign a consent form and explain what it means.

Choosing the right implanted port needle

When choosing an implanted port needle, the size of the needle will be determined by the therapy being delivered:
- 20-G needles for most infusions including blood transfusion or withdrawal
- 22-G needles for flushing.

Remember that you should use only noncoring needles with an implanted port.

Right angle versus straight
A right-angle noncoring safety needle is most commonly used; rarely, a longer needle, such as a straight 2" noncoring needle, is needed to access a deeply implanted port.

Orient the angled needle bevel away from the point where the catheter is attached to the port body. With this position, flushing creates more turbulence and is more likely to remove serum proteins and drug particles from the reservoir.

The LIP performing the procedure obtains consent; occasionally, you may witness the patient's signature. Before the patient signs, make sure that he or she understands the procedure, the purpose of the implanted port, the risk and benefits of the procedure, and any alternative methods other than an implanted port. If not, delay signing until you and/or the LIP clarifies the procedure and the patient demonstrates understanding.

Post-op pointers

Discuss the following postoperative care topics:
- Remind the patient that, after the device is in place, he or she will have to keep scheduled appointments to have the port accessed and flushed. Another option is to teach the patient or a family member how to do this procedure; however, a thorough patency assessment by a professional is needed periodically.
- Tell the patient to report signs and symptoms of systemic infection (fever, malaise, and flulike symptoms) and local infection (redness, tenderness, and drainage at the port or tunnel track site).
- Tell the patient to inform his or her dentist that he or she has an implanted device in case prophylactic oral antibiotics are needed.
- Tell the patient to carry the identification card containing the unique identification number. This will allow subsequent health care professionals to obtain specific information about the patient's particular port.
- Teach the importance of stability of the noncoring port needle and the importance of a blood return from an implanted port.
- Teach the patient to recognize and report signs and symptoms of infiltration, such as pain or swelling at the site, and the importance of stopping the infusion immediately. Stress the need for immediate intervention to reduce damaging the tissue surrounding the port, especially if the patient is receiving vesicant medications.

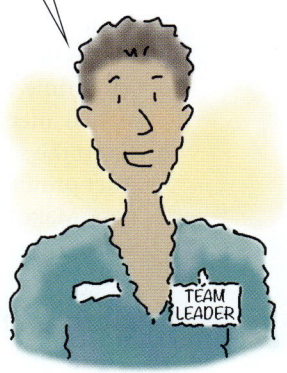

Make sure that the patient understands what's expected of him or her after insertion.

Monitoring the patient

After the implanted port is inserted, observe the patient for several hours. The device can be used immediately after placement. However, swelling and tenderness may persist for about 72 hours, making the device initially difficult to palpate and uncomfortable for the patient.

Site lines

The incision requires routine postoperative care for 7 to 10 days. Assess the insertion site for signs of:
- infection
- bleeding
- redness
- device rotation or port housing movement
- skin irritation.

Implanted port infusion

To administer an infusion using an implanted port, you'll need to set up the equipment and prepare the site.

Preparing the equipment

To set up infusion equipment, follow these steps:
1. Attach the administration set to the solution container and prime with fluid if a continuous infusion is to be started after accessing the implanted port.
2. Insert the set into an electronic infusion pump.
3. After priming, recheck all the connections for tightness. Make sure that all open ends are covered with sealed caps.

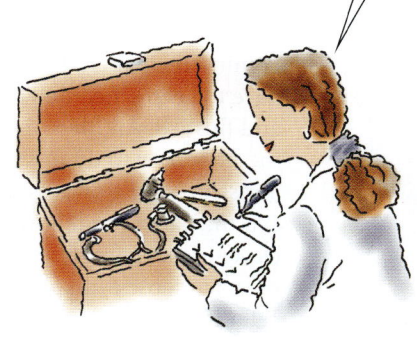

If your facility doesn't have an implantable port access kit, you'll need to gather the necessary equipment.

Preparing the site

To prepare the needle insertion site, obtain an implantable port access kit, if your facility uses them. If a kit isn't available, gather the necessary equipment, including:
- sterile gloves
- alcoholic chlorhexidine skin antiseptic (preferred)
- sterile gauze pads
- transparent dressing
- tape
- mask
- sterile drape
- noncoring needle with extension set and clamp
- foam pad (may be packaged with noncoring needle) or small sterile gauze
- needleless connector for intermittent access or primed administration set and solution container for continuous infusion
- sterile packaged prefilled syringe, 10 mL size with preservative-free normal saline; if not available, an empty sterile 10-mL syringe and a single-dose vial of preservative-free normal saline and vial adapter
- local anesthetic or ice pack according to facility policy and procedure.

Clear the field

When you're ready to prepare the access site, take the following precautions:
- Establish a sterile field for the sterile supplies, and inspect the area around the port for signs of infection or skin breakdown.

- An ice pack may be placed over the area for several minutes to numb the site. You may also apply a local anesthetic cream over the injection port, and cover it with a transparent dressing for the required time. Be sure to remove this cream completely before putting on sterile gloves and preparing the access site. Intradermal anesthetic injection may also be used. Assess for allergies to these agents. Follow facility policy and procedure.

Wash up and get started

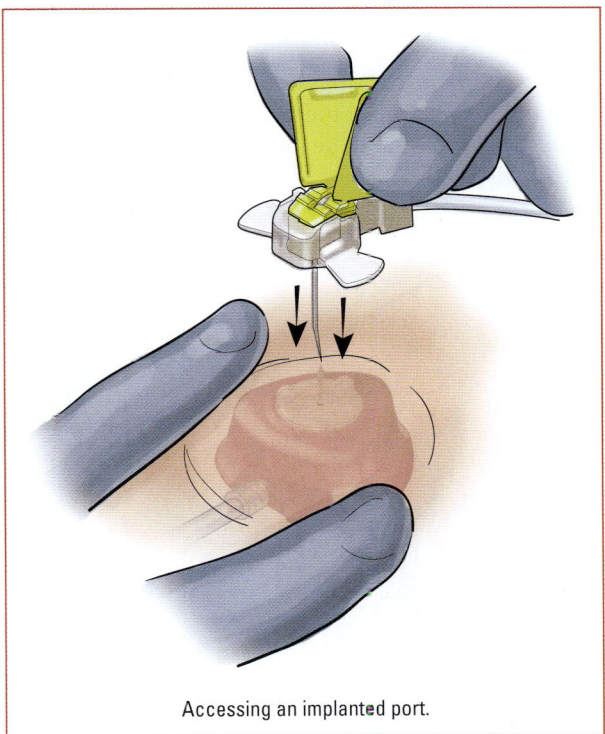

Accessing an implanted port.

To prepare the access site, follow these steps:
1. Don mask.
2. Perform hand hygiene and put on sterile gloves.
3. Attach needleless connector to the extension set of the noncoring needle. Prepare the noncoring needle by attaching the sterile syringe to the extension set and flushing to remove all air. If using a vial and sterile syringe, don one glove to hold the sterile syringe and use the ungloved hand to hold the vial, transferring the saline to the syringe. Place the syringe on the sterile field. Don the second glove.

4. Clean the area with alcoholic chlorhexidine swab using a back-and-forth scrubbing motion for at least 30 seconds. Allow the chlorhexidine to dry completely.
5. Using your nondominant hand with a sterile glove, palpate the implanted port body to locate the center. Stabilize the port body.
6. Push the noncoring needle through the skin and into the center of the port body until you detect the back of the port.
7. Slowly flush the saline into the port, assessing for resistance. Aspirate for a blood return, and complete the saline flush. If resistance is felt and/or there is no blood return, stop the procedure and evaluate the cause.
8. Use the foam pad or sterile gauze to support the wings of the needle if needed. If the wings do not lie flat against the skin, this support is needed for added stability of the wings. The junction of the needle and skin should remain visible.

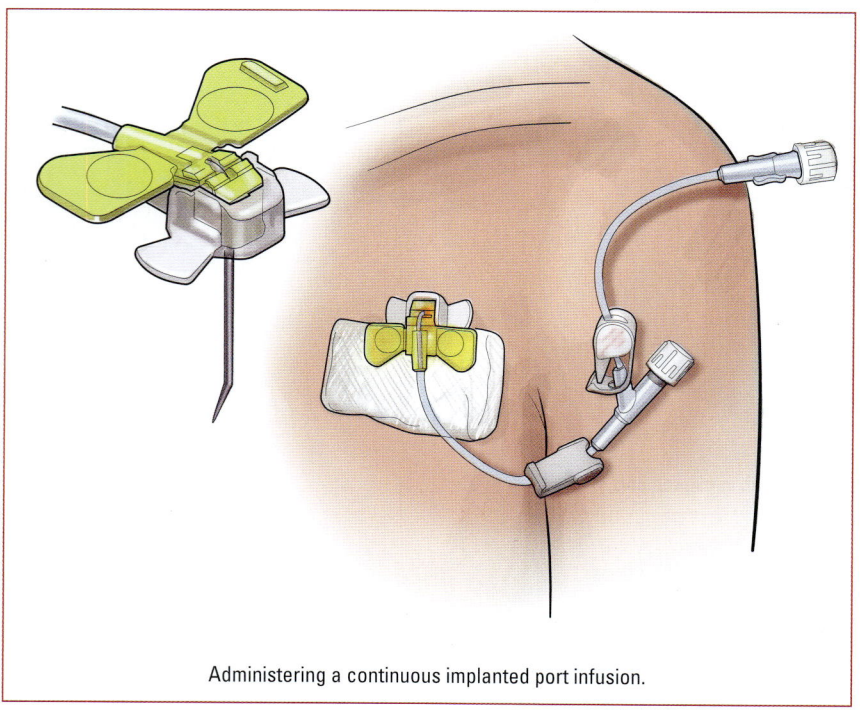

Administering a continuous implanted port infusion.

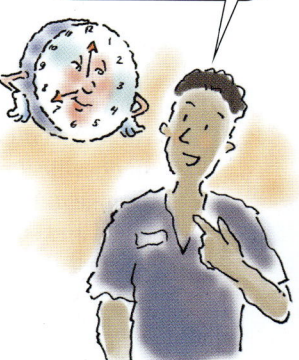

If using transdermal analgesia, remember to apply it for the required length of time before the access procedure.

9. Use sterile tape to secure the needle and place a sterile transparent dressing over the area.
10. Instill locking solution or attach the administration set and begin the infusion.
11. Discard supplies.

Giving injections and infusions through an implanted port

After insertion of the noncoring needle, the implanted port is used like other CVADs for infusions and I.V. push medications. Assessing the catheter and needle patency is critical since neither the port body nor catheter is visible. Obtaining a blood return is extremely important. All CVADs may have no blood return because of a fibrin sheath around the catheter tip or mechanical problem. An implanted port may also have issues with how the port needle was inserted and secured. Inability to obtain a blood return is a sure sign of a problem and the implanted port should not be used until the problem is identified and corrected. The port needle may need to be removed and a new one inserted. Changing the patient's arm or shoulder position with a change in the blood return indicates a mechanical problem like pinch-off syndrome. Ask a more experienced colleague for her assessment. Contact the LIP for orders for more diagnostic tests if the problem continues.

Document the injection according to your facility's policy. Include the following information: the absence of resistance and the presence of a blood return, the type and amount of medication injected, the time of the injection, the appearance of the site, the patient's tolerance of the procedure, and any pertinent nursing interventions.

Maintaining implanted port infusions

To maintain infusion therapy with an implanted port, perform such care measures as:
- flushing the port with the appropriate locking solution if the implanted port is used intermittently
- assessing the site at established intervals, based on the type of fluids or medications being infused and the patient's ability to communicate pain or other problems
- changing the dressing per the facility's protocol or whenever the dressing's integrity is compromised
- managing common equipment problems and patient complications
- discontinuing therapy when ordered, or converting the implanted port to an intermittent system to keep the device patent until it's needed again.

Flushing and locking an implanted port

Follow these guidelines to determine when to flush an implanted port:
- If your patient is receiving a continuous or prolonged infusion, routine or periodic flushing is not necessary. Flushing with normal saline may be needed if fluid flow is interrupted or slowed, if the electronic infusion pump alarm indicates a problem, or if the patient complains of a problem.
- If your patient is receiving an intermittent infusion, flush the port before each infusion to assess patency and remove the previous lock solution. After each infusion, flush with normal saline at the same rate as the medication infusion. Follow with the appropriate locking solution, which could be normal saline, heparin lock solution, or a prescribed antimicrobial lock solution.
- When the port isn't being used, it should be accessed, flushed, and locked about once a month; however, longer periods are documented.

How to administer a continuous implanted port infusion

Follow the step-by-step instructions below to administer a continuous implanted port infusion safely and accurately.

Assemble, remove, flush, connect, and begin
- Assemble the equipment.
- Remove all the air from the extension set of the noncoring port needle by priming it with an attached syringe of saline solution.
- Flush the port system with saline solution. Clamp the extension set, and remove the syringe.
- Connect the administration set, and secure the connections, if necessary.
- Unclamp the extension set and begin the infusion.

Adjust and examine
- Place a gauze pad under the needle hub if it doesn't lie flush with the skin.
- To help prevent needle dislodgment, secure the needle to the skin with sterile tape or sterile surgical strips.
- Apply a transparent semipermeable dressing over the needle insertion site.
- Examine the site carefully for infiltration. If the patient complains of burning, stinging, or pain at the site, discontinue the infusion and intervene appropriately.

Write it down
Document the infusion according to your facility's policy, including the following information: the type, amount, rate, and time of infusion; the patient's tolerance of the procedure; the appearance of the site; and any pertinent nursing interventions.

Getting equipped

To flush the implanted port when it is not being used routinely, first gather the necessary equipment, including:
- 22-G noncoring needle with an extension set
- 10-mL syringe filled with sterile normal saline solution, prefilled, and 0.9% sterile normal saline syringes recommended for flushing all types of CVAD
- 10-mL syringe filled with 5 mL of heparin flush solution (100 units per mL).

Label each syringe carefully so you don't confuse them.

Ready, set, flush

Prepare the injection site, as described in the previous section. Then follow these steps:
1. Attach the 10-mL syringe of normal saline solution to the extension set of noncoring needle, applying gentle pressure to the plunger to expel all air from the set.
2. Palpate the area over the port to locate it, and then, access the port
3. Aspirate a blood return, and flush the port with normal saline solution to confirm patency. Then, flush with the prescribed locking solution (for example, heparin lock 10 units/mL or other antimicrobial lock solution).
4. While stabilizing the port with two fingers, withdraw the noncoring needle.

Obtaining blood samples

You can obtain blood samples from an implanted port with a syringe or directly into a vacuum tube using the discard or mixing method. (See *How to obtain a blood sample from CVAD*, page 157.)

Documenting implanted port infusions

Record your assessment findings and interventions according to your facility's policy. Include such information as:
- type, amount, rate, and duration of the infusion
- appearance of the site
- development of problems, as well as the steps taken to resolve them
- needle gauge and length and dressing changes for continuous infusions
- blood samples obtained, including the type and amount
- patient-teaching topics covered and the patient's response to the procedure.

Special precautions

Routine care measures are subject to a few glitches. Be prepared to handle common problems that may arise during an infusion with an implanted port. Problems may include the inability to:
- flush the port
- withdraw blood from the port
- palpate and access the port. (See *Managing common implanted port problems.*)

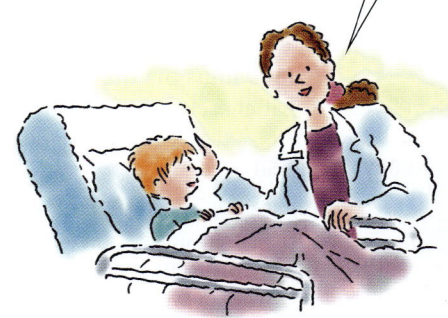

Usually, when a child undergoes implanted port insertion, general anesthesia is used.

A big exception for small patients

Generally, the procedures for implanting and maintaining an implanted port are the same for pediatric, elderly, and adult patients, with one big exception: For pediatric patients, general anesthesia may be used during insertion depending on the situation.

Homework

A home care patient requires thorough teaching about procedures and follow-up visits from a home care nurse to ensure compliance, safety, and successful treatment.

If the patient is to access the port him- or herself, explain that the most uncomfortable part of the procedure is inserting the needle into the skin. After the needle has penetrated the skin, the patient will feel some pressure but little pain. Eventually, the skin over the port may become less sensitive to frequent needle punctures.

All the way back

Stress the importance of pushing the needle into the port until the needle bevel touches the back of the port. Many patients tend to stop short of the back of the port, leaving the needle bevel in the rubber septum. This can cause blockage or slow the infusion rate.

Recognizing risks

A patient with an implanted port faces risks similar to those associated with a traditional CVAD, such as infection, thrombosis, and infiltration/extravasation. Teach the patient or caregiver how to recognize signs and symptoms of these complications. Make sure that they know how to intervene or how to reach the home health agency. (See *Complications of implanted port therapy*, page 185.)

(Text continues on page 187)

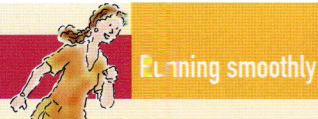

Running smoothly

Managing common implanted port problems

To maintain an implanted port, you must be able to handle common problems. This chart outlines problems you may encounter, their possible causes, and the appropriate nursing interventions needed.

Problem and possible causes	Nursing interventions
Inability to flush or withdraw blood	
Kinked tubing or closed clamp	• Check the tubing or clamp.
Incorrect needle placement or needle that won't advance through septum	• Push down on the noncoring needle in the septum and to verify needle position by aspirating for blood return. • Remove the needle and insert a new noncoring needle in a slightly different location of the septum.
Lack of blood return or resistance to flushing	• Change the position of the arm and shoulder and attempt to flush and aspirate. If this position change produced a blood return, notify the LIP about suspected pinch-off syndrome. Expect an order for a chest X-ray; inform radiology of the suspected problem so that the correct patient position is used in radiology. • If this position change did not produce a blood return, assess the history of port use. Determine if the mostly likely cause is a thrombotic occlusion or a drug precipitate. Notify the LIP with findings. Obtain an order for the appropriate clearance agent, for example, thrombolytic agent for thrombus occlusion. • NEVER forcibly flush the port.
Kinked catheter, catheter migration, or port rotation	• Notify the practitioner immediately. • Tell the patient to notify the practitioner if having difficulty using the port. • Obtain diagnostic studies to determine problem
Inability to palpate the port	
Deeply implanted port	• Note incision near port body. • Use deep palpation technique. • Ask another nurse to try locating the implanted port. • Use a longer noncoring needle to gain access to the implanted port.

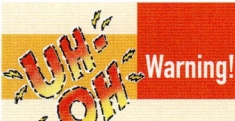

Warning!

Complications of implanted port therapy

This chart lists common complications of implanted port therapy as well as their signs and symptoms, causes, nursing interventions, and preventive measures.

Signs and symptoms	Possible causes	Nursing interventions	Prevention
Site infection			
• Erythema, swelling, and warmth at the port site • Oozing or purulent drainage at port site or pocket • Fever	• Infected incision or pocket • Poor postoperative healing	• Assess the site daily for redness; note any drainage. • Notify the LIP. • Administer antibiotics, as prescribed. • Apply topical treatment as ordered, for example, antibiotic cream and heat.	• Use strict aseptic technique for all port procedures. • Teach the patient to inspect for and report redness, swelling, drainage, or skin breakdown at the port site.
Extravasation			
• Burning sensation or edema in subcutaneous tissue • Absence of a blood return • Pain in neck, shoulder, or chest	• Needle dislodged into subcutaneous tissue • Needle incorrectly placed in port septum • Needle position not confirmed during administration of a vesicant medication; needle pulled out of septum • Damage to catheter between port body and vein entrance • Medial insertion site causing pinch-off syndrome and catheter fracture • Malpositioned catheter tip	• Don't remove the needle. • Stop the infusion. • Apply cold or warm compresses as indicated by the specific vesicant medication that has extravasated. • Notify the LIP with details of the infusing vesicant. • Prepare to administer the antidote according to facility policy and procedure and LIP orders. • Follow up with frequent site assessments	• Ensure correct needle placement before medication administration. • ALWAYS check for a blood return before and during administration of a vesicant medication. • Stop all infusions at the first sign of a problem, such as disappearance of a blood return or patient complaints. • Adequately stabilize the port needle to prevent dislodgement. • Teach the patient how to gain access to the device, verify placement of the device, and secure the needle before initiating the infusion.

Complications of implanted port therapy (continued)

Signs and symptoms	Possible causes	Nursing interventions	Prevention
Vein thrombosis			
• Edema in the ipsilateral extremity, shoulder, neck, or chest • Pain in the extremity, shoulder neck, or chest • Engorged peripheral veins on the extremity, shoulder, neck, or chest • Lack of a blood return if thrombosis is at catheter tip	• Sluggish blood flow rate related to a large catheter placed in a small vein • Known genetic coagulopathies (factor V Leiden) • Chronic diseases associated with hypercoagulable state such as cancer, diabetes, or end-stage renal failure • Pregnancy or oral contraceptives • Surgical and trauma patients • History of multiple CVADs especially with a difficult or traumatic insertion and other devices such as pacemakers • Age extremes • Critical care patients	• Notify the LIP and anticipate order for diagnostic studies and for anticoagulant therapy if vein thrombosis is confirmed. (Do not remove a CVAD when a thrombosis is confirmed if the catheter is in the appropriate position, functioning with blood return, and no evidence of infection.) • Be aware that pulmonary emboli and post-thrombotic syndrome are associated with upper extremity vein thrombosis. • Anticipate anticoagulant therapy for 3 months or more if a CVAD is removed. • Document interventions.	• Assess vein in its natural state and place the right size catheter for the vein (the catheter should occupy no more than 45% of the vein). • Verify that the catheter tip is in superior vena cava near the cavoatrial junction before using the catheter. • Encourage patient to resume normal activities of daily living and adequate hydration.

Discontinuing implanted port therapy

To prepare to discontinue therapy, first gather the necessary equipment, including:
- 10-mL syringe filled with normal saline solution
- 5 mL of appropriate locking solution (for example, heparin lock solution 10 units/mL, antimicrobial lock solution)
- sterile gloves
- sterile 2″ × 2″ gauze pad and tape.

Then, follow these steps:
- After shutting off the infusion, clamp the extension set and remove the I.V. tubing.
- Disinfect needleless connectors by vigorous scrubbing according to facility policy and procedure.
- Attach the syringe filled with saline solution using aseptic technique.

- Unclamp the extension set, flush the device with the saline solution, and remove the saline solution syringe.
- Attach the syringe with the locking solution and instill into the port.
- Clamp the extension set.

Removing the noncoring needle

After instilling the locking solution, remove the noncoring needle by following these steps:
1. First, put on gloves.
2. Place the gloved index and middle fingers from the nondominant hand on either side of the port septum.
3. Stabilize the port by pressing down with these two fingers, maintaining pressure until the needle is removed.
4. Using your gloved, dominant hand, grasp the noncoring needle, and remove it from the port body according to the instructions for use for the specific safety mechanism.
5. Apply a dressing as indicated.
6. If no more infusions are scheduled, remind the patient that he or she will need to repeat this procedure in about a month.

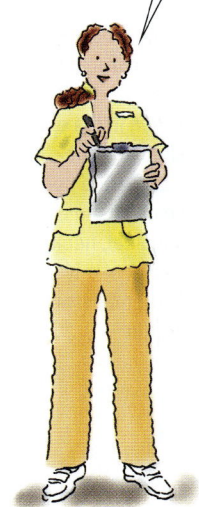

Almost done. I just need to document a few things.

Document

After removing the noncoring needle, document the following:
- removal of the noncoring needle
- condition of the site
- use of the flush and locking solution
- patient's response to the procedure
- patient education
- problems you encountered and resolved.

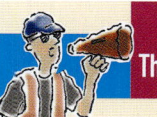

That's a wrap!

Central venous therapy review

Benefits
- Provides access to the central veins
- Permits rapid infusion of medications or large amounts of fluids
- Allows clinicians to draw blood samples and measure central venous pressure
- Reduces the need for repeated venipunctures
- Reduces the risk of vein irritation

Drawbacks
- Increases the risk of life-threatening complications

Central venous therapy review (continued)

Catheter types and uses
- Nontunneled: designed for short-term use, primarily in acute care settings
- Tunneled: designed for long-term use
- PICCs: used for both short- and long-term use
- Implanted ports: used when infusion needs are frequent and greater than 3 to 6 months

Common CVAD insertion sites
- Subclavian/axillary vein
- Internal or external jugular vein
- Brachial vein
- Basilic vein

Insertion site considerations
- Presence of scar tissue
- Possible interference with surgical site or other therapy
- Configuration of lung apices
- Patient's lifestyle and daily activities

Before insertion
- Explain the procedure to the patient and verify that the informed consent has been obtained according to facility policy.
- Place the patient in Trendelenburg position.
- Prepare the insertion site: clip hair and clean the site with alcoholic chlorhexidine solution.
- Assist with sterile drape application.
- Conscious sedation may be used; if so, the patient requires close observation.

During insertion
- Monitor patient response.
- Assist as needed.
- Complete insertion checklist.
- Provide support to the patient.

After insertion
- Monitor for complications.
- Apply a transparent semipermeable dressing.
- Document the insertion.

Complications of central I.V. therapy
- Pneumothorax, hemothorax, chylothorax, hydrothorax
- Air embolism
- Vein thrombosis
- Perforation of vessel and adjacent organs
- Local infection
- Bloodstream infection

Complications of implanted port therapy
- Port pocket infection
- Extravasation
- Thrombosis
- Fibrin sheath formation

Infusion maintenance
- Change the transparent semipermeable dressing whenever it becomes moist, loose, or soiled.
- Change the I.V. solution and tubing every 96 hours for continuous infusion according to facility protocol.
- Flush the catheter before and after each intermittent infusion and as needed for continuous infusion. For any CVAD not in routine use, flush according to facility protocol; however, the CVAD should be removed when no longer part of the plan of care.
- Change the gauze dressing at least every 48 hours. Change transparent membrane dressing every 5 to 7 days.
- Change the needleless connector at the same time as the primary continuous administration set or at least every 7 days for intermittent infusion.

(continued)

Central venous therapy review *(continued)*

Implanted port insertion and maintenance
- Explain the procedure to the patient and make sure the patient has signed a consent form.
- Monitor the patient during and after implantation for complications (infection, clotting, skin irritation).
- Change the dressing whenever its integrity is compromised.
- Flush every 4 weeks if not accessed.

What to document
- Status of the site
- Type of needle used
- Type of device used
- Procedure performed
- Patient's tolerance of the procedure
- Problems encountered and nursing interventions performed
- Type of dressing used
- Patient teaching performed and patient's understanding of teaching

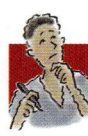

Quick quiz

1. In CV therapy, an access device is inserted with its tip in the:
    A. inferior vena cava or right atrium.
    B. superior or inferior vena cava.
    C. superior vena cava or right atrium.
    D. right atrium or right ventricle.

Answer: B. Depending on venous accessibility and the prescribed infusion therapy, a CVAD is inserted with its tip in the superior or inferior vena cava.

2. The advantages of central I.V. therapy include:
    A. ability to rapidly infuse fluids, administer irritating medication, and measure CV pressure.
    B. minimal or no complications on insertion.
    C. increased patient mobility.
    D. decreased risk of infection.

Answer: A. Central I.V. therapy provides access to central veins as well as the ability to rapidly infuse medications or fluids and measure CV pressure.

3. Which vein is the most commonly used CVAD insertion site?
    A. Femoral
    B. Brachial
    C. Cephalic
    D. Subclavian

Answer: D. The subclavian vein is the most common CVAD insertion site. It provides easy access and a direct route to the superior vena cava and central venous circulation.

4. Clinician responsibilities when preparing a patient for central I.V. therapy include:
    A. explaining the procedure and care measures of the therapy.
    B. selecting the site.
    C. obtaining consent.
    D. inserting the device.

Answer: A. When preparing a patient for central I.V. therapy, the clinician should explain the procedure and its care measures and answer the patient's questions.

5. The risk of using a CVAD for routine blood sampling includes:
    A. extravasation.
    B. vein thrombosis and fibrin sheath development.
    C. development of pinch-off syndrome.
    D. bloodstream infection and anemia.

Answer: D. Hub manipulation increases risk of bloodstream infection. Frequency and technique can lead to anemia.

6. The correct patient position for removal of a CVAD from the jugular or subclavian vein is:
    A. supine with head elevated.
    B. on the side opposite from the insertion side.
    C. supine with head flat.
    D. in a sitting position.

Answer: C. The flat position is necessary to have the exit site at or below the level of the heart to reduce the risk of venous air embolus

Scoring

☆☆☆ If you answered six questions correctly, right on! You took a central route to understanding this chapter.

☆☆ If you answered four or five questions correctly, good job! You followed the text right to the heart of the matter.

☆ If you answered fewer than four questions correctly, don't fret! Instead, center yourself and reaccess the material.

Suggested References

Centers for Disease Control. (2011). *Guidelines for the prevention of intravascular catheter-related infections.* Retrieved from http://www.cdc.gov/hicpac/BSI/BSI-guidelines-2011.html

Chopra, V., Flanders, S. A., Saint, S., Woller, S. C., O'Grady, N. P., Safdar, N., ... Bernstein, S. J. (2015). The Michigan Appropriateness Guide for Intravenous Catheters (MAGIC): Results from a multispecialty panel using the RAND/UCLA Appropriateness Method. *Annals of Internal Medicine, 163,* S1–S39. doi: 10.7326/M15-0744.

Hallam, C., Weston, V., Denton, A., Hill, S., Bodenham, A., Dunn, H., & Jackson, T. (2016). Development of the UK Vessel Health and Preservation (VHP) framework: A multi-organisational collaborative. *Journal of Infection Prevention, 17*(2), 65–72. doi: 10.1177/1757177415624752.

Gorski, L., Hadaway, L., Hagle, M., McGoldrick, M., Orr, M., & Doellman, D. (2016). Infusion Therapy Standards of Practice. *Journal of Infusion Nursing, 39*(1 Suppl.), 159.

Marschall, J., Mermel, L. A., Fakih, M., Hadaway, L., Kallen, A., O'Grady, N. P., …, Yokoe, D. S. (2014). Strategies to Prevent Central Line-Associated Bloodstream Infections in Acute Care Hospitals: 2014 Update. *Infection Control and Hospital Epidemiology, 35*, S89–S107 1p. doi: 10.1086/676533.

Phillips, L., & Gorski, L. (2014). *Manual of I.V. therapeutics* (6th ed.). Philadelphia, PA: FA Davis.

Weinstein, S. M., & Hagle, M. (2014). *Plumer's principles and practice of infusion therapy* (9th ed.). Philadelphia, PA: Wolters Kluwer Health.

Chapter 4

Infusion fluids and medications

Just the facts

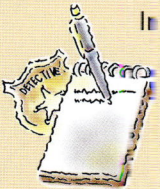

In this Chapter you will learn
- The types of infusion fluids
- Preparation of infusion medications
- Methods of administration of infusion fluids and medications
- Risks associated with infusion medications
- Stability and compatibility of infusion medications
- Calculation of medication dosages
- Flushing and locking of VADs
- Management of patient controlled analgesia
- Types of adverse drug events

Understanding infusion fluids

Infusion fluids fall into two groups—crystalloid and colloid solutions. Crystalloids are substances that form crystals such as electrolytes (for example, potassium and calcium). Crystals are capable of fully dissolving in fluid, allowing the complete solution to move through membranes. Colloid solutions are large molecules that act as plasma volume expanders, pulling fluid from the interstitial spaces. This group includes albumin, dextran, hetastarch, and mannitol and is commonly used to maintain circulating volume after blood loss from surgery or trauma.

Methods for administering fluids and medications can be divided in several ways. A common way to think about delivery is by continuous versus intermittent infusion. Continuous infusion is a constant infusion at a prescribed flow rate (that is, 100 or 125 mL/hour) over hours or days. Intermittent infusion is usually a smaller volume (that is, 50 or 100 mL) of fluid infused periodically (that is, every 6, 8, or 12 hours).

Infusion fluids are available in plastic bag containers of 50 mL, 100 mL, 250 mL, 500 mL, and 1,000 mL. Glass bottles may be used for certain types of fluids if there is an issue of compatibility with the plastic.

Continuous infusion of fluids is ordered when the normal balance of fluids and electrolytes in the body have been altered by illness or injury. (See Chapter 1, *Fluids, Electrolytes, and Infusion Therapy,* page 3.) The reasons for infusing fluids include:
- inability to drink enough fluids to maintain normal fluids and electrolyte balance (for example, nausea)
- need to replace excessive fluid and electrolyte losses (for example, vomiting, diarrhea, hemorrhage)
- inability to absorb adequate fluids and electrolytes through the gastrointestinal (GI) tract
- prescribed medication requiring a large volume for dilution and/or a constant infusion (that is, heparin and potassium chloride).

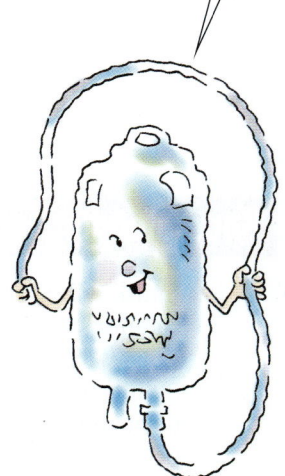

An isotonic solution stays where it's infused—inside the blood vessel.

Bringing back the balance

There are three basic types of infusion fluids:
- isotonic
- hypotonic
- hypertonic.

A few common solutions can be used to illustrate the role of infusion therapy in restoring and maintaining fluid and electrolyte balance. (See *Quick guide to infusion solutions,* page 196.)

Isotonic solutions

The osmolarity of isotonic solutions is similar to intravascular fluids, which is 280 to 295 mOsm/L. The osmolarity of isotonic infusion fluids range from 250 to 375 mOsm/L. Because the solution doesn't alter serum osmolarity, it stays where it's infused—inside the blood vessel (the intravascular compartment). The solution expands this compartment without pulling fluid from other compartments.

Hypertonic solutions

A hypertonic solution has an osmolarity greater than 375 mOsm/L. When a patient receives an infusion of hypertonic solution, serum osmolarity initially increases, causing fluid to be pulled from the interstitial and intracellular compartments into the blood vessels.

When, why, and how to get hyper

Hypertonic solutions may be ordered for patients postoperatively because of the beneficial effects of shifting fluid into the blood vessels
- reduces the risk of edema
- stabilizes blood pressure
- regulates urine output.

Hypotonic solutions

A hypotonic solution has an osmolarity less than 250 mOsm/L. When a patient receives a hypotonic solution, fluid shifts out of the blood vessels and into the cells and interstitial spaces, where osmolarity is higher. A hypotonic solution hydrates cells while reducing fluid in the circulatory system.

Hypotonic solutions may be ordered when diuretic therapy dehydrates cells. Other indications include hyperglycemic conditions, such as diabetic ketoacidosis and the hyperosmolar hyperglycemic state. In these conditions, high serum glucose levels draw fluid out of cells, leaving them dehydrated.

Flood warning

Because hypotonic solutions flood cells, certain patients shouldn't receive them. For example, patients with cerebral edema or increased intracranial pressure shouldn't receive hypotonic solutions because the increased ECF can cause further edema and tissue damage (Table 4-1).

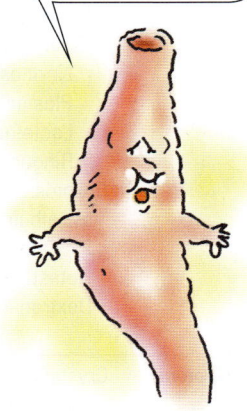

A hypertonic solution causes fluid to be pulled from the interstitial and intracellular compartments into the blood vessels.

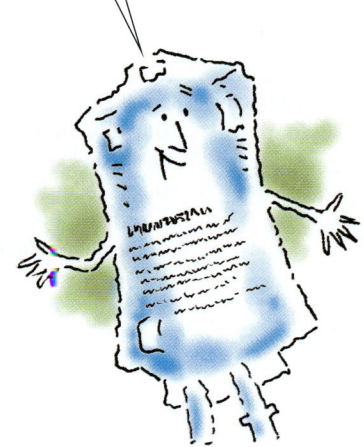

A hypotonic solution causes fluid to shift out of the blood vessels and into the cells and interstitial spaces.

Fluid flow rates

A flow rate that is appropriate for your patient requires an assessment of the patient's needs, including all primary and secondary medical diagnoses. Consider the primary reason for the fluids — replacement or maintenance. When a patient's oral intake is restricted or prohibited temporarily, the goal is usually maintenance of appropriate amounts of water, glucose, sodium, and potassium. Patients with sudden, severe, or prolonged loss of fluids and electrolytes require replacement of those losses. Replacement is provided over 48 hours based on the calculation of the fluid losses. When fluid and electrolyte losses continue (for example, nasogastric suction), the calculation for restoring these ongoing losses plus maintenance

Table 4-1 Quick guide to infusion solutions

This chart lists common examples of the three types of crystalloid and colloid solutions and provides key considerations for administering them.

Solution	Examples	Nursing considerations

Isotonic	Crystalloids:
	• Normal saline (308 mOsm/L)
	• Dextrose 5% in water (D_5W) (252 mOsm/L)
	• Balanced electrolyte solutions:
	  ○ Normosol (295 mOsm/L)
	  ○ Plasma-Lyte (280 to 310 mOsm/L)
	  ○ Lactated Ringer's (275 mOsm/L)
	  ○ Ringer's (275 mOsm/L)
	Colloids:
	• 5% albumin (308 mOsm/L)
	• 25% albumin (312 mOsm/L)
	• Hetastarch (310 mOsm/L)
	• Dextran-70 (310 mOsm/L)
		• Closely monitor the patient for signs of fluid overload, especially if he has hypertension or heart failure.
		• Because the liver converts lactate to bicarbonate, don't give lactated Ringer's solution if the patient's blood pH exceeds 7.5.
		• Avoid giving D_5W to a patient at risk for increased intracranial pressure (ICP) because it acts like a hypotonic solution. (Although usually considered isotonic, D_5W is actually isotonic only in the container. After administration, dextrose is quickly metabolized, leaving only water — a hypotonic fluid.)

Hypotonic	Crystalloids: • Half-normal saline (154 mOsm/L) • 0.33% sodium chloride (103 mOsm/L) • Dextrose 2.5% in water (126 mOsm/L)	• Administer cautiously. Hypotonic solutions cause a fluid shift from blood vessels into cells. This shift could cause cardiovascular collapse from intravascular fluid depletion and increased ICP from fluid shift into brain cells. • Don't give hypotonic solutions to patients at risk for increased ICP from stroke, head trauma, or neurosurgery. • Don't give hypotonic solutions to patients at risk for third-space fluid shifts (abnormal fluid shifts into the interstitial compartment or a body cavity) — for example, patients suffering from burns, trauma, or low serum protein levels from malnutrition or liver disease.
Hypertonic	Crystalloids: • Dextrose 5% in half-normal saline (406 mOsm/L) • Dextrose 5% in normal saline (560 mOsm/L) • Dextrose 5% in lactated Ringer's (575 mOsm/L) • 3% sodium chloride (1,025 mOsm/L)	• Because hypertonic solutions greatly expand the intravascular compartment, administer them by I.V. pump and closely monitor the patient for circulatory overload. • Hypertonic solutions pull fluid from the intracellular compartment, so don't give them to a patient with a condition that causes cellular dehydration — for example, diabetic ketoacidosis. • Don't give hypertonic solutions to a patient with impaired heart or kidney function — his system can't handle the extra fluid.

requires accurate tracking and documentation of fluid output. Medical diagnoses of renal or cardiac failure will influence the volume and rate of infusion fluids for both replacement and maintenance. Electrolytes such as potassium chloride are commonly added to infusion fluids. Wound infection and colon surgery will cause loss of potassium and require replacement. Potassium is always added to infusion fluids, given by infusion and is NEVER given by a manual injection as this method of administration can cause patient death. Adults will usually require 40 to 80 mEq in a 24-hour period based on the losses. A common dose is 20 to 40 mEq added to a liter of fluids; however, this could go up to 80 mEq/L as the maximum concentration. The rate of infusion should not exceed more than 10 mEq/hour. High concentrations of 60 mEq/L or more are categorized as a vesicant and may cause tissue necrosis with extravasation.

Flow rate control is critical in all patients. In hospitalized patients, an electronic infusion pump is commonly used to provide the highest level of accuracy. You will need to know how to calculate flow rates to enter this number as the volume to be infused per hour. When no infusion pump is used, fluid flow rate is by gravity and controlled by restrictions on the administration set from roller clamps. This requires additional calculations based on the number of drops per milliliter the set will delivery, known as the drop factor. (See Chapter 1, *Infusion Flow Rates*, page 32 and *Calculating Flow Rates*, page 33.)

Infusion fluids may be used to deliver intermittent medications by piggybacking or attaching a secondary set to the primary set used for continuous infusion. For these situations, consider the presence of medication added to the primary fluid and the compatibility of these medications when they meet in the administration set. Piggybacking the intermittent medication may not be possible if there are incompatibilities identified. This situation may require a bag of normal saline for piggybacking intermittent medications, frequently known as a carrier fluid. This requires use of additional fluid, so make sure you have an LIP order for the carrier fluid or an established policy for this type of fluid use.

There are specific situations when infusion fluids should never be used. A container of infusion fluids does not contain preservatives. For this reason, the container should only be entered once. Fluids for diluting medications or for filling flush syringes should never be taken from a fluid container (Table 4-2).

Table 4-2 Do's and don'ts with infusion fluids

Do:
- Perform hand hygiene before handling any infusion fluid containers.
- Use aseptic technique when handling all containers and administration sets.
- Check all manufacturer labels and labels added by the pharmacy for accuracy of contents.
- Check expiration dates and beyond-use dates for all fluid containers.
- Begin use of a fluid container within 1 hour after it has been opened and the administration set added.
- Disinfect the injection port before adding any medication to a fluid container.
- Accurately calculate flow rate in milliliters per hour.
- For gravity infusion, know the drop factor on the administration set so you can accurately calculate the infusion rate in drops per minute.
- If refrigerated storage is needed, remove from the refrigerator with enough time to allow for reaching room temperature.

Don't:
- Open a fluid container before time for it to be hung.
- Add the administration set hours before it will be attached to the patient's VAD.
- Add medication to a fluid container while it is infusing as this can result in a rapid infusion if the medication did not mix thoroughly with the fluid.
- Enter a fluid container multiple times, as there is no preservative in these containers.
- Use a fluid container for obtaining solution for diluting medication or VAD flushing.
- Use a microwave or other heating device to warm fluids as there is no way to measure and control the fluid temperature.

Infusion medications

Medications are infused for a variety of reasons including the following:
- The therapeutic effect is best achieved by infusion, as the fluids of the GI tract will destroy the medication before it is absorbed.
- A rapid therapeutic effect is needed (for example, pain control with opioids).
- Greater therapeutic blood levels of the medication are achieved by infusion.
- Oral intake is prohibited.
- An irritating drug may cause pain or tissue damage if given intramuscular (IM).

Medication given directly into the vein, subcutaneous tissue, bone, or other spaces carries additional risk because the medication cannot be recalled after it is given. It is immediately metabolized and its effects cannot be easily reversed. Infusion medications are associated with significant risk to the patient and are reported to be associated

with high rates of serious errors. These factors require the clinician to have complete knowledge of the medication prior to administration including:
- indications and contraindications
- pharmacologic action(s)
- dosing and age-related dose changes as appropriate for the patient
- appropriate type and quantity of fluid for dilution
- stability of the drug
- compatibility of the drug with other fluids and medications in the infusion system
- infusion routes and rates
- side effects and adverse reactions
- necessary patient monitoring parameters (for example, lab values, urinary output volume).

This information should be readily available to each clinician with responsibility for administering infusion medications. A variety of reference books and computer programs on infusion medications are available. Use these valuable resources to learn this information before giving each medication. Do not assume that all infusion medications have the same requirements for safe administration.

Rapid response

I.V. medications enter the bloodstream directly, rapidly achieving therapeutic blood levels. The intraosseous, subcutaneous, and other routes of infusion also reach rapid therapeutic levels. The difference in absorption explains why the oral doses may be larger than the IV doses.

Effective absorption

Drug absorption covers the progress of a drug from the time it's administered through the time it passes into the tissues and becomes available for use by the body. Some oral medications are unstable in gastric juices and digestive enzymes, making absorption uncertain. Some oral medications may also interact with food or other medications that may alter absorption.

Absorption problems also occur with oral medications that are metabolized by the liver where significant amounts of the drug are processed and eliminated before they reach the bloodstream. This process — known as *first-pass metabolism* — may be so rapid and extensive that it precludes oral administration. Because gastric absorption isn't a factor with infusion therapy, drug concentration and administration rate avoid the erratic nature of the oral route.

Identifying and reducing risks

Risks associated with infusion medications include:
- lack of patient information (that is, height, weight, laboratory values)
- lack of drug information for proper dilution or rate of administration
- confusing or ambiguous communication of drug administration methods
- drug preparation without the appropriate labeling, especially in syringes
- drug packaging with confusing labels
- incorrect use of vials and syringes (for example, multiple entries into a single-dose vial)
- absence of clearly written policies and procedures to standardize use of infusion pumps for drug delivery
- lack of staff training on all infusion-related devices and equipment
- deficiency in risk management and quality improvement standards such as infection prevention and adverse event monitoring.

All medication administration involves many facility departments and staff members and is not limited to the nursing staff. Safe preparation and administration of infusion medications require organizational policies and procedures that incorporate all personnel involved in the process.

Ensure that you read and understand all policies and procedures before administering infusion medications and use the drug reference resources available to you. If these resources do not provide all information, many clinicians invest in handbooks so questions can quickly and easily be answered. Hundreds of infusion medications mean you cannot remember all this information, so these resources protect you and your patient.

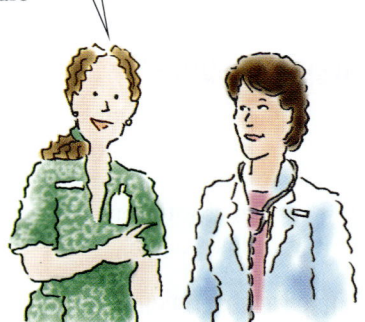

Know your organization's policies and procedures before giving infusion medications.

Continuous or intermittent infusion

Infusion medications may be given by continuous or intermittent infusion. Continuous infusion examples include electrolytes like potassium chloride, vitamins, insulin, heparin, and vasopressors. These are added to the continuous fluids and given by a constant infusion with the flow rate regulated by an infusion pump.

Intermittent medications are given at specific intervals by two methods:
1. manual injection from a syringe, also called I.V. push
2. short infusion by piggybacking into infusing fluids or direct connection to the vascular access device (VAD) hub.

Medications given by I.V. push are prepared in a syringe that is appropriately sized for the volume of medication to be given. Follow the drug manufacturers' instructions regarding additional dilution of any medication given by a manual injection. This preparation should be performed in the laminar airflow workbench in the pharmacy; however, preparation in a clean dry area designated for this purpose may be necessary in some situations. All preparation should be done immediately prior to giving the drug and never done hours before it is needed. If dilution is required, use only a compatible solution from a preservative-free vial (for example, normal saline). Never obtain fluid for dilution from:
- a bag of infusion fluids, regardless of the size of the bag, used for multiple patients
- a multidose vial used for multiple patients; a multiple dose vial must be dedicated to a single patient
- a prefilled saline syringe used for flushing VADs.

The syringe is attached to a needleless injection port on the I.V. administration set or may be attached directly to the needleless connector on the VAD hub. Usually, the rate for giving the medication is by very slow injection as directed by the drug information. A few drugs require a bolus injection, meaning that the drug must be rapidly injected, also directed by the drug information.

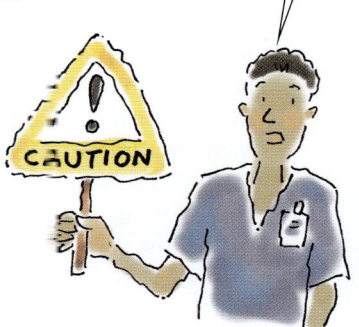

Do NOT transfer a medication from one syringe to another.

Medications given by a short infusion are usually diluted in 50 or 100 mL and given over 30 to 60 minutes. When continuous fluids are also being infused, the intermittent medication is attached to a needleless injection port on the administration set (that is, piggybacking). If no continuous fluids are being given, the administration set is attached to the needleless connector on the VAD hub.

Important issues with infusion medication

There are a few important concepts that are unique to infusion medication including:
- compounding sterile medication
- stability
- compatibility.

Compounding sterile medication

It is imperative that any infused or injected medication be:
- identified with the correct ingredients on the label
- pure or free from physical and chemical contaminates
- the correct strength
- sterile.

Compounding is defined as the combining, mixing, or altering of ingredients of a drug to create a medication tailored to the needs of an individual patient. To meet these requirements for infusion medications, the U.S. Pharmacopeia issued regulations, commonly known as USP <797>, which sets the national standard for the preparation, storage, and transportation of all compounded medications. For many years, hospital pharmacies have provided the services of preparing most infusion fluids and medications. This standard now applies to all health care workers in all health care settings. The days of clinicians compounding complex infusion medications in a small area of the nurses' station are gone!

Multiple steps are frequently required for drug compounding. This increases the risk of touch contamination along with particulate matter such as dust particles floating in the air. The area where drugs are compounded requires a laminar airflow workbench meeting international standards for air quality. This could be a large environment or a smaller freestanding cabinet often seen in infusion centers. USP <797> includes requirements for air flow from heating and air conditioning units, temperature, the traffic flow between adjacent rooms, the control of supplies and utensils into the area, cleaning the workspace and surrounding area, the number of air exchanges per hour, training and competency of personnel, and the attire of personnel working in this space.

Clinicians may be required to prepare an infusion medication under a very specific circumstance — when a medication is required urgently for a specific patient and preparation under strict conditions would add additional risk for the patient due to delays of the drug reaching the patient. In these specific situations, aseptic technique is still required for drug preparation, preparation cannot exceed 1 hour, and administration must begin immediately.

An additional situation where clinicians would be mixing medications may be determined by the length of time the drug remains stable. This applies to alternative care sites such as home care where medication deliveries to the home would result in the loss of stability before the drug is administered.

How is the drug supplied?

Infusion drugs can be supplied four ways:
1. liquid form in a vial or ampule
2. lyophilized powder created by freeze drying or removing the water after it is frozen and under a vacuum
3. premixed from the drug manufacturer, completely diluted and ready to infuse
4. proprietary bag and vial system, containing a lyophilized powder to be diluted with the solution from the infusion bag.

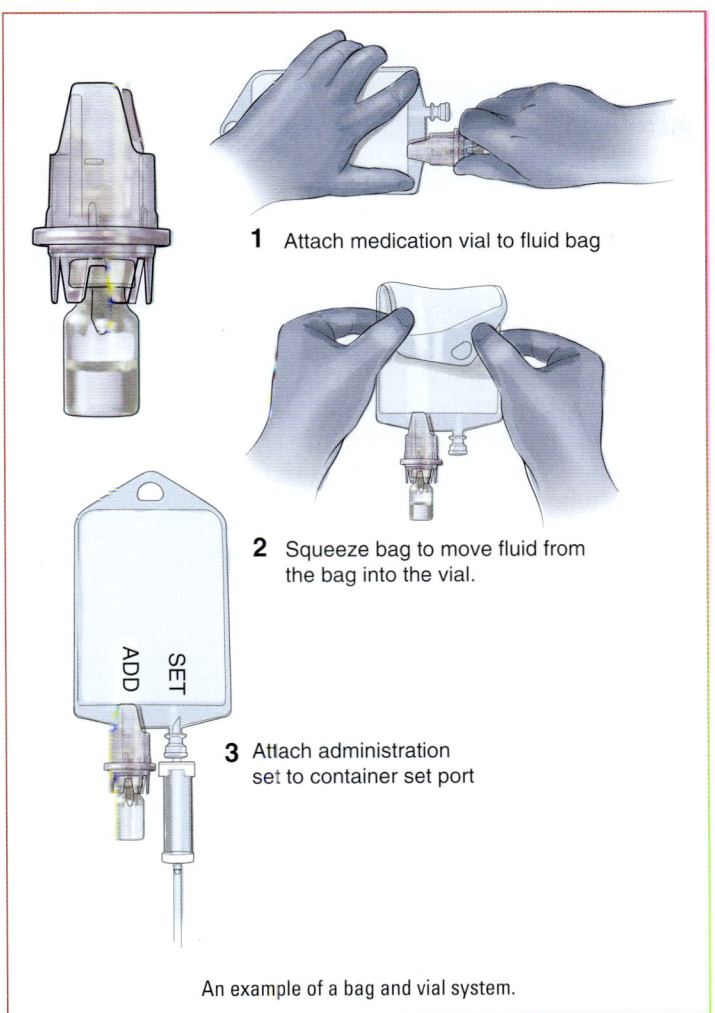

An example of a bag and vial system.

A liquid drug may only require transfer from its vial to a syringe for injection without additional dilution. Follow the drug manufacturer instructions and do not mix these drugs with additional fluid for dilution unless this dilution is recommended by the manufacturer. This adds an unnecessary step and increases the risk of contamination. While it is preferred that these drugs be prepared in the laminar airflow workbench, you may be expected to prepare these drugs before administration to your patient. Preparation of these drugs should be done at the patient's bedside and immediately administered to the patient. If preparation occurs at a location away from the patient such as the medicine room at the nurses' station, the syringe must be labeled with all contents. Distractions in transit to the patient's bedside can cause medication errors.

A lyophilized powder will require additional steps to prepare including drawing up a small amount of compatible diluent into a syringe, injecting this into the vial to dissolve the powder, waiting for it to thoroughly mix, withdrawing the liquid from the vial, and injecting it into a 50- or 100-mL bag of compatible fluids. This number of steps should be done in the laminar airflow workbench with strict attention to aseptic technique.

Premixed medications are prepared by a manufacturer and do not require additional preparation in the pharmacy or at the bedside. These drugs are stable for extended periods and can be attached to the infusion system without any manipulation.

Many manufacturers supply proprietary bag and vial systems. The vial containing the lyophilized powder is designed to fit a specific place on the fluid bag. Once these two components are assembled, fluid is squeezed from the bag into the vial to reconstitute the powder, and then the dissolved medication flows into the bag where it is further diluted with the remaining fluid in the bag. Assembling and immediately using these systems can be done at the bedside; however, these components should not be assembled before they are needed. Aseptic technique is required. Follow manufacturer instructions for the specific steps to assemble and administer medication from these systems.

Stability

Each drug must be able to maintain its pharmacologic properties with stable strength and purity during storage, preparation, and administration. Time is a key element in drug stability. When the active ingredient in a drug preparation loses approximately 10% of its original potency, it is no longer stable. Many factors can affect the stability of a drug including:
- temperature
- moisture
- light
- microbes
- packaging.

Two dates are important to drug stability:
- Expiration date is the date when the drug should be discarded. This date is assigned by the manufacturer and applies to drugs in the original unopened package when stored under the conditions defined by the manufacturer (for example, temperature).
- Beyond-use date (BUD) is the date and time assigned by the pharmacy after the original package has been opened and the drug transferred to another container. This commonly occurs with

infusion drugs that may require reconstitution and transfer to a fluid container for additional dilution. Check the label on the fluid container for the drug name and concentration along with the BUD and be prepared to infuse the drug by this date and time. Dilution and transfer of the drug can alter the physical and chemical properties along with the potential for introduction of microorganisms.

Compatibility

To successfully mix medication in a solution for infusion, everything must be compatible — the drug, diluent, and the fluid container. Polyvinyl chloride used to make many plastic fluid containers causes the greatest concern because a few drugs (for example, insulin, nitroglycerin) can adhere to the internal surface of the container, a process known as adsorption. This process reduces the amount of drug that is being infused to the patient. Infusion of these drugs requires close titration for the desired clinical effect rather than expecting a specific dose to provide a defined clinical response. Containers made of different types of plastics may now be used to infuse the drugs with this problem.

Each drug manufacturer will provide information about the appropriate diluents that are compatible with their drug, and this information is readily available to the pharmacy preparing the medication. If you are expected to prepare a drug in an urgent situation, you will need to check the information for the specific drug or follow instructions provided by your pharmacy. Common fluids like normal saline or 5% dextrose in water are compatible with most drugs; however, don't assume this to be true for all infusion medications. Also balanced electrolyte solutions, such as Ringer's lactate, contain calcium that creates a higher incidence of incompatibility and are not appropriate for some medications.

Combinations of two or more drugs create the greatest concern, because the number of possible combinations is endless. Infusion medications come into contact with other drugs when:
- added to the same fluid container
- mixed in the same syringe
- piggybacked into an injection port on the administration set of an infusing fluid containing another drug
- injected or infused directly into a VAD lumen or administration set without proper flushing between drugs.

The pharmacy will be compounding most infusion drugs and providing them ready for you to infuse. However, you will be

administering them. Planning is necessary to prevent contact between incompatible medications. You will need to consider:
- method of infusion — push or infusion
- number of VADs or the number of available lumens for infusion
- medications mixed in the fluids currently infusing.

Medication should never be added to an infusing fluid container, with or without another drug already in the solution. This process creates an increased risk for contamination of the solution. Additionally, the drug could form a layer on the bottom of the fluid container, preventing the added drug from thoroughly mixing with the remaining fluid and resulting in a rapid infusion of the drug. Finally, the fluid remaining in the container may not be enough volume to provide the correct dilution for the added drug.

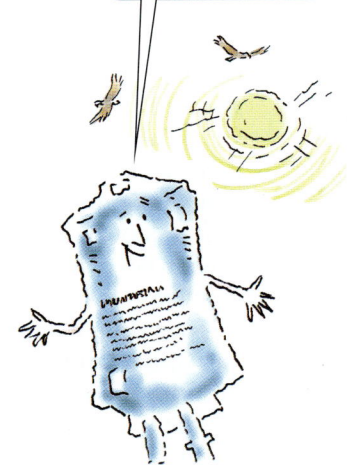

Planning is necessary to prevent contact between incompatible medications.

Each drug given by manual injection or "I.V. push" should be prepared in its own syringe. Do not mix two drugs in the same syringe. For intramuscular injection, adding two drugs to one syringe will prevent the patient from receiving two injections and may be common practice. For infusion techniques, this provides no benefit and prevents control over the correct rate of injection for each drug. If the patient has an adverse reaction, it will be difficult to determine which drug caused the problem.

Many patients, such as those in critical care, may require several continuous infusions, along with multiple intermittent short infusions. This requires planning to ensure that all drugs reach the patient's bloodstream without coming into contact with another incompatible drug. Assessing the number of available lumens on the VAD is critical along with checking a drug resource for recent compatibility information. Before piggybacking an intermittent medication into the administration set, check the primary fluid container for added medication. If present, check the compatibility of these drugs. Proceed with the piggyback infusion only when documented compatibility has been found.

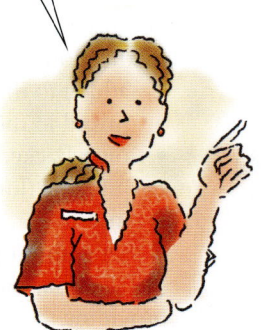

Wall posters with compatibility information may be convenient but may be too old to use!

When administering two medications through the same VAD lumen or the injection port closest to the patient, flushing with normal saline between each medication is the best method for preventing contact between these drugs.

Use appropriate resources

New drugs are constantly being introduced. Testing on compatibility of various combinations is ongoing work from many pharmacy resources, although the speed of drug introduction is faster than publication of the compatibility information. This means that current information must be used to check incompatibility. Some resources are updated monthly or quarterly. Nursing drug handbooks may be updated yearly, but don't rely on any compatibility information that is older than that. The absence of compatibility information on a specific combination of drugs means these drugs should NOT be allowed to contact each other in the infusion system. Compatibility of any drug combination must be documented in the drug references before they could be infused together (Table 4-3).

Table 4-3 Factors affecting drug compatibility

Incompatibility is an undesirable chemical or physical reaction between a drug and a solution or between two or more drugs. The following factors can affect the compatibility of an I.V. drug or solution.

Sequence of mixing
Mixing order is a concern when you are adding more than one drug to an I.V. solution. Chemical changes occur after each drug is added. Changing the sequence in which the drugs are mixed may prevent compatibility.

Drug concentration
The higher the drug concentration, the more likely an incompatibility can develop. Gently invert the fluid container after adding each drug to evenly disperse it throughout the solution. Do this before starting an infusion and before adding another drug to the container.

Contact time
The longer two or more drugs are together, the more likely incompatibility will occur. You should know if two drugs are incompatible before deciding how to give them. For example, your patient is receiving a continuous heparin infusion, and gentamicin sulfate is ordered intermittently every 8 hours. Because these two drugs have an immediate incompatibility, you shouldn't piggyback the gentamicin into the heparin solution. If you do, your patient will not receive a therapeutic dose of gentamicin. This situation will require two separate peripheral catheters or a multiple lumen CVAD

Temperature
Higher temperatures promote chemical reactions. The higher the temperature of an admixture, the greater the risk of incompatibility. For this reason, preparation must occur right before administering it or refrigerate it until needed.

Light
Prolonged exposure to light can affect the stability of certain drugs. Nitroprusside sodium and amphotericin B, for example, must be protected from light during administration to maintain their stability.

pH
Generally, drugs and solutions that are to be mixed should have similar pH values to avoid incompatibility. Wide variations in pH will have the greatest likelihood of incompatibility. The pH of each I.V. solution is listed on the manufacturer's label. You will find the pH of each drug on the package insert.

Types of Incompatibility

Specific incompatibilities fall into three categories:
- physical
- chemical
- therapeutic (See Factors affecting drug compatibility, page 207.)

Physical incompatibility
A physical incompatibility is an undesirable change that can be seen, such as a visible precipitate. Precipitate is formed when substances dissolved in a solution turn into solid particles. This often occurs because of a change in the pH of one or both drugs. pH is the measurement of hydrogen ions in a solution and represents the degree of acidity or alkalinity. A scale of 1 to 14 is used to assess the pH with 7 being neutral. Solutions with a pH above 7 are alkaline; those below 7 are acidic. Checking the pH of drugs may give a clue about incompatibility if their values are on opposite ends of the scale.

Preservatives in the drug itself or the diluent may also be the cause of a physical incompatibility. Parabens, phenol, and benzyl alcohol are examples of preservatives in these medications. A vial labelled as "bacteriostatic" will contain some type of preservative.

Other signs of physical incompatibility seen in the solution include:
- Haze
- Gas bubbles
- Cloudiness.

High-alert infusion medications

Reports of medication errors along with published studies have identified many infusion drugs that are now defined as high-risk medications. These drugs require special attention in their preparation and administration. Examples of common drugs in the group include:
- heparin
- thrombolytic agents such as alteplase, and reteplase
- insulin
- narcotics such as morphine or hydromorphone
- promethazine
- potassium chloride and phosphate concentrations.

Know your facility's policy and procedure for these and any other drugs identified to be high risk. Special practices are used such as preventing access to the vials of these drugs. For instance, vials of potassium chloride are no longer stored outside the pharmacy in most facilities. Confusion between vials of sodium chloride and potassium chloride have resulted in significant patient harm. Additionally, the automatic dispensing cabinets for drugs and the electronic medication administration record may have special alerts for these drugs.

Your facility may require an independent double check by two clinicians before some of these drugs are administered. Make sure you are doing this process correctly. This process should not be overused due to time constraints on staff. Additionally, over-reliance on double checks can lead to ignoring other error-producing problems in the system.

Two people are needed for this process, and they must work separately to verify all details of medication name, dose calculations, dilution, and rate of infusion. One example is the pharmacist checking these details followed by the nurse also checking the same details without influence from the pharmacist. Working independently allows a greater number of mistakes to be identified.

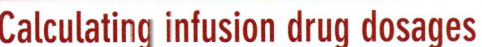

Be careful with special-alert drugs

Calculating infusion drug dosages

In many cases, you must calculate an ordered dosage to verify that the dosage is within the recommended range. Always begin by obtaining an accurate weight and height as this is the basis for all calculation.

Weighing in

With some drugs (I.V. immune globulin, for instance), dosage is based on the patient's weight in kilograms. To convert a patient's weight from pounds to kilograms, simply divide the number of pounds by 2.2. (Remember, 2.2 lb = 1 kg.)

Coming to the surface

With other drugs (such as antineoplastic agents), the dosage may be based on the patient's body surface area (BSA). A common method is to have the electronic medical record system at your facility perform this calculation by entering the correct height and weight. If your system does not provide this data, you can find BSA calculators online such as http://www.medcalc.com/body.html. Accuracy depends upon choosing the correct form of measurement. You can choose pounds or kilograms for weight and inches or centimeters for height. A third method for determining BSA is to use a nomogram. The calculated figure from all these processes will be expressed as square meters (m^2). This number is then used to calculate the exact medication dosage.

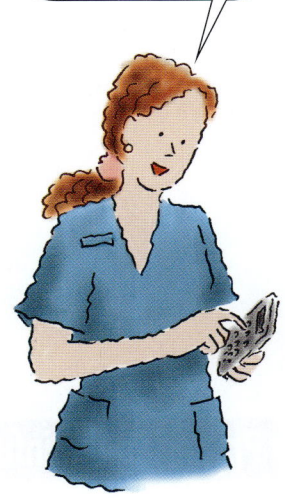

Hmmmm, let's see...to convert pounds to kilograms, just divide the number of pounds by 2.2. That was easy!

Infusion fluids and medications

Using a nomogram for adults

To estimate an adult's body surface area (BSA) with a nomogram, find your patient's weight in the right column and his height in the left column. Mark these two points; then draw a line between them. The point where the line intersects in the middle column gives you the BSA in square meters (m2).

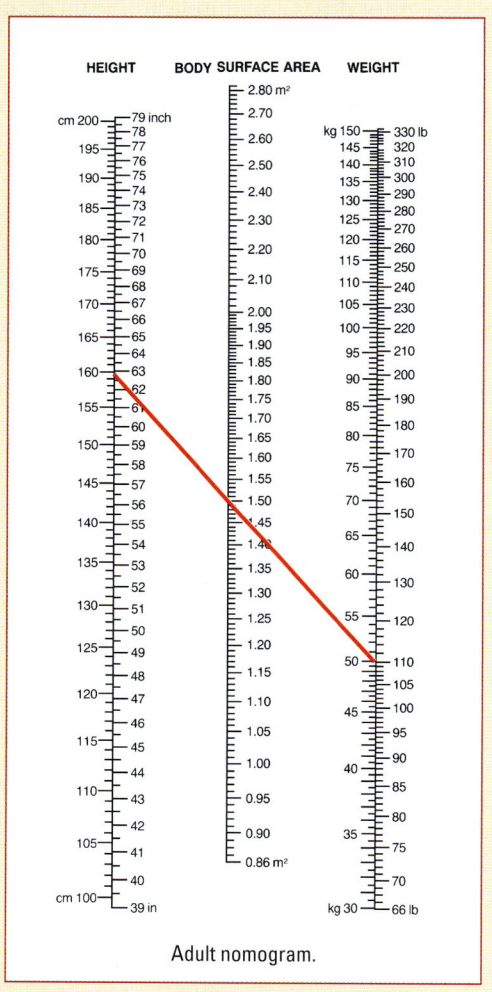

Adult nomogram.

Preparing the infusion medications

The most common situation in which you will be preparing infusion medication is when there is an urgent patient need and waiting to obtain the prepared medication from the pharmacy poses a risk to the patient. In this situation, the pressure is on to get the medication to the patient. However, you are still required to:
- use aseptic nontouch technique to prevent contamination

- prepare the medication in a designated area that is clean, dry, away from obviously contaminated areas like sinks, and outside a high-traffic area to reduce distractions and interruptions
- apply a label with the contents of the solution container.

Safety first

When you are preparing a medication, be sure to take some basic safety measures:
- Always practice good hand hygiene before touching any of the components you will be using. If your hands are contaminated with body fluids, always wash with soap and water. Otherwise use the hand antiseptic gel or foam products provided and follow their instruction for the length of contact time.
- Maintain aseptic no-touch technique throughout the complete procedure. This means knowing the specific sterile components of all devices to be used and preventing contact with areas that are not sterile.
  - Needle or a needleless transfer device — either device may be used for reconstitution and transfer of medication as there is no exposure to blood or body fluids at this point. Needleless transfer devices have many different designs. Make sure you know the instructions for using the specific brand provided. When you are inserting the needle or needleless transfer device into the vial and withdrawing it, make sure that it only touches the vial's rubber stopper after disinfection with the alcohol pad. Also, make sure that you don't inadvertently contaminate the needle or needleless transfer device with your

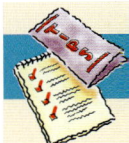

Education edge

Know what's sterile; know what is not

- Vial — only the internal surfaces are sterile. The rubber stopper under the cap is not sterile and requires scrubbing with an alcohol pad before entry.
- Ampule — only the internal surfaces are sterile. Disinfect the ampule with an alcohol pad and wrap the neck of the ampule with a gauze pad as sharp glass edges are exposed when it is broken. Additionally, a filter needle or filter straw should be used to aspirate contents because tiny glass pieces can fall into the liquid medication. Once the fluid has been aspirated into the syringe, remove and discard the filter needle. Do not use this filter to administer the mediation.
- Syringe — the internal fluid pathway and the male luer tip of the syringe are sterile.

finger. To keep your hands steady, brace one against the other while you are inserting and withdrawing the needle or needleless transfer device.

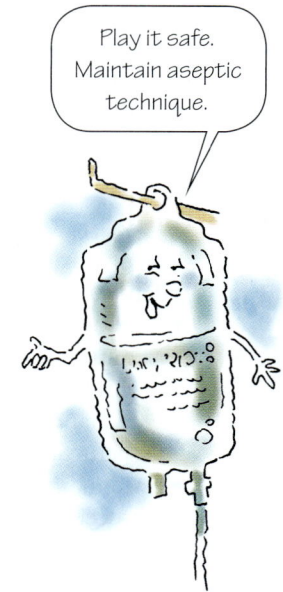

Play it safe. Maintain aseptic technique.

- Administration set — the internal fluid pathway and both ends of the set (the spike and the male luer-locking end) are sterile. As you remove the set from its packaging, make sure the caps are still seated over each end. If not, do not use the set.
- When drawing up the drug before adding it to the solution container, use a syringe that's large enough to hold the entire dose. If you need to use a needle to add the medication to the I.V. bag, make sure the needle is at least 1″ long to penetrate the inner seal of the port on the I.V. bag.

Reconstituting powdered drugs

Many drugs are supplied in powder form and have to be reconstituted with liquid diluents. Common diluents include:
- normal saline solution
- sterile water for injection
- dextrose 5% in water.

Always check the drug manufacturer's instructions about the appropriate type or amount of diluent. Some drugs should be reconstituted with diluents that do not contain preservatives.

A few drugs come in double-chambered vials that contain powder in the lower chamber and a diluent in the upper one. To combine the contents, press the rubber stopper on top of the vial to dislodge the

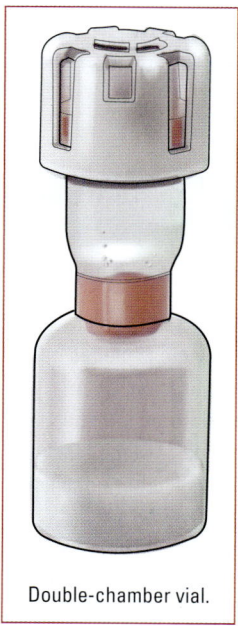

Double-chamber vial.

rubber plug separating the compartments. The diluent then mixes with the drug in the bottom chamber.

Sources of diluent for powdered medication include a single- or multiple-dose vial of fluid. A single-dose vial usually contains 10 mL, will NOT contain any preservative, and can only be entered once to aspirate the contents into a syringe. A multiple-dose vial may contain 30 to 50 mL of fluid, and it will have a preservative as indicated by the word "bacteriostatic" on the label. This preservative is effective against common bacteria but not against viruses and fungi. The use of the word "multiple" may be confusing as these vials should never be used for multiple patients. A multiple-dose vial should be dedicated to a single patient. Numerous cases of infections have been associated with entering a multiple-dose vial with a contaminated needle or syringe.

A bag of infusion solution should NEVER be used as a common source for obtaining fluid to dilute medication or for flushing solution, regardless of the size of the bag or how long it will be used. There have been numerous outbreaks of bloodstream infection associated with this practice.

A commercially prepared prefilled flush syringe should only be used for flushing the VAD before and after medication administration. These prefilled syringes should never be used for diluting medication. The gradation markings on these syringes are only 0.5 and 1 mL and would not provide the specific dose measurement as a traditional empty syringe. In addition, these syringes are only considered sterile where the fluid is located. The syringe barrel beyond the rubber gasket on the plunger rod is clean but not considered sterile. Finally, there is no way to alter the label on these syringes to indicate that a medication has been added. Transfer of contents of this syringe to another syringe should not be done, as it is very easy to contaminate the syringes in this transfer.

Each syringe and needle should be use one time ONLY and then discarded. They should NEVER be used on more than one patient or to draw up additional fluids.

Reconstituting procedure

To safely reconstitute powdered drugs, gather your equipment and then follow these step-by-step guidelines:
- Perform hand hygiene.
- Draw up the amount and type of diluent specified by the drug manufacturer.
- Scrub the rubber stopper of the drug vial or the neck of an ampule with an alcohol swab, and then discard the pad.

- Insert the needle or needleless transfer device connected to the syringe of diluent into the stopper at a 45- to 60-degree angle. Angling the needle minimizes coring or breaking off rubber pieces, which would then float inside the vial.
- Inject the diluent.
- Mix thoroughly by gently inverting the vial. If the drug does not dissolve within a few seconds, let it stand for 10 to 30 minutes. If necessary, invert the vial several times to dissolve the drug. Do not shake vigorously (unless directed) because some drugs may froth.

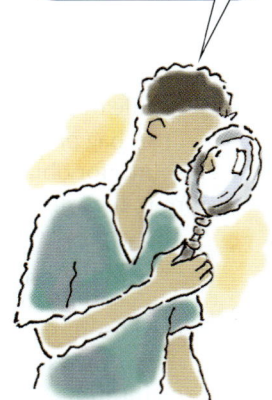

Be sure to inspect for signs of physical incompatibility — particles and cloudiness.

Next steps

The drug is now reconstituted to a liquid form and may require transfer to a small volume bag (50 or 100 mL) of normal saline or dextrose 5% in water for additional dilution and infusion. Disinfect the injection port on the bag by a vigorous mechanical scrub with an alcohol pad. Then inject the needle into this port or attach the needleless transfer device and inject the medication into the solution. After injecting the drug, grasp the top and bottom of the bag and quickly invert it twice. Do not squeeze or shake the bag.

Check it out

Check the expiration date on the drug and the diluent on the original package to be sure they are not expired. Inspect the drug, diluent, and final solution for particles and cloudiness, which are visible signs of incompatibility in the admixture. Remember, incompatibility is more likely with drugs or I.V solutions that have a wide variation in pH.

Liquid drugs: Additional dilution or not?

Liquid medication may be provided in:
- single-dose ampules or vials
- multidose vials
- prefilled syringes
- disposable cartridges.

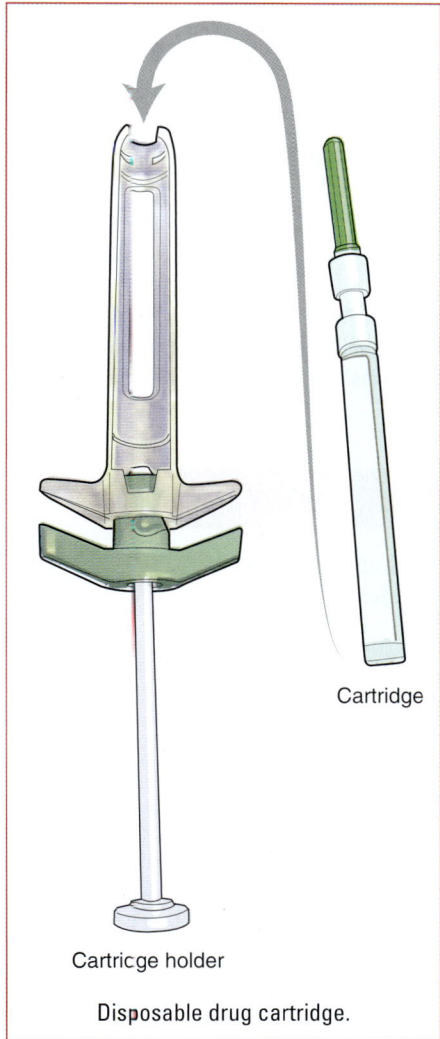

Cartridge

Cartricge holder

Disposable drug cartridge.

Liquid drugs do not need reconstitution. Additional dilution should only be done if the following occurs:
- Recommended by the drug manufacturer. Follow the instructions in the package insert or drug literature.
- The published evidence supports this additional dilution.
- Your facility has written policies and procedures for this dilution.

Multiple reports of medication errors have occurred due to unnecessary dilution. Eliminate this risk by administering these drugs as indicated in the drug manufacturer's instructions.

Labeling solution containers

The fluid container or syringe you prepare must have a label showing:
- patient's full name
- date
- name and amount of the I.V. solution used to dilute the medication
- name and dose of the drug
- rate of infusion
- beyond-use date.

Administration of all drugs prepared for urgent use must begin within 1 hour of when the preparation began. These drugs cannot be prepared in advance of their need due to risk of the growth of organisms.

Administering the medication

Medications can be infused by several methods including:
- through a continuous infusion of fluids by:
  - piggybacking
  - backpriming
  - manual injection or push
- through a locked VAD
  - primary intermittent infusion
  - manual injection or push.

First, assess the current infusion being delivered. If there is no continuous infusion, then the VAD has been locked after the previous medication was administered.

Selecting the right equipment

If you are starting a new continuous infusion and giving a medication, you will need to obtain the primary continuous administration set along with a piggyback or secondary set. For medication alone through a locked VAD, you will need only a regular administration set used for this purpose in your facility. Some facilities use the same set for both primary continuous and intermittent infusions, although it will be used differently.

Electronic infusion pump

Most facilities require all infusions — both continuous and intermittent infusions — be given on an infusion pump to ensure an accurate infusion rate. Make sure you are familiar with administration sets to be used on the pump, how to load the set into the pump, and how to program the pump. Usually, you will be entering the rate in milliliters per hour and the total volume to be infused. When this volume has infused, the pump will beep with an "infusion complete" alarm. There are other alarms on these pumps, so make sure you know how to interpret and manage these.

If you have a primary intermittent medication, the pump administration set may hold a third or half of the total volume to be infused, leaving a significant portion of the medication in the set. This situation requires use of a "carrier" fluid such as normal saline. Follow your facility policy and procedure for this situation. Usually, this will require setting up a continuous infusion of normal saline and then piggybacking the intermittent medication into the pump set. The normal saline is used to purge the air from the set and programmed to infuse after the medication container is empty, flushing the residual medication volume into the patient's bloodstream. The set is then disconnected and the VAD is locked until the next dose.

Filters

Some drugs require filtration during infusion. This requires having a filter in the administration set. The most common filter size with be 0.22 microns and will remove all particulate matter, air, and most microorganisms. When a medication requires filtration during infusion, this information should be provided by the pharmacy on the fluid container label or the electronic medication administration record. (See Chapter 1, *In-line Filters*, page 29.)

A few final steps

Before you administer medication by any method, a few additional steps are necessary:
- Use two methods to identify your patient. This may include checking his full name and facility identification number on his wristband; asking the patient to identify himself verbally, if possible; or asking the patient to provide his birthdate or address or some other information you can verify. Many facilities will use bar code technology for medication administration. Follow your facility's policy and procedure, and use extra caution when the patient can't identify himself.
- Check the patient's history of allergies and be aware that some medication names may be confusing. The brand name of some types of penicillins may not use the word "penicillin." For example, piperacillin sodium and tazobactam sodium are a combination antibiotics that are broad-spectrum penicillin.
- Make sure that you know the key information about the drug you are giving. You should know the purpose of the drug, normal dosage, expected side effects, adverse reactions, contraindications, and correct rate of administration and what aspects of monitoring are required for that drug. Check the provided drug resources

including the drug package insert, an infusion medication reference book, or computer-based drug information. If you have questions or concerns about the appropriateness of the drug for your patient, discuss these concerns with the pharmacists, the LIP, and/or your supervisor before administration.
- Know the risks associated with each drug. Are you giving a drug labeled as a hazardous medication? (See Change to See Chapter 6, *Protect yourself*, page 279.)
- Know the vesicant or irritant properties of the drug so you can correctly monitor the infusion site and intervene appropriately if the medication escapes into the subcutaneous tissue.
- Be sure to explain the procedure to the patient and answer any questions they have about the medication.
- Follow guidelines for protecting yourself from bloodborne pathogens. These guidelines require you to wear gloves (and possibly a gown and mask) when exposed to body fluids.
- Follow all guidelines for preventing intraluminal contamination and a subsequent bloodstream infection. This includes protecting the male luer end of the administration set with a sterile end cap when not in use and disinfection of the needleless connector or injection site by a vigorous scrub with a disinfectant before use.
- Assess the functionality of the VAD before each drug is administered. This includes observation of the site for all signs and symptoms of complications; palpation of the site for changes in temperature or induration (hardness); manually flushing the VAD to detect resistance and aspiration for blood return at the needleless injection site closest to the VAD; and paying careful attention to any patient complaints about the VAD or surrounding area.
- Assess the entire infusion system for cracks or leaking connections.
- Check the medication container for cloudiness or particulate matter in the solution.
- Check the beyond-use dates on the medication container. Notify the pharmacy if the BUD has expired.

Medications through a continuous infusion

Check the primary continuous infusion for any medication(s) that may be in this fluid container. Always make sure that the medication you are giving is compatible with the medication in the fluid container. If you detect an incompatibility, you may need to insert a second peripheral catheter or infuse through a separate lumen on the CVAD.

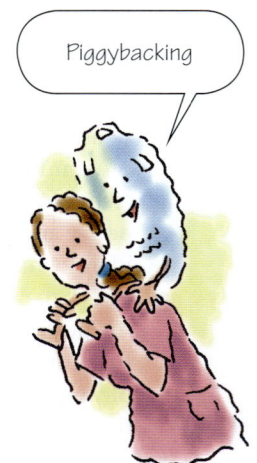

Piggybacking

Piggybacking medications

- Check patency at the needleless injection site closest to the VAD. Do not disconnect the set from the VAD hub. Assess for the history

of infusion pump alarms as their presence may indicate a problem with the patency of the VAD.
- Attach a piggyback or secondary set to the needleless injection site closest to the drip chamber on the administration set or above the infusion pump. When the primary continuous infusion is regulated by gravity and a manual roller clamp, you should have a back check valve inside the administration set, just above the upper injection site. This valve stops the flow from the primary line during infusion of the secondary drug and resumes the primary flow after drug infusion is completed. This administration set will require that you use a hook provided with the secondary set for the primary container.
- Disinfect the needleless injection site with an alcohol pad using a vigorous mechanical scrubbing motion. Scrub for the length of time designated by your facility's policy and procedure, usually 15 seconds. Allow the site to dry. Discard this alcohol pad.
- Connect the secondary set to this injection site. If needed, place the primary continuous fluid container on this hook and suspend it from the IV pole. Hang the secondary set from the IV pole.
- Program the infusion pump for the rate and volume needed for the secondary medication. Open the clamp on the secondary set and start the infusion.
- With a gravity infusion regulated by the roller clamp, the primary fluid begins flowing when the piggybacked medication is infused. Close the clamp on the secondary tubing, check the flow rate of the primary fluid and readjust as needed.
- Allow the secondary set to remain connected to the primary set after the infusion is complete. When these sets remain connected, the entire system may be used for 96 hours. Do not disconnect the primary continuous set from the VAD until it is time to change it. Disconnection for activities such as ambulating or toileting interrupts the prescribed infusion of needed fluids and medications and may increase the contamination of the system.

Tangle proof

Multiple continuous infusions may be necessary along with several intermittent infusions. Disconnection of these administration sets can easily mean a misconnection when it is reconnected. Many events of misconnections have been reported including attaching the tubing from a blood pressure cuff or oxygen delivery to the infusion line. Always trace all administration sets from one end to the other before making any connection. Label the sets with its contents below the drip chamber and on the male luer-locking end that is connected to the VAD hub.

Backpriming medications

When there are multiple secondary medications prescribed for your patient, you may be able to use the same secondary set to give all medications. Check the compatibility between each drug first. There will be a very small amount of drug from the previous dose left in the secondary set.

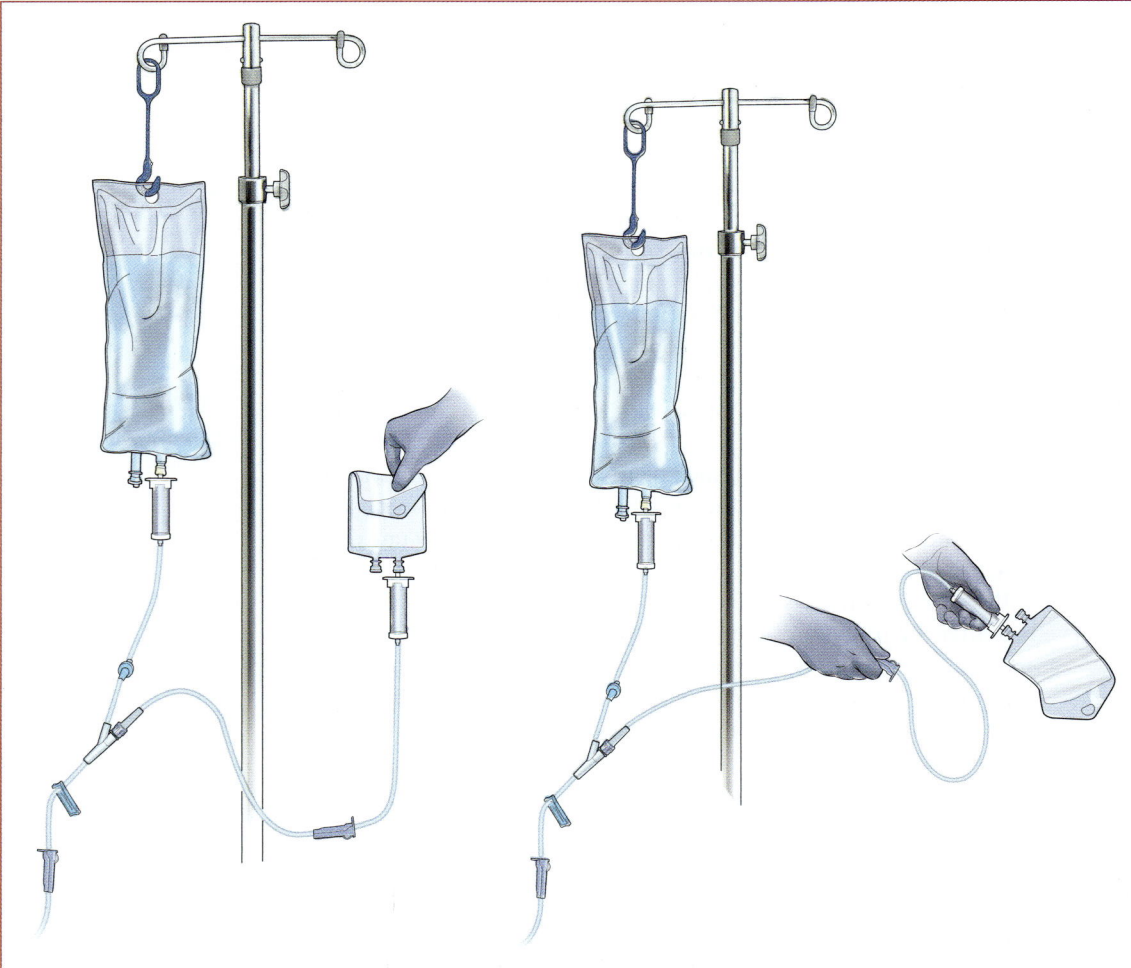

Backpriming a secondary set. **A.** Lowering the empty medication container below the primary fluid container. **B.** Opening the clamp to allow air and primary fluid to backflow through the piggyback set.

- Lower the empty medication container from the previous dose below the primary fluid container and open the clamp. This allows the primary fluid to backflow into the empty container, removing all air from the piggyback set. Remove and discard the

empty container, being careful to not allow the exposed spike to touch anything.
- Remove the cap from the container of the next medication and insert the spike.
- Suspend the secondary set from the IV pole and the primary fluid container on the hook, if needed.
- Regulate the secondary medication as needed.
- At the end of each medication, do NOT disconnect the secondary set. Leave it attached to the primary set so it can be used for the next dose.

Manual injection or push medications

- Choose the needleless injection site closest to the VAD and disinfect it.
- If there is medication in the primary continuous fluid that is incompatible with the medication to be manually pushed, and there is no other available lumen to use, stop the infusion. Attach a saline-filled syringe, aspirate for a blood return, and administer the saline by a slow push to clear the lumen of the incompatible medication.
- Detach the saline flush syringe and scrub the injection site again.
- Attach the medication-filled syringe and manually inject at the rate required for the drug being given. Use your watch or clock to time your rate of injection. Detach this syringe.
- Attach a second saline-filled syringe and flush to remove the medication remaining in the set. The rate of this saline flush should be the same as the rate used to deliver the medication. Detach this flush syringe and regulate the primary fluid flow.
- If there is no issue of compatibility, one saline-filled flush syringe is needed to assess VAD patency.

Medications through a locked VAD

When the patient no longer needs continuous infusion of fluids, the VAD is locked to maintain its patency between intermittent infusions. Both peripheral and central VADs may be locked. The locking solution is commonly normal saline or heparin 10 units per mL. The chosen lock solution depends upon the characteristics of the needleless connector in use and your facility policy and procedure. A common mnemonic to easily remember the sequence of solution is SASH or SAS:

S = saline
A= administer the medication
S= saline
H = heparin lock solution, if needed

Primary intermittent medication

- Suspend the medication container from the IV pole and purge the air from the administration set by allowing the medication to fill the set.
- Disinfect the needleless connector on the VAD hub.
- Attach a 10-mL saline-filled syringe. Flush 1 to 2 mL while observing for any resistance. If you have any difficulty, STOP and investigate the cause. NEVER forcefully flush any VAD for any reason as this can cause catheter damage or embolism to the patient's lungs.
    - Assess the external catheter and attached extension set. It could be a simple kink or a closed clamp. Next, you may need to remove the VAD dressing as the catheter itself could kink under the dressing near the insertion site. If no reason for the resistance is found, the cause could be inside the vein.
    - If you suspect a problem inside the vein, additional action is required. A peripheral catheter may be obstructed from clotted blood inside the lumen. Remove the catheter and insert a new one in a different location. A CVAD could have many problems including:
        - tip migration to a smaller vein or even complete erosion through the vein wall
        - pinch-off syndrome when the subclavian vein is the insertion site (See Chapter 3, *Common infusion problems*, page 158.)
        - intraluminal causes of CVAD occlusion (See Chapter 3, *Occlusions*, page 159.)
        - vein thrombosis (See Chapter 3, *Managing Common Problems with CVADs*, page 161.)
- If no resistance is felt, aspirate by slowly pulling back on the syringe plunger. Do NOT pull in a fast manner as this could prevent backflow of blood. Notice the color and consistency of the blood to assure that it is whole blood. Frothy or pinked tinge fluid is not what you want to see.
- Proceed with flushing the remainder of the saline into the VAD. Detach the syringe.
- Disinfect the needleless connector using a vigorous mechanical scrub with an alcohol pad.
- Remove the end cap from the administration set and attach it to the needleless connector. Regulate the flow rate of the medication according to the rate on the label.
- Note the expected time for completion of this infusion and return to assess it frequently. You must be present when the infusion runs out so you can disconnect the administration set and flush and

lock the VAD. Otherwise, blood can reflux into the VAD lumen where it will form a clot and obstruct the lumen.
- After the infusion is complete, detach the administration set. This administration set may be used for up to 24 hours but do not allow the male luer end to touch anything. Attach a new sterile end cap to protect it until the next use. Do not reuse the flush syringe tip cap for this purpose. Do not attach the male luer end to an injection site on the same set.
- Attach a 10-mL saline-filled syringe and flush the medication from the lumen of the VAD. Detach the syringe.
- If heparin lock solution is needed, attach this syringe and inject the contents into the VAD lumen.

Most commercially available prefilled saline and heparin syringes are designed to prevent syringe-induced blood reflux into the lumen. If using a traditional syringe filled by your pharmacy or yourself, it will cause syringe-induced blood reflux. This reflux is caused by compression of the gasket at the bottom of the syringe plunger. When you release pressure on the plunger, the gasket expands, pulling blood back into the VAD lumen. To prevent this from happening, do not flush all solution into the VAD on the last syringe. Leave at least 0.5 mL of fluid in the final syringe to prevent the gasket compression.
- Negative fluid displacement needleless connector — always close a clamp on the VAD or extension set first, and then disconnect the syringe to prevent blood reflux.
- Positive fluid displacement needleless connector — always disconnect the syringe first, and then close the clamp on the VAD or extension set to allow the positive displacement mechanism to work.
- Neutral displacement needleless connector — syringe and clamping can be in either sequence.

Manual injection or push medications
- Follow the same steps to disinfect the needleless connector, and assess for resistance and aspiration for a blood return.
- Attach the medication-filled syringe and inject it at the rate on the label. Use your watch or clock to time your rate of injection.
- Detach the medication syringe and attach the saline-filled syringe. Flush the saline using the same injection rate as medication. Follow with the heparin lock solution if needed.
- Use the same method for preventing syringe-induced and needleless connector reflux as described above.

Know statement
- Know which type of needleless connector you are using. This dictates the sequence of disconnecting the syringe.

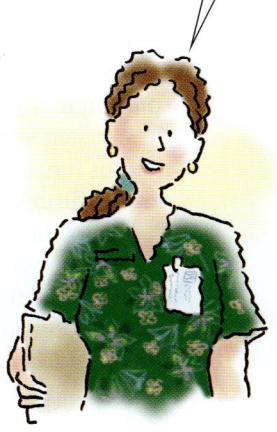

Disinfect all needleless connectors and injection sites before each entry using a new alcohol pad each time.

Flushing and locking the locked VAD

The purpose of flushing the VAD is to:
- assess patency of the lumen before infusion
- prevent contact between incompatible medications given through the same lumen
- ensure that all medication reaches the bloodstream and does not remain inside the VAD lumen.

The most common fluid for flushing is preservative-free normal saline, but always make sure that the medication is compatible with normal saline. An example of a group of drugs that are incompatible with normal saline is amphotericin B and all the amphotericin B lipid-based products. When giving these drugs, dextrose 5% in water must be used for flushing the VAD lumen. There is just one concern — don't allow the dextrose solution to remain inside the lumen for locking purposes as the dextrose will provide nutrients for the growth of microorganisms. Always follow the dextrose solution with normal saline.

The volume of normal saline flush is usually 2 to 5 mL for a peripheral catheter and up to 10 mL for a CVAD. If infusing viscous fluids, such as parenteral nutrition or blood, 20 mL may be needed to thoroughly flush all residual fluid from the lumen.

Flushing is performed before and after each infusion medication and may be done at other times such as when the infusion rate slows down or an infusion pump has occlusion alarms. NEVER use force when flushing any catheter!

The purpose of locking is primarily to maintain the patency of the lumen without infusing fluids. A smaller quantity of locking solution is instilled so that it remains inside the lumen. The volume is slightly more than the internal volume of the VAD lumen. Two to three mL is sufficient for all VAD lumens. Normal saline is the preferred locking solution for short peripheral catheters, so this is done with the same saline-filled syringe used to flush the catheter. For CVADs, the lock solution may be normal saline or heparin 10 units per mL. Locking is the last step when giving an intermittent medication without a continuous infusion. Locking is not necessary when fluids are continuously infusing.

Facility policy and procedures may call for flushing and locking at specific intervals (for example, every 8 or 12 hours) in addition to when the medication is given. Evidence does not support the need for this additional flushing and locking and it requires additional hub manipulation that could introduce more organisms into the lumen. When all fluids and medications have been stopped, and the VAD is not being used for any type of infusion, it is imperative that the VAD be removed to reduce the risk of bloodstream infection. The only exception to this would be those CVADs requiring surgical insertion and removal (that is, tunneled cuffed catheters and implanted ports) that will be needed for periodic infusions in the future.

Another purpose for locking a CVAD lumen may be to treat or prevent a bloodstream infection. A variety of solutions may be prescribed for this purpose including many antibiotics in very high concentrations. These antibiotics may or may not be mixed with heparin solution. Other locking solutions include ethanol, citrate, tauroline and ethylenediaminetetraacetic acid (EDTA) used alone or in combination. These solutions are not commercially available and must be compounded by the pharmacy.

Always follow your facility policy and procedure for flushing and locking each VAD.

Patient-controlled analgesia (PCA)

PCA therapy allows your patient to control IV delivery of an analgesic (usually morphine) and maintain therapeutic serum levels of the drug. The computer-controlled PCA pump delivers medication through the administration set that is attached directly to the VAD hub. The patient can then push a button to receive a dose of analgesic. A timing unit prevents the patient from accidentally overdosing by imposing a lockout time between doses — usually 6 to 10 minutes During this interval, the patient won't receive any analgesic despite pushing the button.

Occasionally, a patient may receive PCA therapy through an epidural catheter or subcutaneously. A smaller ambulatory version of the PCA pump is available for use in hospice, palliative, and home care

Picking patients for PCA therapy

PCA therapy is indicated for patients who require parenteral pain control. Patients commonly use it after surgery and those with chronic diseases, particularly patients with terminal cancer or sickle cell anemia.

To receive PCA therapy, a patient must:
- have severe pain, either constant or intermittent
- be able to understand and comply with instructions and procedures
- be capable of manually pressing the button to activate the drug delivery
- not be sedated from other medications.

Some patients have increased risk with PCA use and require close monitoring. Oversedation is possible in patients with:

- a history of sleeping disorders such as obstructive sleep apnea
- cardiac or respiratory disease
- kidney or liver failure
- older adults
- thoracic or abdominal surgery
- lengthy duration of anesthesia during surgery
- presence of morbid obesity.

A history of opioid abuse and/or addiction is not a contraindication for use of PCA in a postoperative patient. Pain management in these patients requires a comprehensive interprofessional approach.

A patient with any alteration in pulmonary function requires careful evaluation for the use of PCA. Opioid-induced respiratory depression (OIRD) is a serious concern in patients with a history of respiratory disease and/or thoracic surgery. Frequent assessment of respiratory function is necessary in observing for:
- respiratory rate of less than 10 per minute or very shallow breaths
- increasing levels of sedation
- snoring or other noises during respiration.

When these conditions are identified, the patient should be aroused and instructed to take deep breaths. Intermittent or continuous pulse oximetry monitoring and end-tidal carbon dioxide monitoring can help to identify changes in respiratory patterns and prevent serious OIRD.

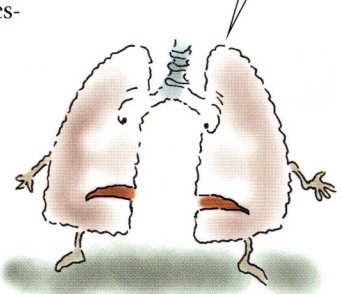

Patients with any alternation in pulmonary function need to be carefully evaluated for PCA use.

PCA "pluses"

Patients receiving PCA therapy use fewer opioids for pain relief than other patients. Also on the upside, PCA therapy provides these advantages:
- It eliminates the need for I.M. analgesics.
- It provides individualized pain relief; each patient receives the appropriate dosage for his size and pain tolerance.
- It decreases the time between the onset of pain and the administration of the analgesic.
- It gives the patient a sense of control over pain.
- It allows the patient to sleep at night while minimizing daytime drowsiness.

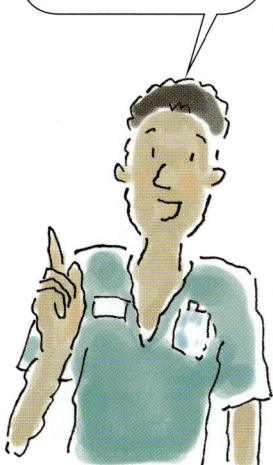

Patients who receive PCA therapy get individualized pain relief and feel a greater sense of control over their pain.

PCA "minuses"

The main adverse effect of opioid analgesics is respiratory depression. Therefore, you must routinely monitor your patient's respiratory rate.

In addition to the effects on the respiratory system, opioid analgesics can lower blood pressure. Also, if the opioid analgesic makes your patient nauseated, he may need an antiemetic drug.

A complete order

The LIP order for PCA should include the:
- loading dose, if any, to be programmed into the PCA pump
- lockout interval, during which the PCA device can't be activated (for example, every 6 to 10 minutes)
- maintenance dose, if a continuous infusion of opioid analgesia is needed
- individual dose or the amount the patient will receive when the device is activated (for example, 1 mg morphine)
- maximum amount the patient can receive within a specified time (usually the amount the patient can receive on demand or the maintenance dose or a combination of both over 60 minutes).

PCA by proxy

In general, only the patient should control the button to deliver the dose of analgesic, based on the concept that the patient will be too sedated to deliver excessive doses. Currently, this practice is changing to allow for authorized agent-controlled analgesia (AACA). The American Society of Pain Management Nursing has identified the benefits of these additional agents when the patient cannot participate in controlling the drug delivery. These agents must be someone who is competent to learn the process and consistently available and may include the nurse, a parent, or family caregiver.

Focusing on the features

PCA pumps are available with a variety of features:
- Some pumps provide continuous infusion and bolus doses. Others provide only bolus doses.
- PCA pumps that provide continuous infusion and bolus doses may offer several volume settings.
- The pump may have a panel that displays the amount delivered or, if necessary, an alarm message.
- You can program certain pumps to record the concentration in milligrams (mg) or milliliters (mL), allowing greater flexibility in choosing rates. Make sure the pump is correctly programmed!
- With some pumps, you can vary the length of the lockout interval from 5 to 90 minutes.

- Pumps can be programmed to store and retrieve information such as the total dose allowed in a specified length of time.
- Most pumps can provide the total volume infused to include the opioid analgesia in intake and output measurements.

Managing PCA therapy

With PCA, the patient self-administers drug delivery by pressing a button on a handheld controller that is connected to the pump. Before the device can be used, it must be programmed to deliver specified doses at specified time intervals.

Independent double checks are necessary for:
- starting a new PCA pump
- changing the prescribed dose or lockout interval
- replacing a filled medication container with a new one.

These checks must be done by two people separate and independent of each other.

Giving an added boost

If the patient is using a pump that provides continuous infusion and bolus doses, make sure that he understands that he's receiving medication continuously, but that he can give himself intermittent bolus doses for incidental pain (from coughing, for example) using the patient control button.

If you program the pump to deliver a continuous infusion plus intermittent doses, remember this rule: The cumulative doses per hour administered by a PCA pump should not exceed the total hourly dose ordered by the LIP. For example, if a total of 6 mg of morphine over 1 hour is prescribed, the order may begin therapy with a continuous infusion of 3 mg/hour, allowing intermittent doses of 0.5 mg every 10 minutes.

Not the controlling type? That's okay

A PCA pump that provides continuous infusion and intermittent doses will provide analgesia regardless of whether the patient uses the control button. This type of PCA is useful for helping patients cope with steady pain that gradually increases or decreases, incidental pain, or pain that's worse at different times. If the patient's pain is intermittent, he may not need continuous infusion.

Check the record first

Before allowing the patient to self-administer opioid analgesics with a PCA pump, review his medication regimen. Concurrent use of two central nervous system (CNS) depressants may cause drowsiness, oversedation, disorientation, and anxiety.

Explain and reassure

Explain to the patient how often he can self-administer the pain medication. Reassure him that the lockout interval will prevent him from administering medication too frequently.

Determining doses

A patient-specific plan for monitoring the patient should be determined by their risk factors and the analgesic being given. Your assessment of the patient's condition and activity level will aid the LIP to determine the initial loading dose and time interval between intermittent doses. Your ongoing frequent assessment may indicate a need to contact the LIP for a change in the prescribed intermittent dose or lockout interval.

Looking into the lockout interval

Here are general guidelines for determining an appropriate lockout interval. These guidelines apply to pumps that provide bolus doses only and pumps that provide bolus doses plus continuous infusions:
- For I.V. doses, set the lockout interval as prescribed by the LIP, usually 6 to 10 minutes.
- For subcutaneous doses, a common lockout interval is 30 minutes or more.
- For epidural doses, a common lockout interval is 60 minutes or more.

What to monitor (and be sure to record!)

During therapy, monitor and record:
- amount of analgesic infused
- patient's respiratory rate, counted for a full minute
- patient's assessment of pain relief using the pain scale for your facility
- use of a sedation scale to determine the patient's level of consciousness.

If the patient doesn't feel that pain has been sufficiently relieved, notify the LIP for a change in the dosage.

Remember to monitor the patient's vital signs, especially when first starting therapy. Encourage the patient to practice coughing and deep breathing. These exercises promote ventilation and prevent pooling of secretions, which could lead to respiratory difficulty.

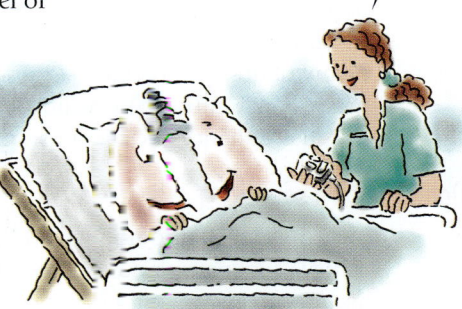

Coughing and deep breathing help prevent respiratory difficulties caused by PCA administration.

PCA complications

The primary complication of PCA administration is respiratory depression. If the patient's respiratory rate declines to 10 or fewer breaths per minute, call his name, touch him, and have him breathe deeply. If he is confused, restless, or can't be aroused, stop the infusion, notify the LIP, and prepare to give oxygen. Administer an opioid antagonist, such as naloxone, if prescribed.

Possible complications include:
- anaphylaxis
- nausea
- vomiting
- constipation
- orthostatic hypotension
- drug tolerance.

A note about nausea

If prescribed, give the patient who experiences nausea an antiemetic such as dolasetron. If the patient has persistent nausea and vomiting during therapy, the LIP may change the analgesic.

Patient teaching

Make sure that the patient and caregiver fully understand:
- how the pump works
- when to contact the clinician
- signs and symptoms of adverse reactions
- signs and symptoms of drug tolerance.

Tell the patient that he'll be able to control his pain and that the pump is safe and effective. Also, remind him that an opioid analgesic relieves pain best when it's taken before the pain becomes intense.

Because an opioid analgesic may cause orthostatic hypotension, tell the patient to get up slowly from his bed or a chair. Instruct him to eat a high-fiber diet, drink plenty of fluids, and take a stool softener, if one has been prescribed. Caution him against drinking alcohol because this may enhance CNS depression.

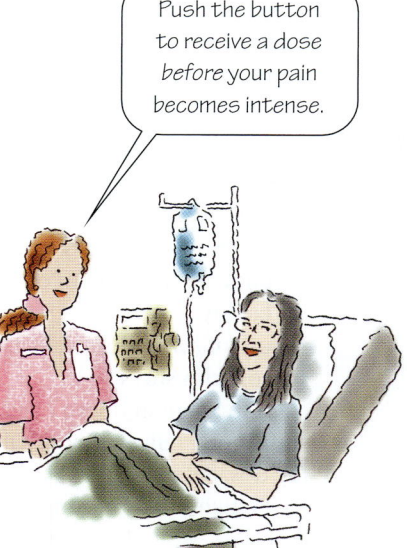

Push the button to receive a dose before *your pain becomes intense.*

Don't keep it a secret

The clinician should notify the LIP if the patient fails to achieve adequate pain relief. In home care, the patient and/or caregiver should have written information about when and who to contact in case of problems.

The patient's caregiver should report signs of overdose, such as:
- slow or irregular breathing
- pinpoint pupils
- loss of consciousness.

Teach the caregiver how to maintain respiration until help arrives should the need arise.

Did it work?

Evaluate the effectiveness of the drug at regular intervals. Ask these questions:
- Is the patient getting relief?
- Does the dosage need to be increased because of persistent or worsening pain?
- Is the patient developing a tolerance to the drug?
- Is the patient's condition stable?

Managing complications of fluids and medication

Complications can be caused by the VAD or the medication itself. VAD complications are discussed in previous chapters. For peripheral VAD complications, see Chapter 2, *Complications of therapy*, page 107. For CVAD complications, see Chapter 3, *Risks of I.V. therapy via the central venous system*, page 164.

Some complications may not have a clear cause. For instance, phlebitis can be caused by:
- mechanical reasons such as site selection for a peripheral catheter in an area of joint flexion
- chemical reasons such as the dilution and rate of medication infusion, or the size of the catheter being too large for the vein and obstructing the blood flow that would provide additional dilution for the medication
- microorganisms introduced during VAD insertion or through the lumen when the medication is given.

Infiltration and extravasation have similar overlapping causes. Remember to learn the nature of the medication you are giving Is it an irritant or a vesicant? An irritant will increase the risk of inflammation to the internal lining of the vein wall and possibly lead to thrombophlebitis. A vesicant can cause tissue destruction once it escapes from the vein and comes into contact with subcutaneous tissue.

Adverse events

Drugs given by all infusion techniques and into all sites quickly produce therapeutic blood levels. This requires vigilance in monitoring your patient for these outcomes along with educating the patient about what to expect. A variety of adverse events can happen:
- side effects
- adverse reactions
- hypersensitivity reactions.

Side effects

Side effects are usually unintended consequences of the medication. They occur in addition to the prescribed purpose of the medication. Common side effects include gastrointestinal disturbances such as nausea, vomiting, and diarrhea from antibiotics. They are usually expected because they have been reported during the studies on the drug and are included in the drug literature. Sometimes, these side effects may prove to be beneficial for other conditions. During pregnancy, steroids like dexamethasone can be harmful, but this drug can enhance pulmonary maturation in the fetus when premature labor could result in incomplete growth and development. In this situation, the harmful effects are used for a beneficial outcome.

Adverse drug reactions

Adverse drug reaction or adverse drug event is an unexpected and often dangerous reaction to a medication. These reactions may or may not be caused by an immune response. Examples include liver toxicity from methotrexate and red man syndrome (RMS) from vancomycin or opioids. RMS is a pseudoallergic reaction or an anaphylactoid reaction. The signs and symptoms are similar to an allergic reaction but not associated with the antibody-antigen complex.

Idiosyncratic reactions are adverse drug reactions that commonly involve the skin, liver, and blood cells. These reactions may be delayed, may reappear rapidly if the drug is stopped and then restarted at a later time, and are not related to dose. The word "idiosyncratic" means it is specific to an individual and very difficult to predict.

Hypersensitivity

Hypersensitivity to infusion drugs may also be known as allergic reactions (Table 4-4). Expanding knowledge of the immune system allows for greater clarification of these reactions. The term

Table 4-4 Types of hypersensitivity

Type; other names	Cause	Reaction time	Drugs involved	Signs and symptoms
I: Immediate, anaphylaxis	IgE antibody	Seconds to a few minutes	Antibiotics, neuromuscular-blocking agents, monoclonal antibodies, proton pump inhibitors	Erythema, angioedema, hypotension, bronchospasm, upper airway symptoms, itching, raised wheals, nausea and vomiting, tachycardia or bradycardia, abdominal pain
II: Cytotoxic or antibody-dependent cytotoxicity	IgM or IgG antibodies	Minutes to hours	Vancomycin, acetaminophen, sulfonamides, phenothiazines	Hemolytic anemia, thrombocytopenia, granulocytopenia
III: Immune complex hypersensitivity	IgG antibodies	Several hours	Penicillins, cephalosporins, ciprofloxacin, monoclonal antibodies	Erythema, Edema, Serum sickness, Vasculitis
IV: Delayed, cell mediated	T cell	24 to 72 hours	Antibiotics, anticonvulsants, quinolones	Induration, Perivascular inflammation

"anaphylaxis" and "anaphylactoid" are commonly used terms indicating a severe allergic reaction. Although the clinical signs and symptoms are very similar, they have very different causes. Anaphylaxis is a systemic, immediate, severe reaction to potent substances that causes histamine release from mast cells and basophils. This reaction is frequently linked to IgE immune globulins but may be caused by IgG and other immune proteins. Anaphylactoid reactions produce the same immediate and severe reactions with the same signs and symptom; however, the release of histamine from the mast cells and basophils has a different cause. Red man syndrome is an example of an anaphylactoid reaction due to direct chemical stimulation of the mast cells and basophils from the drug itself. Red man syndrome can be caused by vancomycin, opioids, pentamidine, and atropine.

More than just the drug!

Infusion medications contain more than just the active ingredient itself. Excipients are additives to provide long-term stability, to reduce viscosity, or to enhance its solubility. Sulfites, parabens, and benzyl alcohol are preservatives. All of these additional components could be responsible for an adverse reaction. Complications specific to the fluid and medication are listed in Table 4-5.

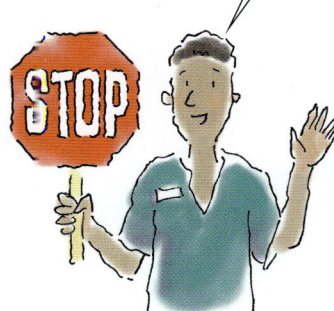

At the first sign of hypersensitivity, STOP the infusion (but don't remove the VAD).

Table 4-5 Managing complications of infusion fluid and medications

Complication	Signs and symptoms	Nursing interventions
Circulatory overload, pulmonary edema	Neck vein distention or engorgement Respiratory distress, cough Oxygen saturation <90% Moist crackles in the lungs Increased blood pressure, heart rate, full bounding pulse Weight gain Anxiety, restlessness	Prevention • Monitor intake and output when receiving infusion fluids. • Monitor and control fluid flow rate accurately. Management • Position the patient in semi-Fowler's position as tolerated. • Reassure the patient to reduce anxiety. • Notify the LIP. • Decrease or stop infusion as ordered. • Administer oxygen as ordered. • Administer diuretics as ordered.
Hypersensitivity/allergic reaction	Itching Red rash Flushing Tearing eyes, runny nose Rapid heart rate, low blood pressure Dizziness, weakness, syncope Anxiety Bronchospasm Wheezing Rapid progression to life-threatening airway constriction, cardiac arrest	• Prevention • Assess history of previous reactions to drugs, food, and others (that is, latex). • Administer drugs with a known risk of infusion reactions (that is, biologic agents) in a setting where immediate treatment is available. • Assess immediate availability of drugs to treat these reactions. • Educate patient about signs, symptoms, and reporting history of these reactions. • Administer first dose of drugs in a controlled setting. Management • Stop the infusion immediately; do not remove VAD. • Maintain a patent airway. • Monitor vital signs. • Activate rapid response as needed. • Notify the LIP. • Administer an epinephrine SC as ordered. • Administer antihistamine, and/or steroid as ordered. An anti-inflammatory and antipyretic may also be prescribed.
Speed shock	Severe headache Syncope Flushed neck and face Tightness in chest Irregular pulse Shock Cardiac arrest	• Prevention • Know drug information before administration. • Use an infusion pump for high-risk drugs. • Do not bypass drug library or alert settings when using a "smart" pump. • Assess the infusion rate of continuous fluids and administer push and piggyback medications at the correct rate. Management • Stop the infusion immediately but do not remove the VAD. • Activate the rapid response team. • Notify the LIP. • Administer antidote as prescribed.

Documentation

After you administer a drug by any infusion route, always document the procedure, including:
- date and time for starting each fluid container
- rate of fluid infusion and the method used to control the rate
- drug(s) added to the primary continuous fluids
- intermittent drug and dosage
- diluent for each intermittent drug
- rate of infusion or injection for each drug
- VAD site and/or lumen used for each primary infusion and each drug given
- condition of the VAD site and presence of a blood return
- duration of administration
- patient's response, including adverse reactions
- your name.

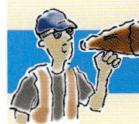

That's a wrap!

Infusion fluids
Types of infusion fluids:
- crystalloid
- colloid
- isotonic
- hypertonic
- hypotonic.

I.V. fluids are given for:
- replacement of fluid losses
- maintenance of fluid balance.

Infusion medications
Benefits:
- achieve rapid therapeutic drug levels
- are absorbed more effectively than drugs given by other routes.

Risks are caused by:
- lack of patient and drug information
- confusing or ambiguous drug information
- inadequate labeling after preparation
- incorrect use of vials and ampules
- absence of clear information on use of infusion pumps for drug delivery
- inadequate staff training and other risk management methods.

Important issues for infusing medications include:
- stability
- compatibility including physical, chemical and therapeutic types.

Infusion medication administration methods
- Through a continuous infusion of fluids by
  - piggybacking
  - backpriming
  - manual injection or push.
- Through a locked VAD
  - primary intermittent infusion
  - manual injection or push.

236 Infusion fluids and medications

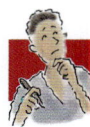

Quick quiz

1. I.V. medication may be indicated when:
    A. the patient needs a slower therapeutic effect.
    B. the medication can't be absorbed by the GI tract.
    C. the medication given orally is stable in gastric juices.
    D. the medication isn't irritating to muscle tissues.

Answer: B. I.V. medication has a rapid effect and may be indicated if the medication can't be absorbed by the GI tract, is unstable in gastric juices, or causes pain or tissue damage when given I.M. or subQ.

2. What's the preferred route of medication in emergencies?
    A. I.V.
    B. SubQ
    C. I.M.
    D. Oral

Answer: A. The I.V. route allows therapeutic levels to be achieved rapidly.

3. Loading dose, lockout interval, and maintenance doses are basic to:
    A. I.V. therapy.
    B. PCA therapy.
    C. continuous I.V. morphine drips.
    D. TPN.

Answer: B. These concepts are basic to PCA therapy.

4. An infusion medication compounded by the clinician is done for:
    A. all medications.
    B. only those given by manual injection or push.
    C. only those used in intensive care.
    D. only urgent situation when the need is immediate.

Answer: D. According to the USP <797>, all compounding of medications is done in a laminar airflow workbench in the pharmacy. The only time a clinician should be performing this step is when the patient need is urgent and there is no time to obtain the medication from the pharmacy.

5. Before giving any infusion medications into a VAD, assess:
    A. the integrity of the dressing.
    B. the flow rate on the fluids.
    C. the absence of resistance when flushed and the presence of a blood return.
    D. the settings on the infusion pump.

Answer: C. According to the Infusion Nurses Society Standards of Practice, flushing to determine any resistance to flow and aspiration for a blood return is required for a complete assessment of VAD patency.

Scoring

⭐⭐⭐ If you answered all six questions correctly, wow! Whether you used a direct, intermittent, or continuous approach, you caught the essence of this chapter.

⭐⭐ If you answered four or five questions correctly, great! You're right in line—no significant absorption problems.

⭐ If you answered fewer than four questions correctly, don't panic! There are six more quick quizzes to go.

Suggested References

Dolan, S. A., Arias, K. M., Felizardo, G., Barnes, S., Kraska, S., Patrick, M., & Bumsted, A. (2016). APIC position paper: safe injection, infusion, and medication vial practices in health care. *American Journal of Infection Control, 44*(7):750–757.

Gorski, L., Hadaway, L., Hagle, M., McGoldrick, M., Meyer, B., & Orr, M. (2016). *Policies and procedures for infusion therapy* (5th ed.). Norwood, MA: Infusion Nurses Society.

Gorski, L., Hadaway, L., Hagle, M., McGoldrick, M., Orr, M., & Doellman, D. (2016). Infusion therapy standards of practice. *Journal of Infusion Nursing, 39*(1S), 159.

ISMP. (2015). *Safe practice guidelines for adult IV push medications.* Horsham, PA: Institute for Safe Medication Practices.

Phillips, L., & Gorski, L. (2014). *Manual of I.V. Therapeutics* (6th ed.). Philadelphia, PA: FA Davis.

Weinstein, S. M., & Hagle, M. (2014). *Plumer's principles and practice of infusion therapy* (9th ed.). Philadelphia, PA: Wolters Kluwer Health.

Chapter 5

Transfusions

Just the facts

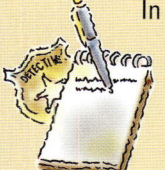

In this chapter, you'll learn:
- blood composition and physiology
- signs of common transfusion complications and appropriate responses to them
- administration of blood components
- special considerations for pediatric and older adult patients.

Understanding transfusion therapy

The circulatory system is the body's main mover of blood and its components. It is made up of the heart, which pumps blood, and a large road map of veins, arteries and capillaries that the blood travels through, known as the bloodstream. The bloodstream carries oxygen, nutrients, hormones, and other vital substances to all other tissues and organs of the body. When illness or injury decreases the volume, oxygen-carrying capacity, or vital components of blood, transfusion therapy may be the only solution.

Purpose of transfusion therapy

Blood products are transfused for a number of reason which include:
- restoring and maintain fluid volume
- improving oxygen-carrying capacity
- replacing deficient blood components
- assisting with coagulation.

Blood composition

The average adult body contains about 5 L of blood. Even though blood looks like a simple liquid, it is actually a complex fluid. Blood is made up of three types of cells that are suspended in a watery fluid. There is no manufactured fluid on the market that can take the place of blood; some fluids can replace

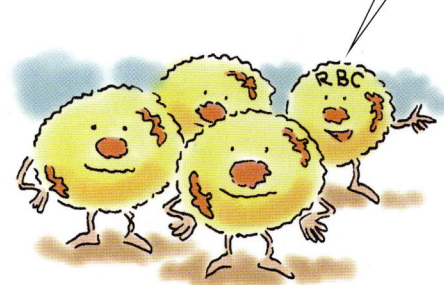

A transfusion may be the only solution when illness or injury, such as from hemorrhage, trauma, or burns, decreases the oxygen-carrying capacity of the blood.

volume, but they cannot improve oxygen-carrying capacity or replace deficient components.

It's elementary!

Three cellular components make up about 45% of the blood volume. They are:
- erythrocytes, or red blood cells (RBCs)
- leukocytes, or white blood cells (WBCs)
- thrombocytes (platelets).

The red cells in the blood provide oxygen for the body. When a person breathes in, air surges into the lungs. The blood harvests the oxygen from the air and carries it on hemoglobin, a molecule on the red cell. As blood travels, it releases this oxygen throughout the body. If blood is unable to provide enough oxygen for the body, a red cell transfusion may be ordered.

The oxygen-carrying capacity of blood may be depleted as a result of respiratory disorders, sepsis, carbon monoxide poisoning, acute anemia due to blood loss, or sickle cell anemia or other chronic diseases.

The liquid component of blood is called plasma. It is mostly water with many elements that are dissolved or suspended in it. Some of these include:
- proteins (i.e., albumin, globulin, and fibrinogen).
- lipids
- electrolytes
- coagulation factors.

A plasma transfusion does not restore the oxygen-carrying capacity of blood, but it does provide water and other products the body may need.

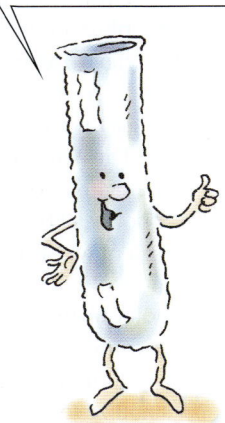

About 55% of the total blood volume is plasma, the liquid component of blood. The remaining 45% consists of formed, cellular elements — RBCs, WBCs, and platelets.

Blood components

Most commonly, after blood is donated, it is divided into component parts for storage. Blood that is left intact is called whole blood. The components of whole blood are:
- Packed red blood cells (RBCs)
- Plasma
- Cryoprecipitate
- Platelets
- Granulocytes.

There are several benefits to separating blood into its component parts:
- The recipient doesn't receive unnecessary fluid volume.
- Compatibility is easier to assure.
- The risk of a reaction is reduced.
- Individual components have more benefit when given separately.
- The blood supply will last longer.
- More patients will benefit.

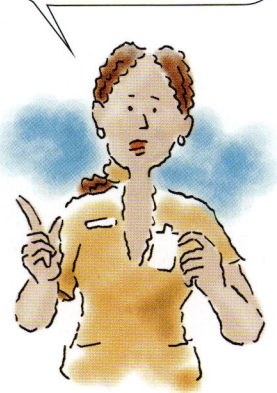

Don't get confused: platelets are cells, and coagulation factors are proteins. Both are necessary to make the blood clot, but they are not the same thing!

Feed me!

After blood is removed from the body, it is essential to provide an environment that will support the life of the cell and assure that the transfusion will be therapeutic. Immediately after collection of whole blood, a nutrient admixture called CPDA-1 is added directly to the bag. This solution allows a unit of whole blood to be stored at 6°C for 35 days and retains 70% viability of the red cells by the time the unit expires.

There are four main ingredients, each with a specific job to do:
- citrate: binds with calcium in blood to prevent clotting of the unit
- phosphate: helps maintain pH
- dextrose: provides nutrition to cells
- adenine: supports structural integrity of cells by promoting synthesis of adenine triphosphate (ATP).

The percentage of red cells to CPDA must be accurate to provide the right amount of preservative without altering the pH. Therefore, the amount of blood withdrawn must be within a specific parameter. The unit of whole blood in CPDA can be stored for up to 35 days at a temperature of 6°C. After phlebotomy, the plasma is often expressed off of the unit of whole blood leaving only the red cell mass in the original phlebotomy bag. Because a portion of the CPDA is removed with the plasma, an additional nutrient admixture (e.g., AdSol®) is added to the red cells to stabilize the environment. This solution extends the viability of the cells so that packed red blood cells can be stored for 42 days at 6°C.

(Text continues on page 242)

Whole blood and its component parts

Component	Comments	Indication	Storage
Whole blood	• Contains all cells and plasma • High risk of transfusion reaction • Rarely administered except from autologous donor • 1 unit = 450 mL; hence the term "a pint of blood"	• Needed for oxygen-carrying capacity as well as fluid • If product is fresh, it may provide coagulation factors as well as platelets.	• A nutrient admixture in the collection bag helps preserve the cells. • Contains citrate, phosphate, dextrose, and adenine to support functioning of blood cell • Refrigerate at 1°C–6°C for 21–35 days depending on preservative.
Packed red blood cells (RBCs or PRBCs)	• RBCs contain hemoglobin, the molecule that carries oxygen and gives blood its red color. • Red cells are viable for 120 days in vivo. • "Packing" the cells removes the plasma. • 1 unit = 200–225 mL	Transfusion increases red cell mass to improve oxygen-carrying capacity of blood.	• Second nutrient admixture added after plasma removed to increase storage time. • Contains additional ingredients that further prolong red cell viability • Refrigerate at 1°C–6°C for 42 days.

Whole blood and its component parts (continued)

Component	Comments	Indication	Storage
Glycerized red cells	• Glycerol added to the RBCs allows for freezing without damage to cells.	Same as RBCs	Store frozen for 10 years.
Fresh frozen plasma (FFP)	• Fluid portion of blood • Contains albumin, fibrinogen, and coagulation factors V and VIII and other coagulation factors	• Restores volume • Keeps fluid in vascular space • Increases blood pressure • Corrects coagulation deficiencies associated with massive bleeding • The risk of immune reaction with plasma products is relatively high. Therefore, the use of manufactured plasma derivatives (albumin, IVIG et al) is preferred.	• Store frozen for 12 months. • Must be frozen within 8 hours of collection
Cryoprecipitate	• Derived from FFP that is slowly thawed and rapidly spun • The coagulation factors form a precipitate that can be collected into a separate sterile bag. • Contains fibrinogen, factor VIIIc, factor VIIvWF, factor XIII and fibronectin • Usual dose = 10–20 units	• Treatment of factor VIII deficiency and fibrinogen disorders • Treatment of significant factor XIII deficiency • The risk of immune reaction with plasma products is relatively high. Therefore, the use of manufactured plasma derivatives (for example, factor VIII, factor IX) is preferred.	Store frozen for 12 months
Granulocytes	• White blood cells (actually more clear than white) are collectively known as leukocytes. • Five cell types exist; three are classified as granulocytes, so named because of the granules present in the cytoplasm. • The main granulocyte is the neutrophil, which is the immediate defense against invading organisms.	• Eligible patients meet three criteria: 1. They have a serious infection not responding to antibiotics 2. Their bone marrow is not able to make its own granulocytes 3. The probability that the bone marrow will eventually be able to produce granulocytes again	• Store at room temperature, under constant gentle agitation to reduce formation of white blood cell debris. • White cells are very fragile after removal from the body. • Must be transfused within 24 hours
Platelets	• Small cells that aggregate, or clump, when bleeding occurs to form a plug • Found in red cell mass but not active in stored RBCs • Viable for 8–10 days in vivo	Restore platelet count that is reduced due to trauma, disease, or medication.	• Store at room temperature, under constant gentle agitation, to prevent clumping. • Use within 5 days of donation

Take it away!

Blood can be donated with one of two intentions: to give it to someone else or to store it for personal use.
- Autologous blood is donated and stored for personal use; from "auto" which means "self." The donor and the recipient are the same person.
- Allogenic blood is donated and stored for someone else to use; from "allo" which means "other." The donor and the recipient are not the same person.

Bank on this!

Blood used for transfusion is stored in a blood bank and infused into a patient by a process called transfusion. These products are dispensed by the blood bank with an LIP's order. Banked blood is administered directly back into the bloodstream, usually through some type of catheter placed in a vein. AABB (formerly known as the American Association of Blood Banks) determines how banked blood products will be collected, processed, stored, and used.

The corner drugstore...

Sometimes the plasma portion of blood is manufactured into medications, which will be stored in a pharmacy. Some of these medications include:
- immune globulin (IVIG)
- antihemophiliac factors
- albumin
- certain vaccines.

These products are dispensed by a pharmacy with an LIP's order. The United States Pharmacopeia (USP) sets standards that govern how the products are stored and dispensed. Pharmacy blood products may be administered by an infusion into the vein or by injection (intramuscularly or subcutaneously); none are given by mouth. Package inserts are provided with all pharmacy products to answer questions about administration.

A word of caution...

Banked blood products are very different from pharmaceutical blood products. Banked blood is a biological substance, meaning that it is part of a living organism.

One potential risk of blood transfusion is the transmission of pathogens from the donor to the recipient. These pathogens include viruses, bacteria, fungi and parasites. Every unit of blood is carefully screened for these pathogens before being accepted into the blood supply. Any unit that tests positive or is suspicious is immediately discarded. Testing is very accurate these days. The decrease in autologous donations shows that the public has become more confident in the safety of our blood supply.

The first transmissible pathogen to be discovered in donor blood was syphilis in the 1930s. Today, all units of blood are tested for syphilis, but the risk of transfusion-associated infection is considered nearly obsolete; no cases of transmission have been reported in over 40 years. Other bacteria may enter donated blood from the patient's skin or from bacteria present in the donor's bloodstream. Use of aseptic technique when drawing blood, screening donors for the possibility of infection, and use of quality-control measures on all components have greatly reduced the risk of bacterial transmission.

Hepatitis B virus (HBV), hepatitis C virus (HCV), human immunodeficiency virus (HIV) and human T-lymphotropic virus (HTLV) have been a concern for blood safety since the late 1970s. Although the potential for transmission of these viruses has not been eliminated, the risk is extremely low due to new testing processes that are available.

One virus that does not disqualify a unit of blood from entry to the blood bank is cytomegalovirus (CMV). The majority of blood donors have been exposed to this virus. If all blood that was CMV positive were destroyed, the blood supply would be very limited. Luckily, contact with the CMV virus is a problem for only a few people. If it is determined that the recipient should not receive CMV-positive blood, a unit will be dispensed that does not contain the virus.

Zoonotic diseases are caused by a variety of pathogens that can be transferred from animal to human. Not all animal diseases can make this transfer because the pathogens may not be able to adapt to the human host. Of those that do, there are several methods of transfer. The most common is transfer from the bite of a contaminated mosquito or tick, known as a vector. The vector feasts on the infected animal and then transfers the pathogen through its saliva when it bites a human.

Arboviruses are zoonotic viruses that are transmitted by insect bite. More than 570 arboviruses exist worldwide, but only a few are of current concern to the U.S. blood supply. West Nile virus has been identified in the U.S. since 1999. The virus infects birds and is transferred to humans by mosquito bite. The risk of transfusion-acquired infection is very low thanks to testing that was developed in 2003. In 2016, cases of Zika virus were identified in Dade County, Florida. The mosquito that is capable of carrying the virus can be found in many areas throughout the U.S. Transfusion-transmission has not been reported in the U.S. No technological testing is available to detect the virus in donor blood; therefore, patient screening is the most beneficial method of maintaining blood safety.

Ebola virus is a zoonotic disease that is not transferred by an insect vector. Direct contact with the infected body fluid is the means of transmission. In 2015, two American missionaries who were infected with Ebola were returned to the U.S. for treatment. Two members of the team caring for these individuals became infected but recovered. No other episodes of U.S.-originating Ebola have been reported, and the risk of infection through blood transfusion in the U.S. is considered very low. Would-be donors who have visited endemic countries may be deferred from donating blood.

Insects also carry parasites, which can be transferred to human hosts. Chagas's disease is caused by the protozoa *Trypanosoma cruzi*. The vector is the triatomine (kissing) bug that lives in housing made of adobe, straw, thatch, and mud. Chagas's has an asymptomatic period that may last years before exhibiting serious, sometimes fatal complications. This long period of latency means that an infected person does not "feel sick" and may not be deferred as a donor. Over the last few years, the U.S. population has seen an increase of residents from endemic countries. These new donors may pose a silent risk for transfer. Fortunately, testing is available to detect the parasite.

Babeoisis is caused by another protozoan parasite that is transferred by deer tick, the most common vector in the U.S. The protozoan resides and replicates in the red blood cell. Asymptomatic donors may transfer the disease. There is no test for babeiosis; individuals with confirmed disease are asked not to donate. Lyme disease, it should be noted, is a bacterium that is not found in the red cells and appears to have no risk of transfusion transmission.

Pharmaceutical blood products do not carry the same risk of disease transmission as do banked blood products. Blood used for pharmacological purposes can be treated in advance to deactivate viruses and render them harmless.

When transfusing blood, remember to protect yourself from exposure to transmissible diseases, such as viral hepatitis and human immunodeficiency virus. The AABB recommends the use of gowns and gloves when handling blood. If splashing is a potential, then a face shield should be worn as well.

Compatibility

Recipient blood is choosy about donor blood. The recipient must have blood that is similar to the donor's blood. This similarity is referred to as compatibility. A variety of lab tests collectively called type and cross-match is done to assure that this compatibility exists. If blood is given to a recipient who is not compatible with the donor, there can be very serious consequences!

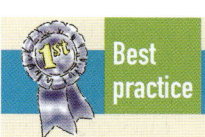

Best practice

Protect yourself with gown and gloves when initiating a blood component.

Type and cross-match is performed to prevent or reduce the risk of an antigen/antibody reaction. Antigens are molecules that may cause the body to form an immune response. Antibodies are immune proteins that react against antigens.
- Typing — checks for major antibody/antigen incompatibility (ABO and Rh)
- Cross-matching — checks for other antibodies in your blood that may react to antigens in the donor blood

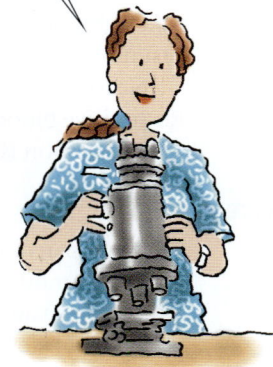

Antigens are found on blood cells; antibodies are found in plasma.

The ABO System

Two blood antigens may be naturally present in blood: A and B. These antigens are inherited and blood type is based on which of these are present on the red blood cells.

Whichever antigen you naturally have, there is also naturally present the antibody to the opposite antigen. Therefore:

If a person has	... then he or she is considered	And he or she also has
A antigen	Type A	B antibody
B antigen	Type B	A antibody
Both A and B antigen	Type AB	No antibody
Neither antigen	Type O	Both A and B antibody

So what happens if you give someone who has type A blood a unit of type B blood? The B antibody in the recipient's blood will immediately attack the B antigen in the donor blood. Because the antigen is located on the red blood cell, the attack will cause destruction (lysis) of all of the donor red blood cells (hemolysis). The by-product of this massive lysis will overwhelm the kidneys, and death may occur. This is known as a hemolytic reaction and is the most severe immediate reaction of a blood transfusion.

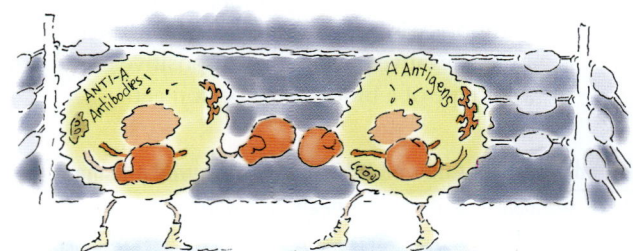

Rh system

The other major antigen group in blood is the Rhesus system, named after the Rhesus monkey and more commonly referred to as Rh. The letter D identifies this most common antigen in this group. If you are

Rh positive, a variant of D antigen is present on the red cells. If you are Rh negative, you have no D antigen on the red cell.

There is no naturally occurring antibody to Rh because that would cause a person to destroy his or her own blood! Rh-negative individuals will only form D antigen if they come in contact with Rh-positive blood. Because the antibody does not form immediately, the second unit of Rh-positive blood is more likely to cause a reaction than the first unit.

Nearly 95% of Blacks, Native Americans, and Asians have Rh-positive blood as well as 85% of Caucasians. The remainder of the population is Rh negative.

A pregnant pause

What happens when an Rh-negative woman has an Rh-positive baby? The mother's blood will start to form the antibody against the D antigen in the baby's blood. Because these antibodies form slowly, there will probably not be a problem with the first pregnancy. If the mother gets pregnant again and the baby is Rh positive, the antibodies that formed during the first pregnancy will activate and will cause destruction of the baby's blood. Immune globulin is administered to prevent the antibody from activating.

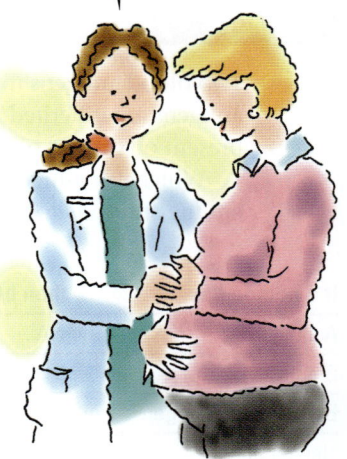

Rh incompatibility rarely affects a first pregnancy, but it could pose a risk for subsequent pregnancies if left untreated.

Blood type compatibility

The antigens that determine a person's blood type are A and B. Whatever antigen is in the blood, the opposite antibody is always present. A person who is Rh positive has D antigen in the blood. D antibody is not naturally present in anyone's blood but will form if an Rh-negative person gets Rh-positive blood. With all this in mind, what type of a blood can a person get?

Blood type		Allowed RBCs		Allowed plasma		Allowed whole blood	
A	Positive	A, O	Pos/Neg	A, AB	Pos/Neg	A	Pos/Neg
B	Positive	B, O	Pos/Neg	B, AB	Pos/Neg	B	Pos/Neg
AB	Positive	A, B, AB, O	Pos/Neg	AB	Pos/Neg	AB	Pos/Neg
O	Positive	O	Pos/Neg	A, B, AB, O	Pos/Neg	O	Pos/Neg
A	Negative	A, O	Neg	A, AB	Pos*/Neg	A	Neg
B	Negative	B, O	Neg	B, AB	Pos*/Ne	B	Neg
AB	Negative	A, B, AB, O	Neg	AB	Pos*/Neg	AB	Neg
O	Negative	O	Neg	A, B, AB, O	Pos*/Neg	O	Neg

- Rh-positive plasma should only be given to an Rh-negative recipient if anti-D is not detected in recipient's blood

Universally accepted!

Because group O negative blood lacks both A and B antigens as well as D antigen, O negative blood can be transfused in limited amounts in an emergency to any patient — regardless of the recipient's blood type — with little risk of adverse reaction. That's why people with group O negative blood are called *universal donors.*

A person with AB blood type has neither anti-A nor anti-B antibodies. This person may receive A, B, AB, or O blood, making him or her a *universal recipient* of red cells. If an Rh-negative recipient has developed anti-D, only negative blood can be given; otherwise, Rh is not a factor when transfusing red cells.

Plasma antibodies

Plasma antibodies are classified into five categories: IgA, IgD, IgE, IgG, and IgM. Of these five, IgA and IgG are divided into subtypes. Not all of these categories and subtypes are associated with transfusion reactions.

Some of these antibodies can activate complement. Complement is made up of protein fragments that are activated in a specific sequence, known as a cascade. If an antibody activates complement, these protein fragments attack the antigen and the cell that the antigen is attached to. In red blood cell reactions, the antibody may simply coat the cells so that they clump together, or it may punch a hole in the cell membrane and cause the cell contents to spill (lysis).

Cross-matching blood identifies how much antibody is present in the body, which can help predict the chance of a reaction if antigen is introduced from the donor blood.

Immunoglobulin	Associated with reaction?	Activates complement?	Lysis
IgA_1, IgA_2	yes	no	-
IgD	no	-	-
IgE	yes	no	-
IgG_1, IgG_2, IgG_3	yes	IgG_1 only	no
IgG_4	no	-	-
IgM	yes	yes	yes

Human Leukocyte Antigen (HLA)

Other antigens exist in the body that are not plasma antigens. One set is those antigens that are a part of the human leukocyte antigen (HLA) system. Many cells in the body have HLA antigens attached to them, including blood cells. The HLA system is actually made up of many different antigens, and each person has his own set. If a foreign HLA antigen enters the body, an HLA antibody will form against it. This is part of the immune system and does not present a danger to an individual.

In a blood transfusion, the donor blood is likely to contain a set of HLA antibodies that the recipient does not have. These donor antibodies may react with the recipient's HLA antigens, and a blood transfusion reaction may occur. Severe reactions are rare but may be fatal. If a patient is susceptible to serious reactions, donor blood should be tested to assure that the donor HLA antibodies match the recipient's HLA antigen profile as closely as possible.

HLA compatibility:
- is responsible for graft success or rejection
- may be involved with host defense against cancer
- may be the culprit when WBCs or platelets fail to multiply after being transfused. (If this happens, the HLA system could trigger a fatal immune reaction in the patient.)

HLA testing is not generally done for transfusion recipients but is essential for organ transplant. For blood transfusion, HLA testing may benefit patients who:
- will be receiving massive, multiple, or frequent red cell transfusions
- will receive platelet and WBC transfusions
- are undergoing organ or tissue transplant
- have severe or refractory febrile transfusion reactions.

Required Compatibility Testing for All Blood Products

	ABO typing	Rh typing	Cross-matching	HLA typing
Whole blood	yes	yes	yes	no
RBCs	yes	yes	yes	no
Platelets	yes	yes	no	patient specific
Plasma	yes	no	no	no
Granulocytes	recommended	yes	yes	yes
Cryoprecipitate	no	no	no	no

Administering transfusions

A license to order

Because blood is used for the treatment of disease, it is registered as a drug by the FDA. The order from an LIP is required prior to transfusion of any blood component. Orders must include type and number of components to be transfused and any special considerations for the handling.

Even the LIP has some limitations. Blood components are ordered when the recipient's serum levels meet a transfusion trigger. The "trigger" is designated by the hospital blood committee and determines conditions that are appropriate for giving blood. For example, if a patient is actively bleeding, a drop in hemoglobin to 10 g/dL may significantly alter cardiac status. However, a patient with chronic anemia may function well with much lower hemoglobin. The trigger is, therefore, based on many considerations. Recipients who do not meet this trigger are generally not recommended for transfusion.

Special handling considerations for which an order is needed include:
- washing RBCs to remove additional leukocytes
- irradiation to prevent T-lymphocyte reactions
- use of a blood warmer
- premedication.

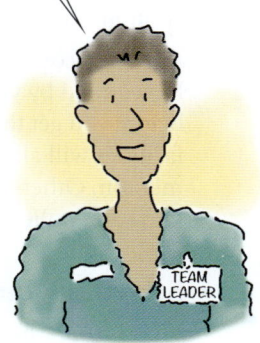

Before obtaining the blood, be sure everything is ready to go!

A license to transfuse

All states allow licensed registered nurses to initiate blood transfusions. The role of the licensed practical nurse or licensed vocational nurse varies from state to state and is usually limited to regulating transfusion flow rates, observing patients for reactions, discontinuing transfusions, and documenting those procedures. Know the rules and regulations from your state board of nursing before performing a transfusion or transfusion-related procedure or delegating chores to another nurse.

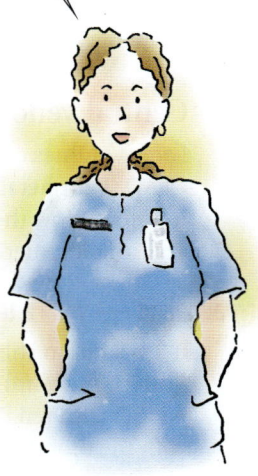

Administering blood and blood components is the registered nurse's responsibility in most states. Know your state rules before you perform or participate in a blood transfusion.

Identifying the patient

Prior to administering blood, a sample of blood is taken from the recipient to do the type-and-cross-match test, as this will verify recipient compatibility to the donor blood. Before drawing this blood sample, the patient must be identified using 2 means of identification. To reduce the risk of error, the tube containing this blood sample must be labeled in front of the recipient.

A method for unique patient identification, commonly a bracelet, is placed on the patient's arm when this sample is obtained. The blood sample and the bracelet will be labeled with the recipient's name, the selected identifier, date and time of collection, and initials of phlebotomist.

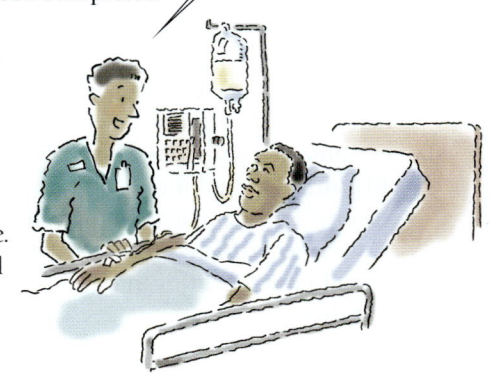

Any identifying bracelet placed on the recipient must be left in place until all ordered units have been transfused.

Do I have your permission to proceed?

Although consents for blood transfusion are not mandated, they may be required by your facility. Be sure the consent has been completed before you get the transfusion process rolling! Some facilities will allow the registered nurse to obtain permission. Others require the LIP to do so. Be sure you know the policy at your facility!

Selecting equipment

Blood components are given by the intravenous route. Blood may be given through any peripheral or central access device.

Peripheral venous catheter

Peripheral veins are commonly used in nonacute transfusion situations. The small diameter of the catheter and peripheral resistance (resistance to blood flow in the vein) can affect flow rates. Although blood can safely be administered through a 24G catheter, flow rate may be slowed and splitting a unit into 2 bags, often called aliquots, may be needed to facilitate infusion over 4 hours for each bag or 8 hours for a complete unit of packed RBCs. A 20 or 22 gauge is generally recommended, and larger catheters may be needed if rapid flow is required. Catheter gauze size is chosen based on the diameter of the patient's veins. Smaller catheters are needed to reduce mechanical vein damage.

Central venous access device (CVAD)

Large volumes of blood products can be delivered safely through any CVAD. Peripherally inserted central catheters (PICC) are more likely to restrict flow than are other types of CVADs due to longer length and smaller internal diameter.

Normal saline — you're the only one for me!

0.9% sodium chloride, aka. normal saline (NS), is the approved solution for the administration of all blood products because NS is compatible with red blood cells. Other intravenous fluids may interact with the blood or with the nutrient admixture that is added for cell preservation. NS may be used to prime the administration set and may be left on one leg of a Y-type blood administration set to flush the set after administration.

Lactated Ringer's (LR) is contraindicated for the infusion of red cell products because it contains calcium. The nutrient admixture used to preserve blood contains citrate that prevents coagulation by binding with the calcium in donor blood. The calcium in LR may reverse this binding action and cause clot formation.

Dextrose 5% in Water (D_5W) is also contraindicated. D_5W is a hypotonic solution, which may make the blood cells swell and then lyse. Fluids containing dextrose may also cause blood cells to stick together forming a clot. The cells adhere to each other like pennies in a roll; this is known as the rouleaux effect.

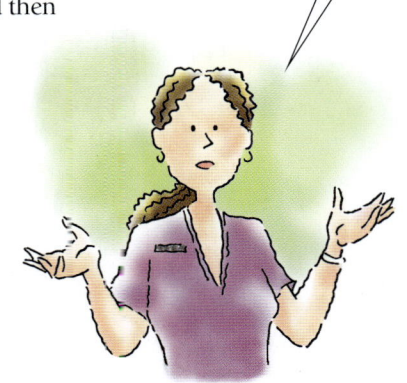

NS should not be added directly into a unit of blood to reduce its viscosity unless ordered by the physician.

Ready to filter through some advice?

During storage of blood, small clots and cellular debris may form. All blood components are filtered through a 170- to 260-micron filter to remove this debris. If low volume components are to be infused, such as single units of platelets or cryoprecipitate, a shorter administration set with a 170- to 260-micron filter should be considered to reduce the amount of product trapped in the administration set.

Banked blood products are leukocyte depleted prior to storage, which greatly eliminates the risk of micro-debris. The use of 20- to 40-micron microaggregate filters is still recommended for transfusion to small infants and for the reinfusion of shed operative blood. However, no benefit has been shown for using microaggregate filters for the banked blood given to the general population.

Prestorage leukocyte depletion also eliminates the need for bedside leukocyte-removal filters. If further leukocyte reduction is needed, different approaches, such as washing, are recommended. Poststorage leukocyte-reduction filters reduce the volume of transfused blood, have poor quality control, and have been associated with transfusion reactions.

Administration sets

The filter that is selected is a part of the administration set. The blood set may be:
- a straight set with only one spike
- a Y set with two spikes
- a short tubing containing a blood filter that may be connected to a standard nonfiltered I.V. set.

The Y set requires the least manipulation, so it is often selected as a measure to reduce contamination of the system. The Y site allows for normal saline to initially prime the set with fluid and flush the blood out of the set at the end of the transfusion. In the event of a transfusion reaction, do not turn on the normal saline, as this will flush additional blood through the set and into the patient's vein. Disconnect the blood set from the catheter, and attach a new I.V. set primed with normal saline.

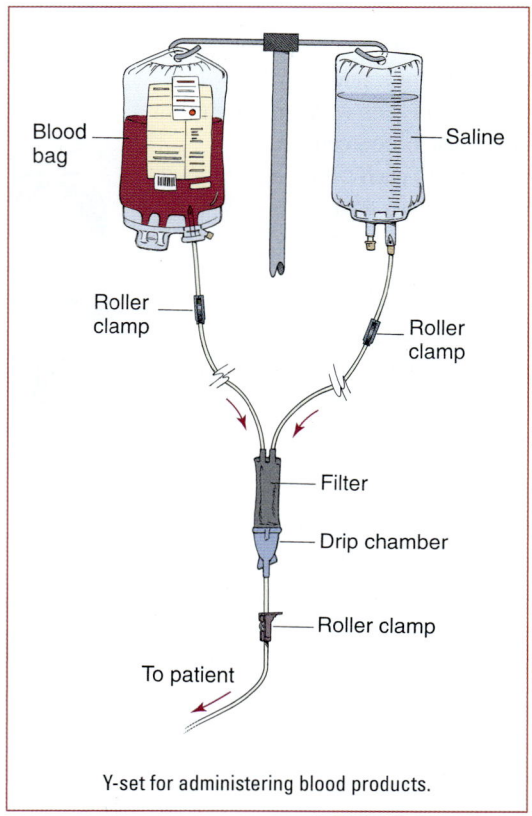

Y-set for administering blood products.

The blood transfusion set may be changed after each unit or at least every 4 hours. The set may be used for more than 1 unit of blood if the total time for the complete transfusion will be no greater than 4 hours. Be sure to know and follow your facility policy about blood transfusion sets.

Let's jump to a pump

Use of an electronic infusion pump can be beneficial to maintain the flow rate. Always check the manufacturer's recommendations to assure the pump is appropriate for the administration of blood components. Only use a blood administration set that is recommended for use with the pump and use according to the manufacturer's directions.

Pumps that are not approved for blood transfusion may put excessive pressure on the cells and cause them to rupture. This can result in hyperkalemia as potassium is released from the damaged cell. The risk is increased when older units of red cells are transfused because the cells are more brittle. Patients receiving blood using an electronic infusion pump should be observed for signs of potassium excess.

The pressure's on!

Pressure bags can help increase flow rate by exerting pressure on the bag. The component bag must fit entirely into the pressure bag's sleeve to assure uniform pressure. Improperly placed component bags cause stress on seams causing them to rip.

Use only a pressure bag with a gauge. Do not exceed 300 mm Hg. Follow manufacturer's recommendations for use. Do not allow the bag to empty completely while under pressure as this can force air into the veins causing an air embolism.

Studies show that the use of a larger gauge catheter will provide adequate rate increase without use of the pressure bag. But ensure that the vein diameter is large enough to accommodate the large gauge catheter.

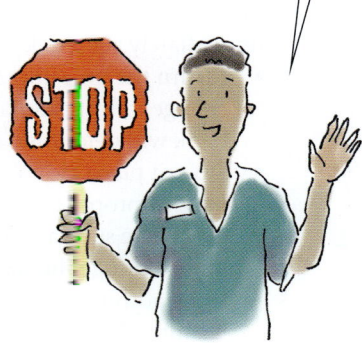

DO **NOT** warm blood by immersion in hot water bath or in microwave oven!!!!! It may lead to fatal hemolysis!!!

When a blanket just won't do

Blood warmers may be used if ordered. Only approved warmers with a temperature gauge are to be used. They are recommended for adults receiving massive, rapid transfusion and for any transfusion to neonates since the cold blood can cause hypothermia. For years, blood warmers were used for patients diagnosed with cold agglutinins disease, but there is no conclusive evidence of the benefit of this measure.

Premedication and vital signs

Any medication to be administered prior to transfusion must be ordered by the LIP. Use of prophylactic medication is controversial since these may mask signs and symptoms of a more serious reaction.

Nonhemolytic febrile reaction (discussed later in this chapter) is the most common reason for premedication. Evidence does not support premedication unless the recipient has previously experienced such a reaction.

You're almost ready. Now, let's make sure the patient is! Your final step before getting the blood is to obtain the recipient's vital signs. If anything seems abnormal, contact the LIP before continuing with the transfusion. Some facilities may have policies restricting transfusion in the presence of elevated body temperature, so make sure you follow those policies.

Vital signs will be taken 5 to 15 minutes after the transfusion has been started and again at the end of transfusion. There is no recommendation for taking them during the transfusion unless a reaction is suspected or as indicated by the patient's condition.

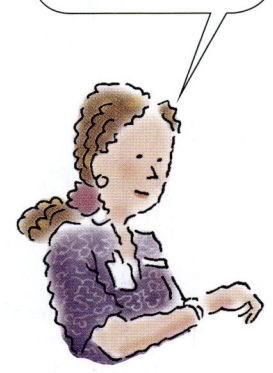

Watch the clock. Premeds are often ordered one hour before starting the transfusion.

Starting the transfusion

If you have completed these steps and everything is ready, you may now get the blood from the blood bank.

Ahh, this is the life!

Blood likes to live in the blood bank. The environment outside of the blood bank is less friendly. If any blood component is obtained from the blood bank and it is decided that the transfusion cannot be immediately started, keep these steps in mind:
- Return the unit immediately to the blood bank. Temperature changes affect the viability and safety of the product. The blood bank will determine if the blood can be safely reissued.
- Do not place blood components in the refrigerator on the nursing unit; improper temperatures can rapidly lyse red blood cells and deactivate substances in other products. The blood or component may no longer be safe for transfusion.
- If the administration set has been added to the blood bag and it cannot be hung, return it to the blood bank where it will be discarded.

I'll second that

Check the blood component against the LIP's order, and be sure all special instructions have been followed. Have a second person trained in this identification process check and sign the blood ticket with you.

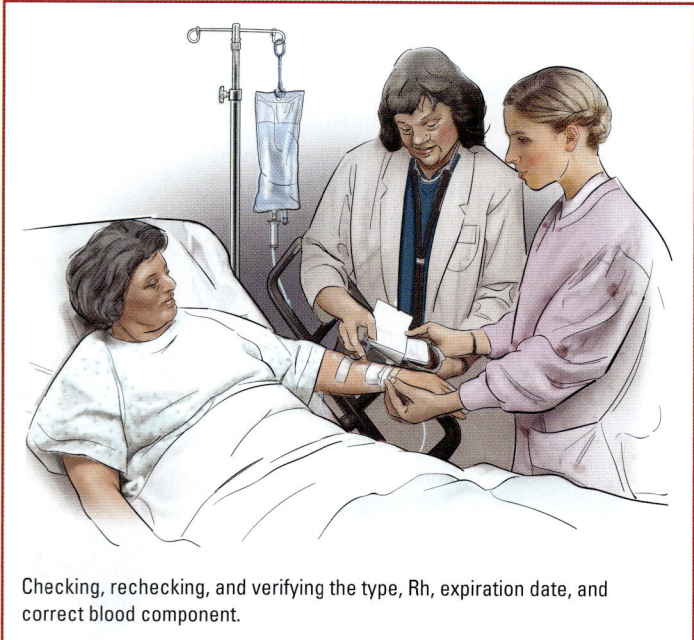

Checking, rechecking, and verifying the type, Rh, expiration date, and correct blood component.

This process must be done at the patient's bedside. All information on the patient's identification bracelet, the attached ticket or forms, and the blood container must match exactly. Look for the following:
- The recipient's identification matches that which is labeled on the bag.
- The information on the blood ticket matches what is on the unit of blood:
  - recipient name and identification number
  - blood component identification number
  - type of component
  - AB type
  - Rh type
  - expiration date.
- Red cell components do not appear to have any clots, discoloration, or gas. Plasma does not appear cloudy or turbid. These are possible signs of contamination.
- The container of blood is intact with no leaks at the seams.
- If possible, have the recipient state his or her name.

Technology such as bar coding may allow for a single person to identify and verify the information if the system in use allows for this. Always strictly follow the policy and procedure from your facility. Attention to all details is required as failure to give the correct unit of blood to the correct patient can have serious, even life-threatening complications.

A slow start is the healthy way to a safe finish

Transfusion containing red blood cells should be started slowly, about 2 mL/min for the first 15 minutes. If there is no sign of a reaction, the rate may be increased as needed to assure the unit is transfused within a 4-hour time period.

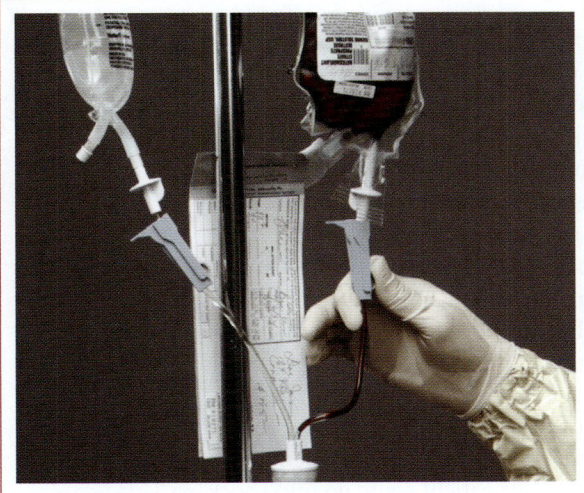

Hanging the bag.

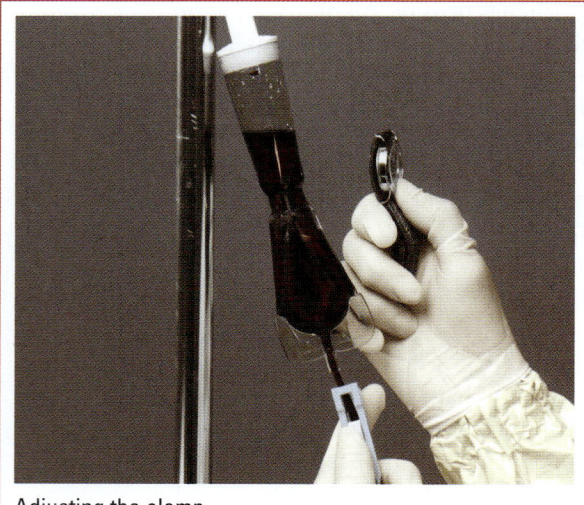

Adjusting the clamp.

Other blood components can be administered at a continuous rate from beginning to end, depending on the recipient's tolerance. Units of fresh frozen plasma are best tolerated over 1 to 2 hours. Rate of transfusion for granulocytes is very recipient dependent since they are often associated with fever and chills. The product should be gently agitated throughout the transfusion to prevent cellular damage. There is no set rate for platelets or cryoprecipitate, but keep in mind the volume in the bag and the recipient's tolerance to fluid. Keep in mind, also, that cryoprecipitate expires 6 hours after thawing.

Transfusion don'ts

A blood transfusion requires extreme care. Here are some tips on what not to do when administering a transfusion:

- Don't add medications to the blood bag.
- Never give blood products without checking the order against the blood bag label — the only way to tell if the request form has been stamped with the wrong name. Most life-threatening reactions occur when this step is omitted.
- Don't transfuse the blood product if you discover a discrepancy in the blood number, blood slip type, or patient identification number.
- Don't piggyback blood into the injection site of an existing infusion set. Most solutions, including dextrose in water, are incompatible with blood. Administer blood only with normal saline solution.
- Don't hesitate to stop the transfusion if your patient shows changes in vital signs, is dyspneic or restless, or develops chills, hematuria, or pain in the flank, chest, or back. Your patient could go into shock, so don't remove the I.V. device that's in place. Keep it open with a slow infusion of normal saline solution; call the LIP and the laboratory.

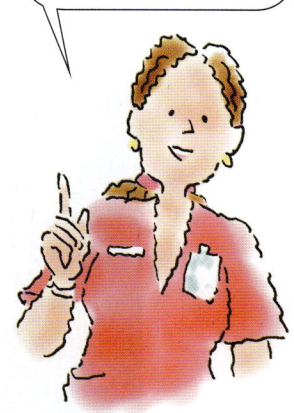

When giving granulocytes, gently agitate the bag several times throughout the transfusion to prevent damage to the cells.

Monitoring a blood transfusion

Although the AABB only recommends vital signs before starting the transfusion, 5 to 15 minutes after starting the transfusion, and at the end of the transfusion, the recipient should be observed throughout the procedure. These are some of the most common signs that something is amiss:
- fever
- chills
- rigors
- headache
- nausea
- facial flushing
- rash
- back pain
- dizziness.

Monitor the blood bag!

Blood transfusions are not generally set up in a piggyback style; that is to say, when the blood bag empties, the saline does not automatically turn on. Air embolism potential does exist if an empty bag continues to infuse, especially if pressure is being used or the transfusion is through a CVAD.

Whether you are administering whole blood, cellular components, or plasma, your primary responsibility is to be sure the patient is the intended recipient. This will help prevent a potentially life-threatening reaction. The administration of all blood products follows the same basic procedure. Always begin by checking, verifying, and inspecting.

Don't forget to document

Make sure that you record:
- date and time of the transfusion
- identification number on the blood bag
- type and amount of blood transfused
- volume of normal saline solution infused
- status of the venous access device
- recipient's vital signs
- signs or symptoms of a reaction (or the absence of signs or symptoms)
- how the patient tolerated the procedure.

Special considerations

Pediatric patients

- Transfusion triggers are the same for infants as they are for adults.
- Depending on size, dose may be ordered as mLs instead of units.

- The number of donors to which the recipient is exposed should be minimized to reduce development of antibodies. Continue with bullet points are they are
    - One unit of blood may be used to obtain several small doses.
    - Platelets should be obtained from a single donor.
    - Fresh frozen plasma (FFP) should only be used for serious bleeding events.
- Rh-negative females should not receive Rh-positive components.
- Washed or fresh blood (<7 days old) is preferred for neonates.
- Blood provided by direct donation (i.e., blood-related family member) should be irradiated prior to transfusion due to the potential risk of a fatal HLA reaction.
- Risk for metabolic disorders and hypothermia is increased.

Older adults
- Be aware of potential for fluid overload.
    - Request the blood bank to split the unit and hang each half over 4 hours to extend total hang time to 8 hours.
    - Administration of FFP may put the recipient at risk for transfusion-associated circulatory overload (TACO).
- Decreased immune response may result in delayed hemolysis (expected rise in hematocrit may not be observed).
- Risk for metabolic disorders and hypothermia is increased.

Terminating the transfusion

After a transfusion is complete, follow these steps:
- Turn on saline to administer all blood held in the administration set.
- Obtain posttransfusion vital signs.
- Access and chart recipient's response.
- Discontinue the peripheral I.V. catheter if appropriate.
- Discard blood container and set in biological waste bag.

Transfusion Complications

Because of careful screening and testing, the supply of blood is safer today than it has ever been. Even so, a patient who receives a transfusion is still at risk for a transfusion reaction. Therefore, it is important to weigh the benefits of a transfusion against the risks. The recipient and family should be informed of these risks. Some facilities have special consent forms for transfusions that include an explanation of the risks.

Transfusion reactions can be categorized as follows:
- Immune — directly related to stimulation of the immune system
    - Immediate — symptoms apparent within 48 hours of initiating the transfusion

        ○ Delayed — symptoms begin 2 to 14 days after the transfusion
    • Nonimmune — does not involve the immune system; arises from other considerations

	Immune	Nonimmune
Immediate	Acute intravascular hemolysis Acute extravascular hemolysis Nonhemolytic febrile reaction Allergy Anaphylaxis Transfusion-related acute lung injury (TRALI) Immune-mediated platelet destruction Posttransfusion purpura	Transfusion-associated circulatory overload (TACO) Hypokalemia Hyperkalemia Citrate toxicity Hypothermia Hemosiderosis Hyperammonemia Bleeding tendencies
Delayed	Graft vs. host disease HLA alloimmunization Refractoriness Delayed extravascular hemolysis Posttransfusion purpura	Bacterial contamination Infection Disease transmission Altered oxygen affinity Nonimmune hemolysis

In the event a transfusion reaction is suspected, stop the blood immediately. Disconnect the blood administration set using aseptic technique because there is a possibility that the blood transfusion will be resumed.
- Connect a new administration set primed with normal saline to the I.V. catheter to maintain line patency.
- Obtain vital signs
- Obtain urine sample.
- Notify the lab to draw a blood sample.
- Notify the LIP of the patient's condition.
- Support the patient symptomatically.

If it is determined that an immune reaction has occurred, the blood transfusion will usually be discontinued. The unused portion of the blood, along with the attached blood ticket, administration set, and NS should be returned to the blood bank for analysis. (See *Overview of Transfusion Reactions*, page 260.)

There are three immune reactions that do not require discontinuing the unit:
- Febrile reaction to granulocytes — fever and rash are common reactions; transfusion may be temporarily halted until symptom control is achieved.
- Nonhemolytic febrile transfusion reaction — after medication, the reaction is sometimes continued but at a slower rate.
- Allergy — further stimulation with the allergen is unlikely to cause further reactions; antihistamines will improve patient comfort. For anaphylactic reactions, the blood must be discontinued.

One last thing...

Because of the inherent risks of blood transfusion and the limited availability of the blood supply, the use of plasma derivatives instead of banked blood is recommended whenever possible. These medications are manufactured from plasma that has been spun off of the red cells at the time of donation. Although a freshly donated unit of whole blood contains all of these fractions — albumin, immunoglobulin, coagulation factors, and others — they are unstable, are available in only small amounts, and quickly break down during storage. Manufactured products increase the yield while greatly reducing the risk of a reaction. When administering these medications, consult the package insert for administration considerations.

Transfusion reactions

(Text continues on page 266)

Reactions that cause lysis

Reaction	Causation	Signs and symptoms (signs and symptoms)	Prevention	Nursing intervention
Acute intravascular hemolysis	• Incompatible A or B antigen on donor red cell • IgM mediated with complement activation • Total lysis of red cells releases large doses of hemoglobin into the bloodstream. S&S related to body's attempt to eliminate this hemoglobin	• Reaction occurs immediately, usually within first 15 minutes of transfusion of first 50 mL of blood • Fever • Severe back pain • Rapid progression of symptoms to renal failure, shock, disseminated intravascular coagulation (DIC) • 10% mortality rate	• Pretransfusion typing • Properly identify patient to assure right blood to right patient • Transfuse blood slowly for the first 15 minutes; closely observe the patient during this time	• Monitor blood pressure. • Treat shock as indicated by the patient's condition, using I.V. fluids, oxygen, epinephrine, diuretics, vasopressor as prescribed. • Obtain labs and urine samples for evaluation. • Observe for signs of hemorrhage resulting from DIC.
Acute extravascular hemolysis	• Incompatible donor antigen other than A or B • IgG mediated • Antibody coats and removes donor cells from system. Cell lysis occurs outside of the bloodstream, in liver, possibly causing increased bilirubin (jaundice).	Anticipated rise in hematocrit is not seen.	Serological testing	• Treat symptoms • May not require intervention

Reactions that cause lysis (continued)

Reaction	Causation	Signs and symptoms (signs and symptoms)	Prevention	Nursing intervention
Delayed extravascular hemolysis	Antibody formation is delayed.	• Anemia after initial rise in hematocrit • May occur 2–10 days after transfusion	Serological testing	None
Nonimmune hemolysis	Faulty administration technique: • elevated temperature of bag • excessive pressure on container • administration of incompatible fluids • addition of medication into system • improper storage of blood on nursing unit	Anticipated rise in hematocrit is not seen	Proper administration technique	No postdiagnostic intervention

Immune responses that do not cause lysis

Reaction	Causation	Signs and symptoms (signs and symptoms)	Prevention	Nursing intervention
HLA (human leukocyte antigen) alloimmunization	Donor antibody to recipient HLA	No indication except for failure to respond to transfusion	Serological testing	None
Non-hemolytic febrile transfusion reaction	Donor antibody to recipient HLA	• May occur ~ 15 minutes after start of transfusion or as much as 2 hours after completion • Temperature elevation of 1.8°F (1°C) • Chills • Headache • Nausea and vomiting • Hypotension • Chest pain • Dyspnea • Nonproductive cough • Malaise	• Premedicate susceptible patients with an antipyretic, an antihistamine, and, possibly, a steroid. • Give HLA-compatible blood to individual with repeated reaction	Relieve symptoms with an antipyretic or antihistamine.
Allergy	• IgE mediated • Allergen in donor plasma to which recipient is sensitive • Urticarial reaction	• May occur immediately or up to 1 hour after start of transfusion • Itching	• Premedicate with an antihistamine if the patient has a history of allergic reactions.	• Administer antihistamines • Transfusion may be continued.

(continued)

Immune responses that do not cause lysis *(continued)*

Reaction	Causation	Signs and symptoms (signs and symptoms)	Prevention	Nursing intervention
		• Hives • Fever • Chills • Facial swelling • Wheezing • Throat swelling	• Observe the patient closely for the first 15 minutes of the transfusion.	
Anaphylaxis	• IgA antigen in donor blood administered to IgA-deficient recipient who has developed antibodies • <5% mortality	• May occur with only a few mLs of blood • Flushing • Urticaria • Abdominal pain • Chills • Fever • Dyspnea/wheezing • Hypotension • Shock • Cardiac arrest	• Serological testing • Transfuse only immunoglobulin A–deficient blood or well-washed RBCs.	Treat for shock by administering oxygen, fluids, epinephrine, and, possibly, a steroid as ordered.
Transfusion-related acute lung injury (TRALI)	• Donor antibody to recipient HLA • Antibody activity occurs in lungs causing endothelial injury, capillary leak, and, subsequently, pulmonary edema	• Occurs immediately or within 6 hours after transfusion • Chills, cough, fever, cyanosis, hypotension, and increasing respiratory distress • Absence of circulatory overload • Leading cause of morbidity and mortality associated with transfusion • 5%–20% mortality	• Donor screening; female donors who have had multiple pregnancies are at highest risk of carrying anti-HLA antibodies	Supportive care including oxygen and mechanical ventilation
Posttransfusion purpura	Previous sensitization due to transfusion or pregnancy	• Typically 7–10 days after a blood transfusion • Dramatic, and sudden self-limited thrombocytopenia		IVIG if needed to correct thrombocytopenia
Transfusion-associated graft vs. host disease (TA-GVHD)	Reproduction of T lymphocytes in donor blood	• Pancytopenia • Hepatocellular damage • Profuse diarrhea • >75% mortality	Irradiation of cellular product for patients who are immunosuppressed	Supportive measures as condition requires

Responses involving microorganism contamination

Reaction	Causation	Signs and symptoms (signs and symptoms)	Prevention	Nursing intervention
Bacterial contamination	• Contamination occurs at the time of donation and microorganisms increase in number during storage. • Reaction is secondary to endotoxin production in unit. • Most commonly occurs with platelets because they are stored at room temperature	• Symptoms usually occur within minutes of starting the transfusion. • Sudden-onset high fever • Chills with rigors • Vomiting • Abdominal cramping • Diarrhea • Shock	• Maintain strict storage control; do not request blood until IV is in place and blood is ready for transfusion. • Inspect blood before the transfusion for gas, clots, and dark purple color.	• Treat with a broad-spectrum antibiotic and a steroid. • Treat for shock. • Support renal function.
Infection	Blood is an excellent medium for the proliferation of bacteria. Any breach in aseptic technique may allow microorganisms to enter the blood and rapidly reproduce.	• Fever • Chills • Nausea • Achiness • Increased white blood cell count	• Change the blood tubing and filter every 4 hours. • Infuse each unit of blood over 2 to 4 hours; terminate the infusion if the period exceeds 4 hours.	• Maintain sterile technique when administering blood products. • Monitor vital signs after infusion. • Onset of symptoms is usually delayed.
Disease transmission	Contamination of unit with microorganisms originating from the donor. Examples include human immunodeficiency virus (HIV), hepatitis B virus (HBV), and hepatitis C virus (HCV).	Disease-specific symptoms	Not detectable at bedside	• Disease-specific • Onset of symptoms may be delayed for days or weeks.

Responses involving rate or volume

Reaction	Causation	Signs and symptoms	Prevention	Nursing intervention
Hypothermia	• Cold blood decreases body temperature, which reduces recipient's metabolism. • May lead to hypocalcemia, metabolic acidosis, and cardiac arrest	• Fever • Tachycardia • Tachypnea • Altered mental status • Shivering	Warm the blood to 95°F to 98°F before massive transfusions (3 units or more) and always for neonates.	• Slow the transfusion. • Warm the patient with blankets. • Obtain an ECG.
Increased oxygen affinity for hemoglobin	Stored RBCs diminish their ability to release oxygen to the cells	Hypoxia observed by reduce pO_2	Give fresh RBCs to patients in ICU or those receiving multiple transfusions.	• Monitor arterial blood gas levels. • Give respiratory support as needed.

(continued)

Responses involving rate or volume *(continued)*

Reaction	Causation	Signs and symptoms (signs and symptoms)	Prevention	Nursing intervention
Transfusion-associated circulation overload (TACO)	Volume overload exacerbated by blood transfusion, especially plasma	• Occurs immediately or within 6 hours after transfusion • Acute respiratory distress • Tachycardia • ↑ blood pressure • Acute or worsening pulmonary edema • Intake and output — positive fluid balance • 1%–8% mortality	• Transfuse blood slowly. • Slow rate according to recipient's age, condition • Caution: plasma administration; • RBC's — split unit to increase transfusion time	• Slow the transfusion. • Give oxygen. • Elevate patient's head to assist with respirations. • Diuretics as ordered

Responses involving metabolic changes

Reaction	Causation	Signs and symptoms	Prevention	Nursing intervention
Hemosiderosis	As aged red cells in donor blood lyse, the free hemoglobin releases iron. The normal excretion rate of iron is low. In susceptible recipients, this increased iron is poorly tolerated.	Initial symptoms are vague: muscle weakness, fatigue, weight loss. May lead to cardiac and hepatic dysfunction	Use newer blood for patients with hemolytic diseases that involve improper iron metabolism.	Perform a therapeutic phlebotomy to remove excess iron.
Citrate toxicity (hypocalcemia)	Excessive citrate in donor blood binds with recipient's calcium so that it is not available in adequate amounts to muscle.	• Tingling in the fingers • Muscle cramps • Nausea • Vomiting • Hypotension • Cardiac arrhythmias • Seizures	Use blood less than 2 days old if administering multiple units.	• Monitor calcium levels. • Slow or stop the transfusion, depending on the reaction. • Expect a worse reaction in hypothermic patients or patients with elevated potassium levels. • Slowly administer calcium gluconate I.V.
Hypokalemia with metabolic alkalosis	Altered pH in stored blood results in alkaline state. Recipient cells uptake serum potassium to release hydrogen and correct the deficiency	K ≤ 3.0 mEq may cause: • muscle weakness • paralysis • respiratory failure • heart arrhythmias.	Use fresh blood in patients with renal impairment	• Obtain EKG. • Administer oral or I.V. potassium if deficit is severe.

Responses involving metabolic changes *(continued)*

Reaction	Causation	Signs and symptoms (signs and symptoms)	Prevention	Nursing intervention
Hyperkalemia	As aged red cells in donor blood lyse, they release potassium. In susceptible recipients, this excessive potassium can cause an elevation in serum potassium.	K > 5.0 mEq/L may cause: • muscle fatigue • weakness • paralysis • nausea • heart arrhythmias.	Use fresh blood for infants or patients with renal impairment.	• Obtain an ECG. • If severe, administer sodium polystyrene sulfonate (Kayexalate) orally or by enema. • Administer I.V. insulin and glucose.
Bleeding tendencies	• Stored red cells have no functional platelets or coagulations factors. With massive transfusion, recipient may become depleted.	• Bruising, nosebleed, petechiae, or similar signs of abnormal bleeding	When giving multiple units of blood, consider need for non–red cell products to help maintain hemostasis.	• Monitor platelet value. • Administer FFP and/or platelets to correct deficiencies.
Hyperammonemia	• Related to age of blood • May lead to encephalopathy and death	Behavioral changes from stupor-like to combative • Sweet mouth odor	For newborns and patients with liver disease, use fresh units or wash cells before transfusion.	Stop blood. Medications to restore metabolic balance; low-protein diet until stable; dialysis if severe

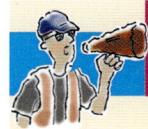

That's a wrap!

Transfusions review

Purpose
• To restore and maintain blood volume
• To improve the oxygen-carrying capacity of blood
• To replace deficient blood components

Compatibility
• ABO blood type: A, B, AB, O
• Rh blood group: Rh-positive, Rh-negative
• HLA blood group: non-ABO antigens that may affect compatibility of donor and recipient

Transfusion products
Whole blood
• Provides plasma and red blood cells from a single donor but not a good source of platelets or coagulation factors

Packed RBCs
• Used to maintain or restore oxygen-carrying capability and capacity

Granulocytes
• Assists in fighting serious infection not responding to antibiotics when bone marrow is *temporarily* incapacitated

Platelets
• Used to control or prevent bleeding

Plasma and plasma fractions
• Used to correct blood deficiencies, control bleeding tendencies caused by clotting factor deficiencies, and increase circulating blood volume

Transfusion reactions
Hemolytic
• Caused by incompatible blood
• May result in renal failure and shock
• May be life threatening

(continued)

Transfusions review *(continued)*

Febrile
- Occurs when the patient's HLA antibodies react against antigens on the donor's WBCs or platelets
- Causes flulike symptoms, chest pain, and hypotension

Allergic
- Caused by an allergen present in the transfused blood
- Symptoms include hives, itching, fever, chills, facial swelling, wheezing, and sore throat

Plasma protein incompatibility
- Occurs when blood that contains immunoglobulin A (IgA) proteins is infused into an IgA-deficient recipient who has developed anti-IgA antibodies
- Symptoms include flushing, abdominal pain, chills, fever, hypotension, shock, and cardiac arrest

Bacterial contamination
- Caused by contamination during collection or processing

- Symptoms include chills, fever, vomiting, abdominal cramping, diarrhea, shock, and kidney failure

Multiple transfusion reactions
- Hemosiderosis
- Bleeding tendencies
- Increased blood ammonia levels
- Increased oxygen affinity for hemoglobin
- Hypothermia
- Citrate toxicity
- Potassium intoxication

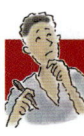

Quick quiz

1. What size micron filter is recommended for transfusing all blood products?
   A. 20–40 microns
   B. 60–80 microns
   C. 170–260 microns
   D. Leukocyte-reducing filter

Answer: C. The standard blood administration set comes with a 170–260 micron filter.

2. Which type of transfusion involves collecting and reinfusing the patient's own blood?
   A. Autologous
   B. Hemapheresis
   C. Plasmapheresis
   D. Homologous

Answer: A. Autologous transfusion involves collecting, filtering, and reinfusing the patient's own blood.

3. A blood transfusion set must be used for no more than:
   A. 24 hours
   B. 12 hours
   C. 4 hours
   D. 2 hours

Answer: C. The set must be discarded after it has been in use for 4 hours, so make sure that all blood ordered can be infused in this period. Otherwise, use a new set for each unit.

4. If you detect signs or symptoms of a transfusion reaction, the first thing you should do is:
    A. obtain vital signs.
    B. notify the blood bank.
    C. notify the practitioner.
    D. stop the infusion.

Answer: D. If you detect signs or symptoms of a transfusion reaction, stop the transfusion and start NS. Then take and record the patient's vital signs.

5. You should start a blood transfusion at a slow rate to:
    A. maintain blood volume.
    B. observe for the effects of a transfusion reaction.
    C. prevent clot formation at the tip of the venipuncture device.
    D. prevent hypothermia.

Answer: B. Always start the transfusion at a slow rate to observe for the effects of a transfusion reaction.

Scoring

☆☆☆ If you answered all six questions correctly, congrats! The information recipient (you) and the information donor (this chapter) are clearly compatible.

☆☆ If you answered four or five questions correctly, good going! The micron filter of your mind has allowed the key particles of information to successfully transfuse.

☆ If you answered fewer than four questions correctly, don't fret. Perhaps the flow rate on your information infusion device was set too low.

Suggested References

AABB Technical Manual (18th ed.). In Mark K. Fung, (Ed.), Bethesda, MD: AABB, 2014.

Agnihotri, A, & Agnihotri, A. (2014). Transfusion associated circulatory overload. Indian *Journal of Critical Care and Medicine, 18*(6), 396–398.

Cook, L. (2013). Infusion-related air embolism. *Journal of Infusion Nursing, 36*(1), 26–36.

Gorski, L., Hadaway, L., Hagle, M., McGoldrick, M., Orr, M., & Doellman, D. (2016). Infusion Therapy Standards of Practice. *Journal of Infusion Nursing, 39*(1S), 159.

Mizuno, J. (2013). Use of microaggregate filters instead of leukocyte reduction filters to purify salvaged, autologous blood for re-transfusion during obstetric surgery. *Journal of Anesthesia, 27*(4), 645–646.

Nightingale, MJ, Norfolk, DR, & Pinchon, DJ. (2010). Current uses of transfusion administration sets: a cause for concern? *Transfusion Medicine, 20*(5), 291–302.

Wang, RR, Triulzi, DJ, & Qu, L. (2012). Effects of prestorage vs poststorage leukoreduction on the rate of febrile nonhemolytic transfusion reactions to platelets. *American Journal of Clinical Pathology, 138*(2), 255.

Watkins, T, Surowiecka, MK, & McCullough, J. (2015). Transfusion indications for patients with cancer. *Cancer Control, 22*(1), 38–46.

Chapter 6

Antineoplastic therapy

Just the facts

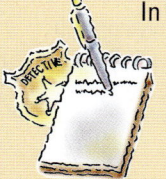

In this chapter, you'll learn:
- ♦ the way in which antineoplastic agents treat cancer
- ♦ types of antineoplastic agents
- ♦ techniques for administering antineoplastic agents
- ♦ adverse effects of antineoplastic agents
- ♦ complications of antineoplastic agents and how to avoid them.

Understanding I.V. antineoplastic agents

Antineoplastic agents, surgery, and radiation are the mainstays of cancer treatment. Antineoplastic agents are most commonly administered into veins (I.V.), using peripheral or central veins — although they are also administered by the oral, subcutaneous (S.C.), intrathecal, intramuscular (I.M.), intra-arterial, intraperitoneal, and intrapleural routes.

Antineoplastic drugs may be administered in the licensed independent practitioner's (LIP) office, an outpatient clinic, the patient's home, a long-term care facility, or hospital. Wherever treatments take place, the same basic principles of I.V. therapy apply. Because of rapid changes in health care delivery leading to a rise in administration of antineoplastic agents outside the hospital setting, emphasis on patient teaching has also increased.

Precision is part of the decision

Suppressing rapidly dividing cancer cells with antineoplastic agents requires effective delivery of an exact dose of these toxic drugs. Administration of these drugs intravenously achieves this effective dosing. Additional benefits include complete absorption and systemic distribution.

It is important to remember that because of the toxicity of these drugs, they are considered to be hazardous and require proper handling from receipt into the facility through disposal.

Which cell is well?

Although antineoplastic agents are intended to control or eliminate cancer cells, they can also damage healthy cells. Healthy cells are attacked because the drugs can't differentiate between healthy cells and cancerous ones. Antineoplastic agents attack all rapidly growing cells. Because hair and nail follicles are rapidly growing cells, patients undergoing treatment with antineoplastic agents typically lose their hair and their nails become brittle.

Multiple cycles of treatment with intravenous antineoplastic drugs will involve frequent peripheral venipunctures and central venous catheter insertion. Consequently, mechanical and chemical vein and tissue damage can occur putting patients at risk for serious complications such as phlebitis, thrombophlebitis, and extravasation.

How antineoplastic medications work

The cell cycle is considered to be the normal life cycle of a cell and is made up of the stages that a cell goes through to reproduce. Healthy and cancerous cells pass through similar life cycles, and antineoplastic agents affect both types. Some of these medications are cell cycle specific, meaning the drugs are effective only during specific phases of the cell cycle. Other drugs are cell cycle nonspecific, meaning that their action is not dependent on a certain segment of the cell cycle. Understanding the cell cycle helps the LIP predict which selection of medications will most likely work effectively together and how often a dose of each one should be administered.

Five phases in the cell cycle have been identified:
1. G0: This stage is considered the starting point for the cycle and is a resting stage. At this point, the cell has not started to divide.
2. G1: This stage lasts 18 to 30 hours. During this stage, the cell synthesizes proteins and increases in size so that new cells will be appropriately sized.
3. S phase: This stage lasts 18 to 20 hours. During this stage, the cell duplicates the chromosomes containing DNA. This will ensure that both new cells produced will have matching strands of DNA.
4. G2 phase: This stage lasts 2 to 10 hours. During this stage, the cell verifies the DNA and prepares to split into two separate cells.
5. M phase: This stage lasts 30 to 60 minutes. During this stage, mitosis occurs, in which the cell splits into two new cells.

The relationship between various antineoplastic drugs and the cell cycle is important to understand. These

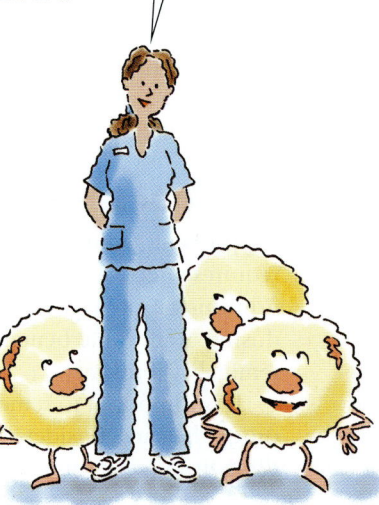

The cell cycle and antineoplastic agents

All cell cycle through five phases. Antineoplastic drugs that are active on cells during one or more of these phases are called cycle specific. The illustration below tells what happens at each phase of the cell cycle and gives examples of cycle-specific drugs that are active during each phase.

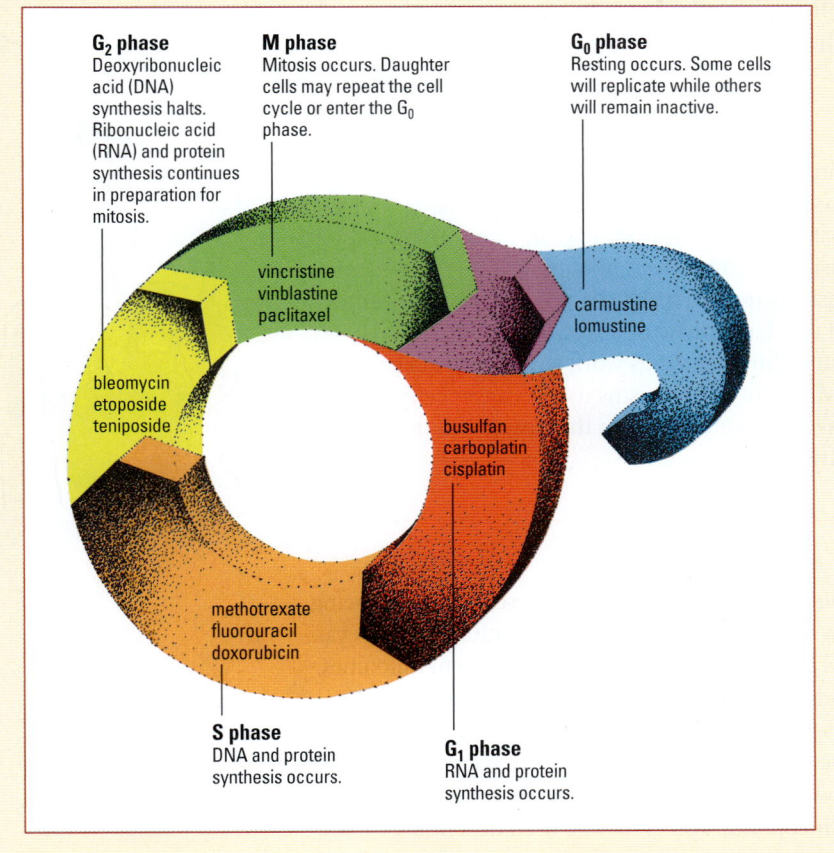

G_2 phase
Deoxyribonucleic acid (DNA) synthesis halts. Ribonucleic acid (RNA) and protein synthesis continues in preparation for mitosis.

M phase
Mitosis occurs. Daughter cells may repeat the cell cycle or enter the G_0 phase.

G_0 phase
Resting occurs. Some cells will replicate while others will remain inactive.

vincristine
vinblastine
paclitaxel

carmustine
lomustine

bleomycin
etoposide
teniposide

busulfan
carboplatin
cisplatin

methotrexate
fluorouracil
doxorubicin

S phase
DNA and protein synthesis occurs.

G_1 phase
RNA and protein synthesis occurs.

medications cannot distinguish between cells that reproduce normally and cancerous cells, thus damage occurs to both normal and cancer cells. The beneficial damage to cancer cells also can mean side effects that can be difficult for the patient to tolerate. All clinicians involved with the patient's care must be able to recognize and manage these side effects, keeping them at a minimum while also maximizing the effect of the drugs on cancerous cells.

Covering all the bases

Because tumor cells are active in various phases of the cell cycle, antineoplastic drug protocols typically employ more than one drug.

This way, each drug can target a different site or take action during a different phase of the cell cycle.

Let's get specific…as well as nonspecific

During a single administration of a cycle-nonspecific antineoplastic drug, a fixed percentage of normal and malignant cells die, while a percentage of normal and malignant cells survive.

When cycle-specific antineoplastic medications are administered, cells in the resting phase survive. (See *The cell cycle and antineoplastic Agents*, page 271.)

Calculating collateral cost

The challenge is to provide a drug dose large enough to kill the greatest number of cancer cells but small enough to avoid irreversibly damaging normal tissue or causing toxicity. Given in combination, antineoplastic drugs potentiate each other, and the tumor responds as it would to a larger dose of a single drug.

In addition, because different drugs work at different stages of the cell cycle or employ different mechanisms to kill cancer cells, using several drugs decreases the likelihood that the tumor will develop resistance to the antineoplastic agent.

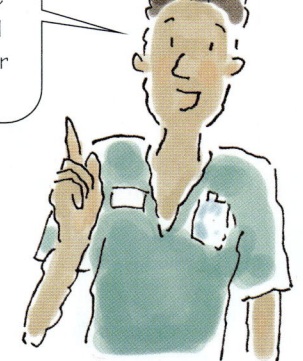

Our challenge is to deliver a drug dose large enough to kill the greater number of cancer cells…

…but small enough to avoid irreversibly damaging normal tissue or causing toxicity.

The selection process

There are many antineoplastic drugs approved for use, with more being approved each year by the Food and Drug Administration (FDA) as various clinical drug trials are completed with successful patient outcomes. Drug selection depends on the patient's age, overall condition, tumor type, and allergies or sensitivities as well as the stage of the cancer. The LIP strives to select the most effective drugs for the first round of antineoplastic drug therapy because this is when cancer cells respond best. Second- or third-line antineoplastic agents may be used depending on the patient's hypersensitivity reaction or the tumor's resistance to the drugs.

Going in cycles

Eradicating a tumor calls for repeated drug doses, which is considered a single course of antineoplastic medication and is repeated on a cyclic basis. The cycle can be repeated daily, weekly, every other week, or every 3 to 4 weeks. Treatment cycles are carefully planned so normal cells can regenerate. The timing of repeat treatment cycles depends on the cycle of the targeted cells and the return of normal blood counts.

Most patients require several treatment cycles before they show any beneficial response. However, every patient differs. Some patients show faster tumor response time than others and some don't respond at all. (See *Determining tumor response*, page 273.)

Determining tumor response

Response evaluation criteria in solid tumors (RECIST) refers to a set of criteria used to assess tumor size in order to assess response to therapy. They were initially introduced in 2000 and were revised in 2009. RECIST criteria categorize cancerous lesions as measurable versus nonmeasurable and target versus nontarget. Measurable lesions can be assessed quantitatively. The target lesion is then selected from the measurable lesions. As a specific number of classified lesions are reevaluated, the patient's tumors can be categorized as improving, stable, or progressive. Improving means that there is a complete response to the therapy and all lesions have disappeared.

Antineoplastic agents

Antineoplastic drugs are categorized according to their pharmacologic action as well as the way in which they interfere with cell production. Antineoplastic agents focused on the cell life cycle and cell reproduction. Recently approved antineoplastic drugs include bendamustine, cabazitaxel, clofarabine, decitabine, eribulin, nelarabine, omacetaxine, pralatrexate, romidepsin, and vorinostat.

The introduction of biological agents has expanded cancer treatment options through knowledge of the human immune system and supporting, enhancing, or altering this system to fight cancer and other diseases. Categories of biological agents include interferons, interleukins, colony-stimulating factors, and monoclonal antibodies. Research into the cancer genome has led to the discovery of new small molecule drugs, also known as targeted therapies. These drugs are highly specific to molecules on the cell wall or inside the cancer cell. (See Chapter 7, *Biological Agents* for discussion of the immune system and how these drugs work.)

Antineoplastic therapy

The traditional approach to cancer treatment is categorized by the drug's pharmacologic action and the effect on the cell life cycle. These categories include alkylating agents, antimetabolites, antitumor antibiotics, topoisomerase inhibitors, and plant alkaloids.

Alkylating agents

Alkylating agents directly damage DNA to keep the cell from reproducing and work in all phases of the cell cycle. They are used to treat many different cancers, including leukemia, lymphoma, Hodgkin disease, multiple myeloma, and sarcoma, as well as cancers of the lung, breast, and ovary. Because these drugs damage DNA, they can cause long-term damage to the bone marrow and occasionally can lead to development of acute leukemia. The risk of leukemia from alkylating agents is "dose dependent," meaning that the risk is small with lower doses, but goes up as the total amount of the drug used gets higher. Alkylating agents are divided into different classes, including:

- nitrogen mustards: mechlorethamine (nitrogen mustard), chlorambucil, cyclophosphamide (Cytoxan), ifosfamide, and melphalan
- nitrosoureas: such as streptozocin, carmustine (BCNU), and lomustine
- alkyl sulfonates: busulfan
- triazines: dacarbazine (DTIC) and temozolomide (Temodar)
- ethylenimines: thiotepa and altretamine (hexamethylmelamine).

The *platinum drugs* are sometimes grouped with alkylating agents because they kill cells in a similar way. They include:

- cisplatin
- carboplatin
- oxaliplatin.

Antimetabolites

Antimetabolites interfere with DNA and RNA growth by substituting for the normal building blocks of these substances. These drugs damage cells during the S phase of the cell cycle. They are commonly used to treat different types of leukemia, cancers of the breast, ovary, and the intestinal tract, as well as other types of cancer. Examples of antimetabolites include:

- 5-fluorouracil (5-FU)
- 6-mercaptopurine (6-MP)
- capecitabine (Xeloda)
- cytarabine (Ara-C)
- floxuridine
- fludarabine
- gemcitabine (Gemzar)
- hydroxyurea

- methotrexate
- pemetrexed (Alimta).

Antitumor antibiotics

These drugs work by altering the DNA inside cancer cells to keep them from growing and multiplying.

Anthracyclines are antitumor antibiotics that interfere with enzymes involved in DNA replication. These drugs work in all phases of the cell cycle and are widely used for a variety of cancers. They typically have a limited lifetime dose due to their cardiotoxicity. Examples of anthracyclines include:
- daunorubicin
- doxorubicin (Adriamycin)
- epirubicin
- idarubicin.

Antitumor antibiotics that are not anthracyclines include:
- actinomycin D
- bleomycin
- mitomycin-C
- mitoxantrone (also acts as a *topoisomerase II inhibitor*).

Topoisomerase inhibitors

These drugs interfere with enzymes called topoisomerases, which help separate the strands of DNA so that they can be copied during the S phase. Topoisomerase inhibitors are used to treat certain types of leukemia, as well as lung, ovarian, gastrointestinal, and other cancers.

Topoisomerase inhibitors are grouped according to which type of enzyme they affect: *Topoisomerase I inhibitors* include:
- topotecan
- irinotecan (CPT-11).

Topoisomerase II inhibitors include:
- etoposide (VP-16)
- teniposide
- mitoxantrone (also acts as an *antitumor antibiotic*).

Topoisomerase II inhibitors can increase the risk of developing acute myelogenous leukemia (AML) 2 to 3 years after the drug is given.

Plant alkaloids

This group may be known as *mitotic inhibitors* because they primarily work by stopping mitosis in the M phase of the cell cycle, although

they also act in G2 phase. They can damage cells in all phases by keeping enzymes from making proteins needed for cell reproduction. Examples of mitotic inhibitors include:
- taxanes: paclitaxel (Taxol) and docetaxel (Taxotere)
- epothilones: ixabepilone (Ixempra)
- vinca alkaloids: vinblastine (Velban), vincristine (Oncovin), and vinorelbine (Navelbine)
- estramustine (Emcyt).

They are used to treat many different types of cancer including breast, lung, myelomas, lymphomas, and leukemias. These drugs may cause secondary nerve damage.

Corticosteroids

Corticosteroids are natural hormones and hormonelike drugs that are useful in the treatment of many types of cancer. When these drugs are used as part of cancer treatment, they are considered chemotherapy drugs. Examples of corticosteroids include:
- prednisone
- methylprednisolone (Solu-Medrol)
- dexamethasone (Decadron).

Steroids are also commonly used to help prevent nausea and vomiting caused by chemotherapy. They are used before antineoplastic drug treatment to help prevent severe allergic reactions, too.

Miscellaneous antineoplastic agents

Some antineoplastic drugs act in slightly different ways and do not fit well into any of the other categories. These include L-asparaginase, which is an enzyme, and the proteasome inhibitor bortezomib (Velcade).

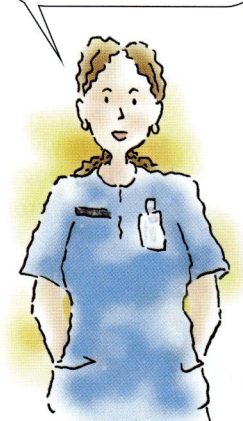

When drugs are given in combinations, they're called protocols.

Multitasking drugs

The LIP orders antineoplastic drugs to control cancer, to cure cancer, to prevent metastasis, or for palliation. Drugs may be given alone or in combinations called *protocols*. (See *Sample antineoplastic protocols*, page 277.)

(Text continues on page 278)

Sample antineoplastic protocols

Antineoplastic drugs are commonly given in combinations called protocols. Here are some protocols typically given for common cancers.

Specific cancers	Protocols	Drugs
Bladder cancer	M-VAC Both generic and trade names may be used in protocol abbreviations.	• Methotrexate • Vinblastine • Adriamycin (doxorubicin) • Cisplatin When a trade name is used, you'll find the generic name in parentheses.
Breast cancer	ACT	• Adriamycin (doxorubicin) • Cyclophosphamide • Taxol (paclitaxel) or Taxotere (docetaxel)
Cervical cancer	CF	• Cisplatin • Fluorouracil
Prostate cancer	CE	• Cisplatin
Gastric cancer	ECF	• Etoposide • Epirubicin • Cisplatin • Fluorouracil
Laryngeal cancer	CF	• Cisplatin • Fluorouracil (5-Fu)
Acute lymphocytic leukemia, induction	DVPA	• Daunorubicin • Vincristine • Prednisone • Asparaginase
Melanoma	CVD	• Cisplatin • Vinblastine • Dacarbazine
Acute myelocytic leukemia	POMP	• Prednisone • Oncovin (vincristine) • Methotrexate • Purinethol (mercaptopurine)
Lymphoma (non-Hodgkin's)	CHOP	• Cyclophosphamide • Doxorubicin/hydroxydoxorubicin • Oncovin (vincristine) • Prednisone
Lung cancer, small cell	CE	• Cisplatin • Etoposide

(*continued*)

Sample antineoplastic protocols *(continued)*

Specific cancers	Protocols	Drugs
Lung cancer, non-small cell	PC	• Paclitaxel • Cisplatin
Lymphoma (Hodgkin's disease)	ABVD	• Adriamycin (doxorubicin) • Bleomycin • Vinblastine • Dacarbazine
Lymphoma, malignant	BEACOPP	• Bleomycin • Etoposide • Adriamycin (doxorubicin) • Cyclophosphamide • Oncovin (vincristine) • Procarbazine • Prednisone • Filgrastim
Multiple myeloma	VAD	• Vincristine • Adriamycin (doxorubicin) • Dexamethasone
Testicular cancer	BEP	• Bleomycin • Etoposide • Platinol (cisplatin)

The search for new cancer treatments is ongoing. Each year, the National Cancer Institute screens thousands of potential new compounds for antineoplastic action.

Preparation for antineoplastic drug administration

Antineoplastic agents are considered hazardous drugs because they can cause adverse reactions or harm to personnel handling them. A drug is considered hazardous if it meets one or more of these characteristics:
- able to cause cancer in humans or animals — a carcinogen
- able to cause fetal defects — a teratogen
- toxic to the reproductive process
- causes organ toxicity at low doses
- able to cause mutation in genetic material — a mutagen
- a new drug that mimics an existing drug to cause one of these criteria.

Due to these risks, there is no acceptable level of exposure to any hazardous drug. Nurses, pharmacists, and other personnel involved in the preparation, administration, and disposal of antineoplastic drugs must complete specialized training and document competencies for all aspects of handling hazardous drugs, proper use of personnel protective equipment, proper use of all equipment and supplies, spill management, appropriate response to known or suspected exposure, and proper disposal of hazardous drugs.

Protect yourself

The National Institute for Occupational Safety and Health (NIOSH) lists antineoplastic medications with other hazardous drugs that are administered in health care settings. Review the protocol at your facility to ensure that the proper precautions are being taken for preparation, administration, and disposal of these drugs. Because these medications are hazardous to prepare, administer, and dispose of, personnel who will be handling these drugs must be educated regarding the toxicities associated with exposure. The effects of such exposure can be immediate, such as burning of the skin and mucous membranes, as well as long-term, such as hair loss. The required precautions associated with antineoplastic drugs must be emphasized along with the proper type of personal protective equipment that must be worn to avoid exposure. Personnel who are pregnant or breastfeeding or who are attempting to conceive should avoid exposure to antineoplastic agents since these drugs are cytotoxic.

All personnel who deal with hazardous drugs in any way must be thoroughly educated on the proper procedures to be used during all handling of these drugs, such as use of a Class II Biological Safety Cabinet, the proper method for administration, and the correct method of disposal in accordance with the guidelines generated by the OSHA and USP <800>. Hazardous waste containers should be made of puncture-proof, shatter-proof, leak-proof plastic. Antineoplastic waste is usually identified with yellow biohazard labels. Use them to dispose of all antineoplastic-contaminated I.V. fluid containers, administration sets, filters, and syringes. Red sharps containers are used to dispose of all contaminated sharps such as needles.

Follow the guidelines

Many health care facilities use existing guidelines as a basis for their policies and procedures regarding antineoplastic drugs. The major sources for these guidelines include the following agencies and associations:
- The American Society of Health-System Pharmacists (ASHP) has published guidelines for the preparation of antineoplastic drugs and recently updated them for 2016.

- The Occupational Safety and Health Administration (OSHA) published standards for controlling exposure to antineoplastic drugs initially in 1995 and revised those standards in 2014.
- The Oncology Nursing Society (ONS) published revised guidelines for nursing education, practice, and administration of antineoplastic drugs in 2014.
- The Infusion Nurses Society (INS) published revised standards of practice for safe delivery of antineoplastic drugs in 2016.
- The United States Pharmcopeial Convention (USP) Standards has issued two chapters that sets safety standards for preparation and administration of antineoplastic agents:
  - USP <797> is the chapter on Pharmaceutical Compounding: Sterile Preparations sets the standard for preparing all sterile medications based on the level of risk involved.
  - USP <800> is the chapter specifically addressing Hazardous Drugs: Handling in the Healthcare Settings. This chapter addresses the protection of all health care personnel in all settings and includes receipt of the drug through administration and disposal. The goal of these standards is to adequately contain all hazardous drugs to protect the patient, health care personnel, and the environment from exposure. This chapter was released in August 2016; however, facilities have been given until July 2018 to become compliant with this document.

Protective measures

Preparation of antineoplastic drugs requires adherence to guidelines regarding:
- drug preparation areas and equipment
- protective clothing
- specific safety measures.

Drug preparation

The facility pharmacy personnel should prepare the antineoplastic drugs. With documented competency and the ability to work in a biological safety cabinet, a nurse may prepare these drugs also. Some states allow a supervised pharmacy technician to prepare these drugs. Regardless of who is preparing these drugs, it is the responsibility of the nurse to verify that the dosage of the medication is accurate before administering the medication. It is important to have an accurate weight and height to calculate the patient's body surface area (BSA). Dosing for most antineoplastic drugs is based on BSA, expressed as meter square or m^2.

Preparation of equipment

Prior to preparing equipment for administration of antineoplastic agents, verify that informed consent was obtained and patient has had all questions answered regarding all aspects of treatment.

Protect the air when you prepare

Perform all drug compounding within a setting designated exclusively for the purpose of preparing hazardous drugs. This setting will include a biological safety cabinet or a compounding aseptic containment isolator (CACI) for the purpose of protecting the person working in the cabinet and the environment. These cabinets must be filtered and vented to the outside with a specific number of times the air is exchanged per hour. The airflow inside the device pulls the aerosolized antineoplastic drug particles away from the person working in the cabinet.

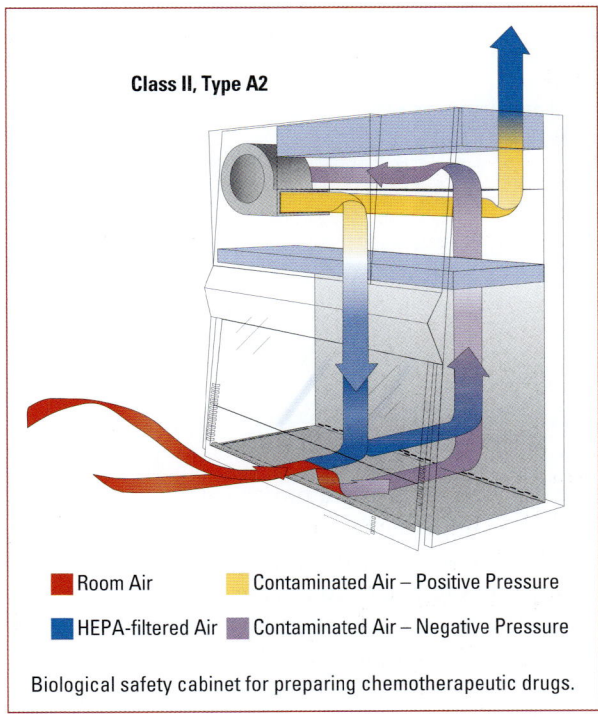

Biological safety cabinet for preparing chemotherapeutic drugs.

Close to you

Have close access to a sink, and eyewash station, alcohol sponges, and gauze pads as well as OSHA-required antineoplastic hazardous waste containers, sharps containers, and antineoplastic spill kits. (See *Equipment for preparing antineoplastic drugs*, page 282.)

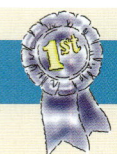

Best practice

Equipment for preparing antineoplastic drugs

These items should be available in your work area when preparing antineoplastic drugs:
- patient's medication order
- prescribed drugs
- appropriate diluent (if necessary)
- medication labels
- long-sleeved gown impermeable to hazardous drugs, closed in the back with closed cuffs
- gloves specially tested and designated for handling hazardous drugs, 2 pairs are worn for administration and changed every 30 minutes or if contaminated with the drug
- head, hair, and sleeve covers
- eye goggles that fully wrap around the eyes
- fit-tested respirator for face protection
- closed system drugs transfer devices (CSTD)
- syringes with luer lock connections and needles of various sizes
- I.V. administration set with luer lock connections
- 70% alcohol
- sterile gauze pads
- plastic bags with "hazardous drug" labels
- sharps disposal container
- hazardous waste container
- antineoplastic spill kit.

The lowdown on gowns and gloves

Administration of antineoplastic drugs requires use of protective clothing. Gowns should be disposable, impermeable to hazardous drugs with long sleeves, closed cuffs, and a closure in the back and without seams that could allow the drugs to enter. Gowns are never worn into other areas outside of the designated compounding area. They must be changed after known contamination and within 3 hours of use.

Gloves designed for use with antineoplastic drugs should be disposable and made of thick latex or nonlatex material and labeled as compliant "chemotherapy" gloves. They must be powder-free because powder can carry contamination from the drugs into the surrounding

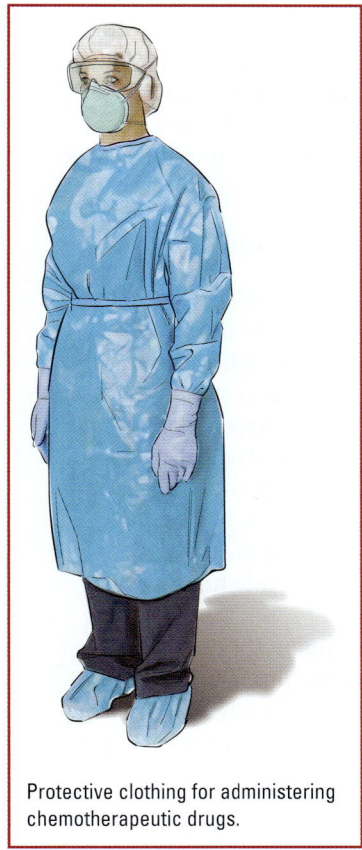

Protective clothing for administering chemotherapeutic drugs.

air. Gloves are changed every 30 minutes while working with hazardous drugs or when they become contaminated with the drug. Two pairs of gloves are used during the administration of these drugs. Wash your hands before putting on the gloves and after removing them.

Eye protection requires goggles that fully wrap around to protect splashes from entering from any direction. Head cover and two pairs of shoe covers are also worn.

Safety measures

Take care to protect staff, patients, and the environment from unnecessary exposure to antineoplastic drugs. Don't leave the drug preparation area while wearing the protective gear you wore during drug preparation. Eating, drinking, smoking, or applying cosmetics in the drug preparation area violates OSHA guidelines.

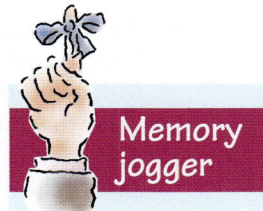

Memory jogger

To remember the clothing you should wear when preparing antineoplastic drugs, think of the three **G**'s:

Gown

Gloves

Goggles.

Laying the groundwork for safety

Put on protective gear before you begin to compound the antineoplastic drugs. Before preparing the drugs, clean the work area inside the cabinet with 70% alcohol and a disposable towel; do the same after you're finished and after a spill. Discard the towel into the yellow leakproof antineoplastic waste container.

Feeling exposed

Personnel protective equipment is the first line of defense against exposure to all hazardous drugs. Accidental exposure during routine compounding and administration and during spill cleanup can result in unintended exposure that can lead to health changes in the exposed personnel. It is imperative that all procedures for handling hazardous drugs be followed closely. If an antineoplastic drug comes in contact with your skin, wash the skin thoroughly with soap and water. This will reduce drug absorption into the skin. If the drug comes in contact with your eye, immediately flood the eye with water or isotonic eyewash for at least 5 minutes while holding the eyelid open.

After an accidental exposure, notify your supervisor immediately. Your supervisor should send you to employee health, where the exposure event will be documented in your employee health record. Medical follow-up may be necessary depending on the type of drug and the quantity of exposure.

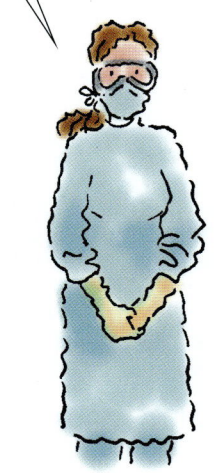

Put on your protective gear before you begin to do anything with antineoplastic drugs.

Better safe than sorry

Here are some other safety precautions to keep in mind:
- Use aseptic, no-touch technique when preparing all drugs.
- Prior to administration, verify the order of antineoplastic drug with two clinicians who are qualified to administer such agents. Verify the drug name, dose, volume, rate of administration, expiration date, infusion pump rate, and the physical appearance of the drug as well as calculation of the correct drug dosage. Two qualified clinicians perform calculation and order verification processes independently, and then, results from each are compared.
- Use only a closed system drug transfer (CSDT) device for connecting syringes and administration sets during compounding and administration of all antineoplastic drugs.
- Wear a facemask and goggles to protect yourself against splashes and aerosolized drugs.
- Place all contaminated needles in the sharps container, and don't recap needles.

- Use only syringes and I.V. sets that have a luer lock connection.
- Label all antineoplastic drugs with a yellow biohazard label.

Closing the system

Connected syringes, vials, I.V. catheter hubs, and injection ports on administration sets can cause small drops to leak from these connections or vapor to spray into the air. The National Institute for Occupational Safety and Health (NIOSH) defines a closed system drug transfer device as a device that prevents transfer of contaminated particles from the outside environment into a system and the escape of hazardous drug or vapor concentrations from the system into the outside environment. These devices are specifically designed for transfer of hazardous drugs during all compounding and administration procedures. They work in two ways. First, they prevent the introduction of contaminants from the environment into the solution. Second, they prevent the release or escape of the hazardous drug or its vapor outside the container, syringe, or administration set. INS, ONS, and USP support their use for the protection of health care personnel from unintended exposure to any hazardous drug. Closed system transfer devices have been shown to reduce the levels of surface contamination where antineoplastic drugs are handled.

Transport tactics

Transport the prepared antineoplastic drugs in a sealable plastic bag that's prominently labeled with a yellow antineoplastic biohazard label.

The spiel on spills

Make sure that your facility's protocols for spills are available in all areas where antineoplastic drugs are handled, including patient care areas. Antineoplastic spill kits should be readily available. (See *Inside an antineoplastic spill kit*, page 286.)

If a spill occurs, follow your facility's protocol, which should be based on OSHA guidelines and USP <800>. This protocol will likely instruct you to follow these steps:
- Put on protective garments, if you aren't already wearing them.
- Isolate the area and contain the spill with absorbent materials from the spill kit.
- Use the disposable dustpan and scraper to collect broken glass or desiccant absorbing powder. Carefully place the dustpan, scraper, and collected spill in a leakproof, punctureproof, antineoplastic designated hazardous waste container.

> ### Best practice
>
> **Inside a antineoplastic spill kit**
>
> Based on Occupational Safety and Health Administration guidelines and your facility's protocols, a antineoplastic spill kit should contain:
> - long-sleeved gown that's water-resistant and nonpermeable, with cuffs and back closure
> - shoe covers
> - two pair of powder-free chemotherapy gloves (for double gloving)
> - respirator mask
> - chemical splash goggles
> - disposable dustpan and plastic scraper (for collecting broken glass)
> - plastic-backed absorbent towels, or spill-control pillows
> - desiccant powder or granules (for absorbing wet contents)
> - disposable sponges
> - two large cytotoxic waste disposal bags.

- Prevent the aerosolization of the drug at all times.
- Clean the spill area with a detergent or bleach solution.

Drug administration

Because dosage, route, and timing must be exact to avoid possibly fatal complications, only nurses who have completed specialized training in administration of antineoplastic agents and who have documented competency when administering antineoplastic drugs should be involved in administering these drugs. To document your competency, obtain the needed education, and then work with a designated preceptor to gain experience with supervision.

There are three steps to follow when administering antineoplastic drugs:
1. Perform the preadministration check and document all steps.
2. Obtain I.V. access, by insertion of a peripheral catheter, by accessing an implanted port, or assessing the patency of an existing CVAD.
3. Give drugs per LIP's order, according to your facility's antineoplastic protocol and standards of practice.

Performing a preadministration check

Before administering an antineoplastic drug, perform the independent double-check of LIP orders and dose calculations, and then compare these results with another nurse.

Count on doing this

The patient's blood count should be checked before beginning the antineoplastic infusion. Many facilities have nursing policies that require the nurse to notify the LIP for approval to administer the antineoplastic drug if the patient's blood count drops below a predetermined value. Antineoplastic drugs that are excreted through the kidneys, such as cisplatin and carboplatin, require checking serum creatinine levels.

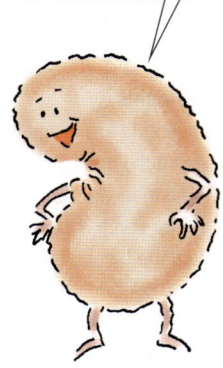

Check serum creatinine levels before giving drugs that excrete through me!

Which drugs? Which route?

Make sure that you understand clearly which drugs are to be given and by which route. Check whether the drug is classified as a vesicant, nonvesicant, or irritant. (See *Risks of tissue damage*, page 288.)

Who's on first?

The sequence of giving multiple antineoplastic drugs may make a difference in how the drugs work and the potential for toxicity. Follow the order of drugs as prescribed. Document the sequence used to administer all drugs, along with the specific site and condition and the specific lumen used for a multiple lumen central VAD.

Confirm and verify

Confirm any written orders for needed antiemetics, fluids, diuretics, or electrolyte supplements to be given before, during, or after antineoplastic administration. Verify the patient's level of understanding of the treatment and adverse effects. Make sure that either the patient or a surrogate has signed an informed consent form for each specific antineoplastic drug they're to receive and for the insertion of the I.V. device, if required. (See *Preventing errors*, page 291.)

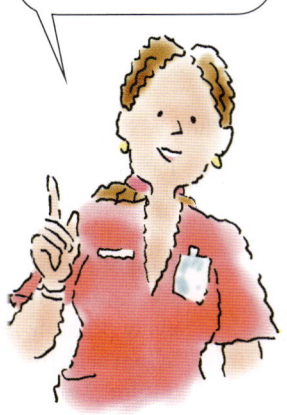

Before administering an antineoplastic drug, know its potential for damaging tissue.

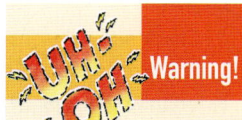

Warning!

Risks of tissue damage

To administer antineoplastic medications safely, you need to know each drug's potential for damaging tissue. In this regard, antineoplastic drugs are classified as vesicants, nonvesicants, or irritants.

Vesicants

Vesicants are drugs that have the potential to cause damage to tissue surrounding the vein if the medication escapes from the vein. The degree of tissue damage depends upon many factors such as the concentration of the drug, and the amount of drug in contact with subcutaneous tissue before it is identified. Some vesicants cause tissue damage by binding to the DNA inside normal cells, while others do not bind with DNA.

DNA-binding vesicant drugs include:
- alkylating agents: nitrogen mustard
- anthracyclines: daunorubicin, doxorubicin, epirubicin, and idarubicin
- other: dactinomycin and mitomycin C.

Non–DNA-binding vesicant drugs include:
- vinca alkaloids: vinblastine, vincristine, and vinorelbine
- taxanes: docetaxel and paclitaxel.

Irritants

Irritants cause a local venous response, with or without external signs of inflammation. Irritants include:
- alkylating agents: carboplatin, carmustine, cisplatin, cyclophosphamide, dacarbazine, ifosfamide, melphalan, oxaliplatin, and thiotepa
- antimetabolites: cytarabine, fludarabine, 5-fluorouracil, gemcitabine, methotrexate, and raltitrexed
- others: bleomycin, etoposide, and irinotecan.

Consult your pharmacist for a comprehensive list of drugs in each category.

Obtaining vascular access

Patients receiving antineoplastic drugs have many vascular access device options. For antineoplastic drugs to be administered for up to 3 months, a short peripheral catheter is probably the best choice if the patient has good peripheral veins. Do not use an existing peripheral I.V. catheter that is more than 24 hours old in order to ensure that every possible precaution has been taken to prevent extravasation. When selecting a peripheral vein, avoid choosing one that is close to a joint. Avoid multiple venipuncture attempts — only 2 attempts per nurse for a maximum of 4 venipuncture attempts. When veins are not easily visible or palpable, do not blindly perform venipuncture attempts. Near-infrared light and ultrasound devices may be needed to insert the catheter. Contact the infusion or vascular access specialists in your facility. (See Chapter 2, *Infusion Through Peripheral Veins*, page 53.)

Central venous access may be required for patients with poor peripheral veins, when the required length of therapy is longer than 3 months, and when the therapy includes vesicants requiring continuous infusion over long periods. Tunneled cuffed catheters, peripherally inserted central catheters (PICC), and implanted ports are central venous access devices used for antineoplastic administration and are used for long-term vascular access. The most appropriate choice of devices is based on a thorough assessment of patient needs in a collaborative process with all health care team members including the patient. Factors to consider include:

1. frequency and duration of therapy
2. patient's age and other chronic diseases
3. history of vascular access devices and infusion therapies
4. characteristics of the therapy (for example, osmolarity, pH, vesicant or irritant nature)
5. need for supportive therapies such as parenteral nutrition or pain management
6. need for stem cell collection, plasmapheresis, and bone marrow reinfusion
7. patient/family's ability to care for the VAD and available resources
8. patient preference.

(See Chapter 3, *Infusion Therapy Requiring Central Venous Access*, page 119.)

Confirm and document that a blood return is present prior to initiating an I.V. infusion of an antineoplastic agent for both peripheral and central VADs. Aspirate from the peripheral catheter using a slow, gentle technique with a small syringe (that is, 3 mL) or place a tourniquet on the arm well above the catheter and try again to aspirate for a blood return. Inability to obtain a blood return from a short peripheral catheter is an indication to remove and insert a new catheter.

A central VAD that does not produce a free-flowing blood return should not be used before diagnostic tests are performed to confirm the pathway of fluid flow. Absence of a blood return could indicate a catheter tip in a suboptimal location; has migrated into a smaller tributary vein, into the jugular vein or contralateral subclavian vein; the tip can completely erode through the vessel wall; or the tip could be encased in a fibrin sheath or complete vein thrombus.

Assessment of VAD patency

Apply a transparent dressing so that the site can be observed for early signs of infiltration, extravasation, and vein irritation. Complete assessment of the VAD patency including observation, palpation, aspiration for blood return, flushing for lack of resistance, attention to the quality of the fluid flow, and listening and correctly responding to all patient complaints will be needed to avoid infiltration and extravasation.

Assess and verify blood return every 2 to 5 mL during an I.V. push medication and every 5 to 10 minutes during an infusion of an antineoplastic agent. Remain with the patient during the entire infusion. The infusion should be discontinued at the first sign of any complication, especially extravasation.

Giving drugs

Before administering an antineoplastic drug, start the infusion of a prescribed I.V. fluid into the I.V. catheter. Continue to visually monitor the site and document its appearance and the patient's response. Recognize that use of an electronic infusion pump does not cause extravasation and can neither prevent extravasation nor even decrease the likelihood that it will occur. Infusion pumps are machines that continue pumping fluid at the set rate without any means to detect the pathway of fluid flow. It is the responsibility of the nurse to monitor the infusion site frequently so that the first sign of an extravasation can be detected immediately; do not rely on infusion pump alarms for this purpose. Severe extravasation injury usually requires surgical debridement, skin grafts, and can cause decreased function with that extremity. Need for amputation is possible, especially when there is arterial damage as well.

Small ambulatory infusion pumps are used for continuous infusion of antineoplastic drugs in alternative settings. The patient may have the infusion started at an infusion clinic or LIP office and then return home for infusion over several hours or days. The patient may return to the oncology clinic or a home health nurse may perform periodic monitoring and discontinue the pump when complete. The patient will need well-written instructions about signs and symptoms to look for and report and the specific phone number to call if there is a problem during the infusion.

Administration variations

I.V. antineoplastic drugs can be administered:
1. by indirect I.V. push through the injection port of an I.V. administration set infusing regular fluids
2. as a continuous infusion for several hours or even days
3. as a short-term infusion over 30 to 60 minutes, usually given piggyback into infusing plain fluids.

Reducing extravasation risks

Follow these guidelines when giving vesicants to avoid extravasation:
• Use a distal vein in the forearm that allows successive proximal venipunctures.
• Avoid using the hand, wrist, antecubital space, damaged areas, or areas with compromised circulation.
• Don't probe for veins as this increases the risk of nerve injury.
• Place a transparent dressing over the site.
• Start with infusion of free flowing normal saline solution or other prescribed I.V. fluids without any added medication.
• Inspect the site for swelling, redness or blanching, and leakage.
• Tell the patient to report burning, stinging, pain, pruritus, or temperature changes near the site.
• After drug administration, flush the line with normal saline solution using a quantity sufficient to clear all drug from the administration set. Check for blood return at frequent intervals regardless of whether the medication is being administered peripherally or through a central venous catheter (every 3 to 5 mL during an I.V. push or every 5 to 10 minutes during an I.V. infusion).

Finish with a flush

No matter which method of administration is ordered, flush the vein with normal saline solution between the administration of each drug. This flushing reduces contact between the drug and the vein wall, and it also prevents contact between two drugs that may be incompatible with each other.

Investigating infiltration and extravasation

Check for infiltration during administration as well as for signs of a hypersensitivity reaction.

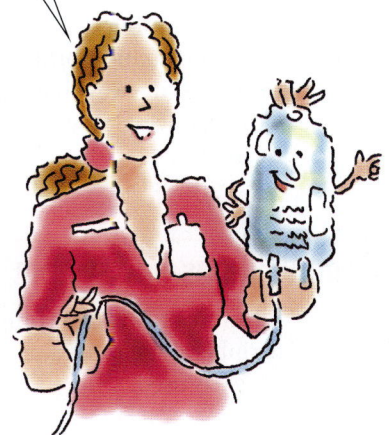

Instruct the patient to report burning, stinging, or pain at or near the site, but recognize that pain may not be present initially. Observe around the site for streaky redness along the vein and other skin changes. Also, listen to what the patient has to say about his level of comfort; sudden discomfort during drug administration or flushing could indicate infiltration. Aspirate for a blood return at frequent intervals and look for blood that is the color and consistency of whole blood. Flushing with saline should be done at the same rate as the medication. The I.V. administration set and VAD will hold varying amounts of the drug so flushing at the same rate ensures that this last volume of drug is given at the correct rate.

For a peripheral catheter, keep in mind the expression, "When in doubt, take it out!"

Concluding treatment

After the infusion is complete, take the following steps:
- Dispose of all used needles and contaminated sharps in the biohazard container.
- Dispose of personal protective gear, goggles, and gloves in the yellow antineoplastic waste container.
- Dispose of unused medications, considered hazardous waste, according to facility policy.
- Wash your hands thoroughly with soap and water, even though you have worn gloves.
- Document the sequence in which the drugs were administered.
- Document the anatomical site accessed for a peripheral catheter (such as lower third of left inner forearm), the gauge and length of the catheter, and the number of attempts for insertion of a short peripheral catheter. When a CVAD is used, document the specific lumen used for administration.
- Document the name, dose, and route of the administered drugs, as well as the volume and type of diluent and rate of drug administration.
- Document the type and volume of the I.V. solutions and any adverse reactions and nursing interventions.
- According to facility policy and procedures, wear protective clothing when handling body fluids from the patient for 48 hours after the antineoplastic treatment.

Complications of antineoplastic drug therapy

The properties that make antineoplastic drugs effective in killing cancer cells also make them toxic to normal cells. No organ or body system is untouched by antineoplastic drug treatment. Therefore, all administration protocols strive to time the treatments and adjust the doses in a way that maximizes the effects against cancer cells while allowing time for normal cells to recover between courses of treatment.

Complications per system

Infusion site–related complications affect the patient's arm if a peripheral site is used or the chest area if a central venous access device is used.

Irritant or flare reaction

Irritation to the vein may be seen during medication infusion. The patient may complain of tightness or aching along the path of the vein and the vein tract may appear red or darkened. Swelling does not occur and blood return is still present unless the irritation is combined with an escape of the infusing fluid into the subcutaneous tissue. Examples of antineoplastic agents known to be irritants include bleomycin, carboplatin, carmustine, dacarbazine, gemcitabine, ifosfamide, and topotecan. Treatment for an irritant reaction includes warm compresses for 15 to 20 minutes several times per day. Greater dilution of the drug by the pharmacy and using a larger peripheral vein with a small catheter will provide more dilution from the blood flow.

Some irritants may also act as mild vesicants if they escape into the subcutaneous tissue. This may cause the local tissue to harden or discolor, along with pain and swelling. Tissue sloughing and necrosis are not common with this group, which includes oxaliplatin, vinorelbine, medphalan, bendamustine hydrochloride, and irinotecan.

A flare reaction is caused by release of histamine from mast cells and basophils. The peripheral vein tract becomes temporarily red, with itching and a rash. There is no pain or swelling and a blood return is present. Treatment involves flushing the vein with normal saline and withholding the antineoplastic agent until signs and symptoms resolve. Hydrocortisone and antihistamines may be necessary for treatment as well as prevention if the antineoplastic drug must be administered in the future.

Extravasation

Extravasation is the inadvertent leakage of a vesicant (a drug that can cause tissue damage) solution into the surrounding tissue. Blistering, tissue sloughing, and necrosis can be the outcome, but this takes days or even weeks to appear. It is critical to recognize this problem early so that the infusion can be stopped quickly to limit the amount of drug that enters the tissue.

Stay hip to these tips

When assessing the patient for extravasation, keep these points in mind:
- Initial signs of extravasation may resemble those of infiltration — swelling, pain, and blanching.

- Symptoms can progress to blisters; skin, muscle, tissue, and fat necrosis; and tissue sloughing. The veins, arteries, and nerves may also be damaged. Depending on the drug and the concentration of the drug in the solution, blistering can be apparent within hours or days of the extravasation, but ulceration and tissue sloughing usually takes days to weeks.

Emergency!

If a vesicant has extravasated, it's an emergency! Know your facility policy and procedure before administering antineoplastic drugs and be prepared to act. Quickly take the following steps, designed to limit the damage:
- Stop the infusion. Detach the administration set; attach a syringe directly to the hub of the peripheral catheter or implanted port access needle and aspirate all contents. Remove the peripheral catheter or port needle. For other types of CVADs, aspirate the contents from the catheter, flush with normal saline, and lock the catheter according to facility policy and procedure.
- Elevate the extremity.
- Apply the appropriate cold or warm compresses based on the drug given.
- Notify the LIP of the event including the drug and the type of catheter involved. For a CVAD, further diagnostic testing will be required to determine the fluid flow pathway, the necessity for removal, and a new plan for vascular access for future cycles of antineoplastic drugs.
- Administer the appropriate antidote according to facility policy and LIP orders. The efficacy of antidotes has not been established through clinical trials and is based on case reports. Most antidotes are injected subcutaneously in multiple small quantities around the periphery of the extravasation. Dexrazoxane, given by I.V. infusion daily for 3 days, is the exception. Studies have shown this to be effective in 98% of anthracycline extravasations.

Follow-up assessment and care are required but dependent upon the patient, venue of care, and facility policies. The response to extravasation treatment should be documented, including skin integrity, presence of pain and other signs and symptoms, mobility of the extremity, and neurovascular assessment. Educate the patient about protecting the site from sunlight and what to report to his health care provider. Referral to a plastic or hand surgeon, for pain management, or physical therapy may be needed.

Extravasation Management Guidelines

Vesicant drug	Apply heat or cold	Additional treatment/antidote
Alkylating agents Mechlorethamine hydrochloride (Mustargen)	Cold for 6 to 12 hours after administration of sodium thiosulfate	**Sodium thiosulfate**: mix 4 mL of 10% sodium thiosulfate with 6 mL sterile water (yields 10 mL of 1/6 molar sodium thiosulfate). For every 1 mg of mechlorethamine suspected to have extravasated, inject 2 mL of the 1/6 molar sodium thiosulfate solution subcutaneously into the extravasation site using a 25 gauge or smaller needle.
Anthracyclines Daunorubicin (Cerubidine) Doxorubicin (Adriamycin) Epirubicin (Ellence) Idarubicin (Idamycin)	• Cold initially for 15–20 minutes four times a day for 3 days. • Remove cold pack at least 15 minutes before dexrazoxane therapy.	**Dexrazoxane (Totect)**: dexrazoxane should be administered over 1–2 hours I.V. at the recommended doses below, daily for 3 consecutive days. Site of administration should be in a large vein away from the extravasation. The first infusion should be initiated as soon as possible and within the first 6 hours after extravasation. • Day 1: 1,000 mg/m^2 • Day 2: 1,000 mg/m^2 • Day 3: 500 mg/m^2 If cooling techniques are being used, withhold cooling 15 minutes before the infusion. Infuse in an extremity or area other than the one affected by extravasation.
Antitumor antibiotics Mitomycin (Mutamycin) Dactinomycin (actinomycin D, Cosmegen)	Cold for 15–20 minutes at a time for at least four times per day for 24 hours	None known
Plant alkaloids Vinblastine (Velban) Vincristine (Oncovin) Vinorelbine (Navelbine)	Heat for 15–20 minutes at a time for at least four times per day for 24–48 hours	**Hyaluronidase**: inject a total of 1 mL (150 units) divided into 5 subcutaneous injections of 0.2 mL in a pinwheel fashion using a 25-gauge needle, changing needles between each injection, into affected area.
Anthracenedione Mitoxantrone (Novantrone)	Cold for 15–20 minutes at least four times a day for the first 24 hours	No known antidotes
Taxanes Docetaxel (taxotere) Paclitaxel (Taxol) Paclitaxel protein-bound particles for injectable suspension (Abraxane)	Cold for 15–20 minutes at least four times a day for the first 24 hours	No known antidotes

Hypersensitivity or anaphylactic reactions

A hypersensitivity or anaphylactic reaction can occur at the initial dose of the drug or on subsequent infusions of the same drug. Some antineoplastic drugs put the patient at high risk for anaphylaxis.

Hypersensitivity reactions can occur at the beginning, middle, or end of the infusion. (See *Signs and symptoms of immediate hypersensitivity*, below.)

The specific treatment for a hypersensitivity reaction will depend on the severity of the reaction. Usually, you'll follow these five steps:
1. Stop the infusion.
2. Begin a rapid infusion of normal saline solution using a new administration set to prevent infusion of additional drug in the original set.
3. Check the patient's vital signs.
4. Notify the LIP.
5. Administer emergency drugs as ordered by the LIP.

What to give and when

Antihistamines are typically given first, followed by corticosteroids and bronchodilators. Epinephrine is given first in severe anaphylactic reactions. After you have administered the drug, monitor the patient's vital signs and pulse oximetry every 5 minutes until he's stable and then every 15 minutes for 1 to 2 hours — or follow facility policy and procedures for acute treatment of allergic reactions.

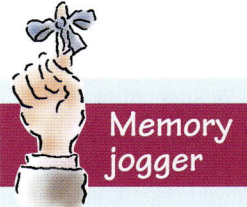

Memory jogger

As soon as you spot an extravasation, think of the three **C**'s:

Cut off (the infusion)

Counteract (effects of the drug)

Contain (the affected area).

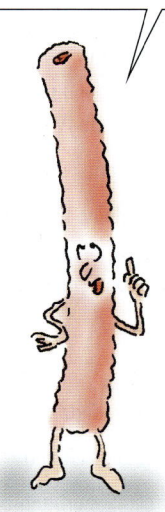

Infiltration and extravasation occur OUTSIDE the vein in the subcutaneous tissue. Irritant and flare reactions happen INSIDE the vein lumen.

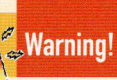 **Warning!**

Signs and symptoms of immediate hypersensitivity

An immediate hypersensitivity reaction to an antineoplastic drug will appear within 5 minutes after starting to administer the drug.

Organ system	Subjective complaints	Objective findings
Respiratory	Dyspnea, inability to speak, tightness in chest	Stridor, bronchospasm, decreased air movement
Skin	Pruritus	Cyanosis, urticaria, angioedema, cold and clammy skin
Cardiovascular	Chest pain, increased heart rate	Tachycardia, hypotension, arrhythmias
Central nervous system	Dizziness, agitation, anxiety	Decreased sensorium, loss of consciousness

Throughout the episode, maintain the patient's airway, oxygenation, and tissue perfusion. Life support equipment should be available in case the patient fails to respond. Document the drugs and dosage as well as the patient's response to the treatment.

What the future holds in store...

The patient should discuss future drug infusions with the LIP. The LIP may reduce the dose of the drug or switch to a drug that targets the tumor type and is less toxic. If the LIP continues the drug at a lower dose, premedication with an antihistamine and perhaps a corticosteroid will be required. Be sure to check with the LIP for preinfusion treatments before subsequent therapy cycles.

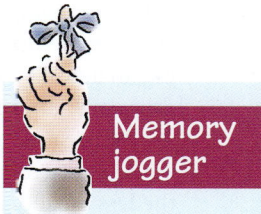

When your patient has an immediate hypersensitivity reaction, guide your response with these pairs of words:

• stop and stay (stop the infusion and stay with the patient)

• check and call (check vital signs and call the LIP).

Short-term adverse effects

The short-term adverse effects of antineoplastic drug therapy include:
- nausea and vomiting
- hair loss (alopecia)
- diarrhea
- myelosuppression
- stomatitis.

These effects are produced by damage to tissues with a large proportion of frequently reproducing cells, including bone marrow, hair follicles, and gastrointestinal mucosa.

All patients are different; not all experience these adverse effects, and some don't have any short-term adverse effects at all.

Nausea and vomiting

Nausea and vomiting can appear in three patterns:
- anticipatory
- acute
- delayed.

Each has its own cause. Because daily antineoplastic treatments may span several weeks, expect to see a mix of these three patterns. Managing them is a difficult balancing act but is crucial because of the effects that nausea and vomiting have on the patient's nutritional status, emotional well-being, and fluid and electrolyte balance.

Anticipatory — it's enough to just think about it

The anticipatory pattern is a learned response from prior nausea and vomiting after a dose of antineoplastic medication. It's most likely to develop in people who experienced moderate to severe symptoms after previous doses of antineoplastic drugs.

These patients tend to have very high anxiety levels.

The key here is pretreatment. Aprepitant (Emend) is usually effective in preventing this type of nausea. The patient takes aprepitant before receiving antineoplastic medication and continues it for 2 days after the medication. However, because some patients have overwhelming anxiety, I.V. lorazepam may be necessary before antineoplastic drugs are administered.

Posttreatment control of nausea and vomiting can help prevent anticipatory nausea. The less nauseous a patient feels after treatment, the less anxiety he'll experience before the next treatment.

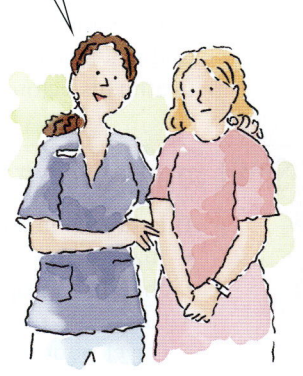

Anticipatory nausea and vomiting may occur in a patient who had unpleasant symptoms after a previous dose of chemotherapy.

Acute — within the first 24 hours

Acute nausea and vomiting occur within the first 24 hours of treatment. A major factor is the emetogenic (vomit-inducing) potential of the drug or drugs administered. For example, cisplatin has a high potential; more than 90% of patients receiving it will experience nausea and vomiting. Bleomycin, however, has a low potential; only 10% to 30% of patients are affected.

Other factors that contribute to the occurrence and severity of nausea and vomiting include the combination of drugs, doses, rates of administration, and patient characteristics. There are many antiemetic drugs available. Ondansetron and granisetron are commonly used today. Other drugs, such as lorazepam or dexamethasone, may also be used.

Delayed but not out of the woods yet

Delayed nausea and vomiting is loosely designated as starting or continuing beyond 24 hours after antineoplastic treatment has begun. Although its cause is less clearly understood than the anticipatory and acute patterns, the arsenal of drugs for treating it is larger. In addition to serotonin antagonists, and corticosteroids, various antihistamines, benzodiazepines, and metoclopramide are usually effective. Some patients are treated with antiemetic drugs for up to 3 days or longer after treatment.

Alopecia

Alopecia results from the destruction of rapidly dividing cells in the hair shaft or root. It may be minimal or severe depending on the type of antineoplastic drug and the patient's reaction.

Let them know it will regrow

Because so many patients find alopecia disturbing, reassurance about resumed hair growth is important. Inform the patient that his scalp may become sore at times due to the follicles swelling. Educate the patient on hair regrowth. Some patients will have hair growing back during the antineoplastic treatments, whereas others will have no hair growth until 2 to 3 months after treatment is complete. Inform the patient that this new hair may be a different texture or color.

Give the patient sufficient time to decide whether to order a wig. Offer to help the patient go to the various websites that pertain to wigs and assist him or her in selecting one. This will also give him time to match the wig color to his natural hair color before total hair loss occurs. The American Cancer Society has helped with the cost of wigs in the past and has even made donated wigs available. Remind the patient that she can take the wig to her usual hairdresser to have it cut and styled to match her own hair prior to the antineoplastic treatments. Put the patient in touch with the American Cancer Society's "Look Good, Feel Better" program that provides instruction on how female patient can wear makeup to camouflage loss of eyebrows and eyelashes during treatment.

Diarrhea

Diarrhea — brought on because the rapidly dividing cells of the intestinal mucosa are killed — occurs in some patients receiving antineoplastic medication. Complications of persistent diarrhea include weight loss, fluid and electrolyte imbalance, and malnutrition. To minimize the effects of diarrhea, use dietary adjustments, antidiarrheal medications, and ointments to the rectal area if irritated.

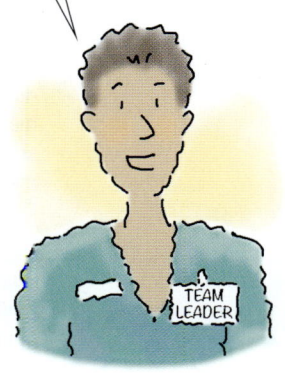

Patients receiving antineoplastic drugs need reassurance about their hair loss.

Myelosuppression

Myelosuppression is damage to the stem cells in the bone marrow. These cells are the precursors to cellular blood components — red and white blood cells and platelets — so their damage produces anemia, leukopenia, and thrombocytopenia. (See *Managing complications of antineoplastic drug usage*, page 300.)

Stomatitis

Stomatitis produces painful mouth ulcers 3 to 7 days after certain antineoplastic drugs are given, with symptoms ranging from mild to severe. Because of the accompanying pain, stomatitis can lead to fluid and electrolyte imbalance and malnutrition if the patient can't chew or swallow adequate food or fluid.

Oral hygiene is key

Treat stomatitis with scrupulous oral hygiene and topical anesthetic mixtures. Because pain may be severe, patients sometimes require opioid analgesics until ulcers heal. Allowing the patient to suck on ice chips while receiving certain drugs that cause stomatitis helps decrease the blood supply to the mouth, decreasing ulcer formation.

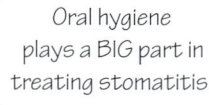

Oral hygiene plays a BIG part in treating stomatitis.

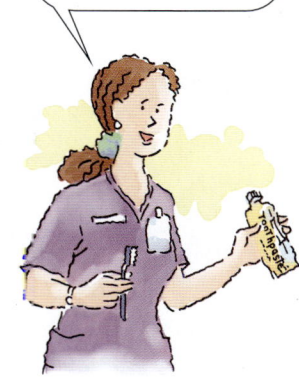

Long-term adverse effects

Organ system dysfunction, especially in the hematopoietic and GI systems, is common after antineoplastic drugs. These effects are usually temporary, but some systems suffer permanent damage that manifests long after antineoplastic medication treatments end. The renal, pulmonary, cardiac, reproductive, and neurologic systems all show various temporary and permanent dysfunctions from exposure to antineoplastic drugs.

Managing complications of antineoplastic drug usage

This chart identifies some common adverse effects of antineoplastic and offers ways to minimize them.

Adverse effect	Signs and symptoms	Interventions
Anemia	Dizziness, fatigue, pallor, and shortness of breath after minimal exertion; low hemoglobin and hematocrit; may develop slowly over several courses of treatment	• Monitor hemoglobin, hematocrit, and red blood cell count; report dropping values; remember that dehydration from nausea, vomiting, and anorexia will cause hemoconcentration, yielding falsely high hematocrit readings. • Be prepared to administer a blood transfusion or erythropoietin. • Instruct the patient to take frequent rests, increase intake of iron-rich foods, and take a multivitamin with iron as prescribed.
Leukopenia	Susceptibility to infections; neutropenia (an absolute neutrophil count less than 1,500 cells/µl)	• Watch for the nadir, the point of lowest blood cell count (usually 7 to 14 days after last treatment). • Be prepared to administer colony-stimulating factors. • Include the following information in patient and family teaching: good hygiene practices, signs and symptoms of infection, the importance of checking the patient's temperature regularly, how to prepare a low-microbe diet, and how to care for vascular access devices. • Instruct the patient to avoid crowds, people with colds or respiratory infections, and fresh fruit, fresh flowers, and plants.
Thrombocytopenia	Bleeding gums, increased bruising, petechiae, hypermenorrhea, tarry stools, hematuria, coffee ground emesis	• Monitor platelet count: under 50,000 cells/µl means a moderate risk of excessive bleeding; under 20,000 cells/µl means a major risk and the patient may need a platelet transfusion. • Avoid unnecessary I.M. injections or venipunctures; if either is necessary, apply pressure for at least 5 minutes, and then apply a pressure dressing to the site. • Instruct the patient to avoid cuts and bruises, shave with an electric razor, avoid blowing his nose, stay away from irritants that would trigger sneezing, and do not use rectal thermometers. • Instruct the patient to report sudden headaches (which could indicate potentially fatal intracranial bleeding).
Alopecia	Hair loss that may include eyebrows, eye lashes, and body hair	• Minimize shock and distress by warning the patient of the possibility of hair loss, discussing why hair loss occurs, and describing how much hair loss to expect. • Emphasize the need for appropriate head protection against sunburn and heat loss in the winter. • For patients with long hair, suggest cutting the hair shorter before treatment because washing and brushing cause more hair loss.

A devastating effect

One devastating long-term effect of antineoplastic drug treatment is secondary malignancy. Certain alkylating agents given to treat myeloma, Hodgkin's disease, and malignant lymphomas can cause this. A secondary malignancy can occur at any time. The prognosis is usually poor.

Teaching and documentation

To give your patient some sense of control in the face of overwhelming odds, explain each procedure you do and teach him strategies for dealing with fear, pain, and the unwelcome adverse effects of antineoplastic drug usage.

Keep in mind that a positive attitude and a strong emotional support system will enable your patient to better endure — if not overcome — the disease and its treatments.

Building a strong chain of communication

Documentation is important for more than just legal reasons. Because the treatment for cancer can be prolonged, numerous health care providers and facilities may be involved over an extended period. Without clear and concise documentation of treatments given, actions taken, and patient responses, the chain of communication can break down. When communication is impaired, the patient will most certainly experience additional needless suffering. Ensure that the patient has verbalized understanding of the medications that he or she will be receiving. Also, document evidence of the patient's anxiety or depression and his or her use of coping methods.

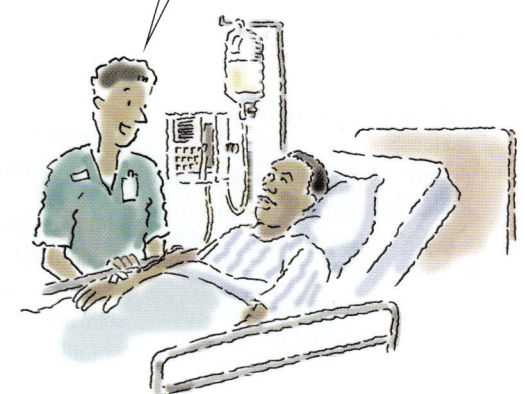

Help your patient gain control by explaining each procedure.

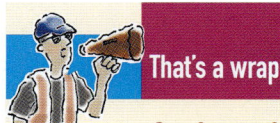

That's a wrap!

Antineoplastic infusions review

Antineoplastic infusion
- Usually calls for more than one drug to target different cancer cell phases
- Works best when the most effective drug is chosen as the first line

Antineoplastic drugs
- Categorized according to their action and how they interfere with cell production
- May be cycle specific (act during specific phases of a cell cycle) or cycle nonspecific (act on reproducing and resting cells)
- Enhances the body's ability to destroy cancer cells
- Involves administration of monoclonal antibodies, which target tumor cells, or immunomodulatory cytokines, which affect immune response

Administering antineoplastic infusions
- Perform a preadministration check.
- Prepare antineoplastic drugs using appropriate protective measures.
- Biological safety cabinet, use of proper attire, closed system drug transfer devices.
- Establish peripheral I.V. access if needed using smallest gauge possible.
- Connect the I.V. fluid container of normal saline solution or other prescribed fluid to the I.V. catheter before giving the drug.
- Closely monitor the patient and I.V. site. Don't proceed without a blood return. Check for a blood return at frequent intervals and stop the infusion if the blood return is lost.
- Properly dispose of equipment.
- Document the procedure.

Antineoplastic drugs and tissue damage
- Vesicants — cause blisters and severe tissue damage
- Nonvesicants — do not cause irritation or tissue damage
- Irritants — cause a local venous response, with or without external signs of inflammation

Infusion site complications
Infiltration
- Results from nonvesicant leaking into surrounding tissue
- Causes swelling, blanching, and possible flow rate change

Extravasation
- Results from vesicant leaking into surrounding tissue
- Causes swelling, pain, and blanching or redness and can result in blistering of the tissue; may progress to a necrotic ulcer

Vein flare
- Results from irritant drug
- Causes vein to become red and surrounded by hives

Adverse effects of antineoplastic drug usage
- Alopecia (hair loss) — may be minimal or severe
- Anaphylactic reaction — may occur any time during drug administration
- Diarrhea — may lead to weight loss, electrolyte imbalance, and malnutrition
- Myelosuppression — damage to precursors of WBCs, RBCs, and platelets
- Nausea and vomiting — may be anticipated, acute, or delayed
- Secondary malignancy — usually occurs after use of alkylating agents

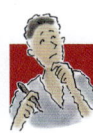

Quick quiz

1. Which is *not* an advantage of administering antineoplastic drugs by the I.V. route?
    A. The drugs are completely absorbed.
    B. The chances of acute nausea and vomiting are decreased.
    C. The dose is highly accurate.
    D. The drugs are systemically distributed.

Answer: B. Administering antineoplastic drugs I.V. doesn't decrease the chance of nausea and vomiting.

2. A drug that's cycle specific will attack normal and malignant cells during specific phases of cell development, EXCEPT for which phase?
    A. Resting phase
    B. Mitosis phase
    C. Deoxyribonucleic acid synthesis phase
    D. Ribonucleic acid synthesis phase

Answer: A. Cycle-specific drugs are effective only during specific phases of the cycle. When cell cycle–specific antineoplastic drugs are administered, cells in the resting phase survive.

3. Administering antineoplastic drugs requires wearing:
    A. disposable gloves.
    B. two pairs of latex surgical gloves.
    C. any type of latex gloves.
    D. two pairs of antineoplastic gloves, also known as "chemotherapy" gloves.

Answer: D. Antineoplastic gloves help prevent inadvertent exposure because they're thick and powderless and extend to the elbow.

4. Who's authorized to write antineoplastic drug orders?
    A. The attending licensed independent practitioners (LIP)
    B. The nurse
    C. A fourth-year medical student
    D. A pharmacist

Answer: A. Only a licensed independent practitioners (LIP) is allowed to write a antineoplastic drug order.

5. To treat extravasation, the first step is to:
    A. give an antidote.
    B. notify the licensed independent practitioners (LIP).
    C. stop the infusion.
    D. notify the pharmacy.

Answer: C. The first step in treating extravasation is to stop the infusion. Check your facility's policy to determine whether the I.V. catheter should be removed. Notify the licensed independent practitioners

(LIP) and pharmacy after stopping the infusion. Treatment for extravasation should always be in accordance with manufacturer's guidelines and should be appropriate according to facility policy.

Scoring

★★★ If you answered all five questions correctly, congratulations! Now treat yourself to some extra time in your resting phase.

★★ If you answered three or four questions correctly, not bad! You are getting into the flow of things.

★ If you answered fewer than three questions correctly, don't get discouraged! Sometimes, it takes a few learning cycles before the information starts taking effect.

Suggested References

Boulanger, J., Ducharme, A., Dufour, A., Fortier, S., & Almanric, K. (2015). Management of the extravasation of anti-neoplastic agents. *Supportive Care in Cancer, 23*(5), 1459–1471.

Chalian, H., Töre, H. G., Horowitz, J. M., Salem, R., Miller, F. H., & Yaghmai, V. (2011). Radiologic assessment of response to therapy: Comparison of RECIST versions 1.1 and 1.0. *Radiographics, 31*(7), 2093–2105. doi:doi:10.1148/rg.317115050

Department of Health and Human Services Centers for Disease Control and Prevention National Institute for Occupational Safety and Health. (2014). *NIOSH list of antineoplastic and other hazardous drugs in healthcare settings 2014*. Retrieved from http://www.cdc.gov/niosh/docs/2014-138/pdfs/2014-138_v3.pdf, on February 12, 2016.

Eisenberg, S. (2012). Biologic therapy. *Journal of Infusion Nursing, 35*(5), 301–313. doi:10.1097/NAN.0b013e31826579aa

Gorski, L., Hadaway, L., Hagle, M., McGoldrick, M., Orr, M., & Doellman, D. (2016). Infusion therapy standards of practice. *Journal of Infusion Nursing, 39*(1S), 159.

National Institute for Occupational Safety and Health. (2016). Occupational exposure to antineoplastic agents and other hazardous drugs. *Workplace Safety and Health Topics.*

Neuss, M., Polovich, M., McNiff, K., Esper, P., Gilmore, T., LeFebvre, K., ... Jacobson, J. (2013). 2013 Updated American Society of Clinical Oncology/Oncology Nursing Society antineoplastic administration safety standards including standards for the safe administration and management of oral antineoplastic. *Oncology Nursing Forum, 40*(3), 225–233.

Polovich, M., Olsen, M., & LeFebvre K. (Eds.). (2014). *Chemotherapy and biotherapy guidelines and recommendations for practice* (4th ed.). Pittsburgh, PA: Oncology Nursing Society.

Povoski, S. (2016). Long-term central venous access. *Cancer Management.* Retrieved from http://www.cancernetwork.com/cancer-management/long-term-central-venous-access, on August 29, 2016.

USP. (2008). *USP <797> guidebook to pharmaceutical compounding — Sterile preparations*. Rockville, MD: United States Pharmacopeia.

USP. (2016). *USP <800> hazardous drugs — Handling in healthcare settings*. Rockville, MD: The United States Pharmacopeial Convention.

Chapter 7

Biologic therapy

Just the facts

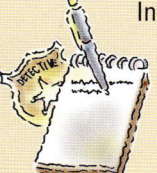

In this chapter, you will learn:
- what biologic therapy is
- the basic function of the immune system
- the diseases treated with biologic therapy
- types of biologic therapy
- safe administration of biologic therapy
- adverse effects of biologic therapy
- future directions
- complications of biotherapy drugs and how to avoid them.

Introduction to biologic therapy

Mapping the human genome and modern genetic engineering opened up a new world of biologic agents for the treatment of many diseases. Originally, this group of agents, known as "immunotherapy," was used to modulate the human immune system and has greatly expanded over the years. Many names may be used to describe this type of therapy, including immunotherapy or biological response modifiers, but biologic therapy seems to be an accepted, all-inclusive term.

Working together

Biologic therapy refers to treatments that stimulate, enhance, or suppress the human immune system. These agents are created from human blood and blood components, bacteria, or viruses, plus other forms of biotechnology. Biologic agents are similar to and processed like other proteins in the human body. This means that the human response and the adverse reactions to these agents are different from other pharmaceutical drugs.

Know your immune system!

To understand biologic therapy, an understanding of the immune system is needed. This knowledge will help to recognize your patient's

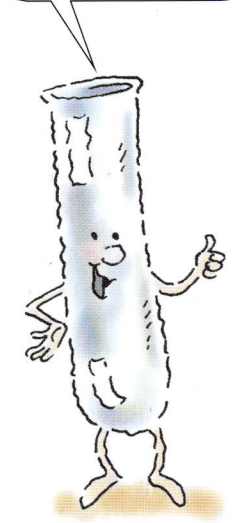

Biologic therapies are created from human blood and blood components, bacteria, or viruses and are genetically engineered to work with the immune system.

biological response to the therapy. Biologic therapy is used to treat immunodeficiency and autoimmune disorders and cancer.

The immune system

To understand biologic therapy, it helps to know some basic information about the immune system, a complex network of organs, tissues, and specialized cells. Tonsils, adenoids, appendix, Peyer's patches, spleen, thymus gland, bone marrow, lymph nodes, and lymphatic vessels comprise the immune system.

Two lines of defense

The human body has two basic types of defense. The first line of defense is the physical barrier involving the skin, mucous membranes, and the lining of the respiratory tract. This line of defense produces a nonspecific response because it works regardless of the invader.

The second line of defense is the immune system. This complex system recognizes foreign invaders and then develops the specific weapons to fight them. It is even able to remember what the invader looked like so that the next time its response will be even swifter. An immune response is triggered when the immune system encounters a substance, called an antigen, it recognizes as "foreign." These foreign invaders could be bacteria, viruses, fungi, parasites, or cancer cells.

There are two basic types of immune response protecting the body from foreign invaders:

- *Innate or nonspecific immunity* includes the protection from skin and mucous membranes, mechanical barriers such as coughing or sneezing and chemical barriers such as tears and sweat, and white blood cells providing a general—or nonspecific—level of immune protection.
- *Adaptive or acquired immunity* provides a specific response to the antigen. The presence of the antigen triggers humoral immunity from B lymphocytes, memory B cells, and other plasma cells, causing the production of antibodies, also known as immunoglobulins (Ig). Cytotoxic T cells, natural killer cells, and macrophages (large white blood cells) produce cell-mediated immunity that can directly destroy microbes or abnormal cells. Cells of adaptive immunity produce cytokines that include interferons, interleukins, and growth factors.

Understanding how immune system cells exchange messages and find ways to make these messages clearer and stronger are the goals of research in immunology. Each of these components, and each step in the immune response, represents a potential avenue for the development of a cancer, an immune deficiency, or an autoimmune disorder.

Three important components are critical to normal immune response including white blood cells (WBC), which signal, identify, and attack invaders cells; cytokines, which are small proteins that influence behavior of nearby cells; and immunoglobulins, which are large proteins that recognize and destroy antigens.

White blood cells

There are five types of white blood cells (WBCs):
1. Neutrophils are primarily located in the bloodstream, are the most abundant type of WBC, and are the first to respond to invading microorganisms.
2. Eosinophils are located in the respiratory and digestive tract and are involved with the allergic response.
3. Basophils are the rarest type and release histamine and heparin in response to allergens.
4. Lymphocytes are concentrated in areas of the body that commonly encounter hostile invaders such as the stomach and intestines, lungs, and lymph system. Types of lymphocytes include:
   - B lymphocytes, which mature from stem cells in the bone marrow, then migrate to the spleen in their maturation process. They secrete antibodies, the proteins that recognize and attach to antigens, and target tissue that should be destroyed.
   - cytotoxic T cells that directly attack infectious or cancer cells.
   - helper T cells that assist in suppressing or regulating the immune system's response by signaling other immune system cells.
   - natural killer (NK) cells, which produce powerful chemical substances that rapidly bind to and kill invading pathogens and suppress tumor formation. They attack without first having to recognize a specific antigen.
5. Monocytes circulate in the bloodstream. When they settle in tissue, they engulf and digest the invaders. In this phase, they are known as macrophages, and the process is known as phagocytosis.

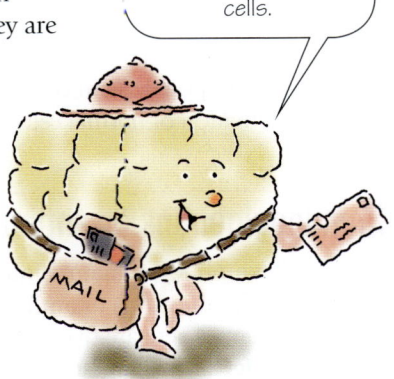

Cytokines

Cytokines are small proteins released by cells that are responsible for communication and interaction between cells. These messenger proteins include interferons, interleukins, tumor necrotic factor, colony-stimulating factors, and chemokines.

Interferon

Interferon (IFN) occurs naturally in the body and is grouped by different types, depending on their receptors on cell surfaces. IFN is produced by viral stimulation and is capable of protecting other cells from infection. IFN may act directly on cancer cells by slowing growth and encouraging normal cell behavior.

Interleukins

Interleukins (ILs) deliver messages to leukocytes to stimulate growth of immune cells, especially T- and B-cell lymphocytes. ILs are labeled numerically with 37 different types produced by the human body. ILs stimulate the growth and activity of many cancer-killing immune cells, including NK cells and cytotoxic T cells. They also can suppress rejection in transplants and increase the production of macrophage inflammatory cytokines.

Colony-stimulating factors

Colony-stimulating factors (CSFs) encourage the growth of bone marrow stem cells especially WBCs. They are needed to fight infections, but they often are destroyed by cancer treatments such as antineoplastic drugs or radiation.

Tumor necrosis factor

Tumor necrosis factor (TNF) is a cell-signaling protein primarily produced in the acute phase of systemic inflammation. It is produced by many types of cells including macrophages, natural killer cells, and mast cells. Faulty regulation of TNF is associated with many diseases such as cancer, major depression, psoriatic arthritis, Alzheimer's disease, and inflammatory bowel disease.

Chemokines

These cytokines control leukocyte migration and organize WBCs and hematopoietic stem cells. They are involved with inflammation, transformation of normal cells into cancer cells, and autoimmune processes.

Immunoglobulins or antibodies

B lymphocytes mature into plasma cells, which manufacture immunoglobulins (Ig) or antibodies as part of the humoral immune system. There are five types of immunoglobulins:
1. IgG is the largest group that phagocytize antigens.
2. IgM is produced first when an antigen is detected.

3. IgA acts in the sites where environmental substances enter the body such as the nose and lungs.
4. IgD is present in small amounts. Although the specific function is not confirmed, it is thought to act with basophils and mast cells.
5. IgE activates the release of histamine from mast cells and is associated with immediate allergic or hypersensitivity reactions.

Not foolproof!

It is generally believed that the immune system's natural capacity to detect and destroy abnormal cells serves numerous functions in the prevention and control of many disease processes, but this is not a foolproof system. Some cancer cells are able to evade detection by using one or more strategies. For example, cancer cells can undergo genetic changes that lead to the loss of cancer-associated antigens, making them less "visible" to the immune system. For autoimmune diseases, cell communication involves multiple interrelated pathways. Obstruction of a single pathway may not be sufficient to produce clinical improvement. Additionally, these multiple pathways may be part of the reason for adverse reactions from some biologic agents. The goal of biologic therapy is to overcome these barriers to produce an effective immune response targeted for the patient's need.

Clinical indications for biologic therapy

Biologic therapies are used to treat diseases where there is either an excessive or deficient immune response. These therapies work in a precise manner on the body's immune system by altering the way cells grow, mature, and respond. This approach is unique because it manipulates the body's natural resources instead of introducing toxic substances that aren't selective and can't differentiate between normal and abnormal processes or cells.

Cancer

Biologic agents eliminate, regulate, or suppress conditions that allow uncontrolled cell growth and make cancer cells more vulnerable to destruction by the immune system. These agents can block or reverse the process that changes a normal or precancerous cell into a cancerous cell and enhance the body's ability to repair normal cells that are damaged by antineoplastic drugs or radiation therapy.

Direct and indirect

Biologic therapy may or may not target cancer cells directly. Cancer vaccines may be preventive as is the case with vaccines for human papillomavirus and hepatitis B, with a goal to prevent cervical, oropharyngeal, and liver cancers. Vaccines may also treat cancers directly by shrinking tumor growth, stopping the return of cancer, or eliminating cancer cells not killed by other treatments. Other biological therapies, such as antibodies or segments of genetic material (RNA or DNA), do target cancer cells directly. Biologic therapies that interfere with specific molecules involved in tumor growth and progression are also referred to as targeted therapies. Biologic therapies may be used to treat the side effects of other cancer treatments. In noncancer patients, biologic agents decrease inflammation or risk of infection, but these agents used for cancer treatment change the cancer cells' biology so that they become weak and die.

Two basic categories

There are two basic categories of biologic therapy for cancer:
1. Immunotherapy uses a variety of methods and agents to create a hostile environment for the existence or growth of cancer in the body.
2. Cytotoxic therapy destroys the cancer cells or makes it difficult for them to grow and reproduce. Another term for this approach is tumor cell modulation.

Immunotherapy

Although many avenues of active and passive immunomodulation, and selective and nonselection approach have been tried, nonspecific active methods and passive immunotherapy have the most success. Nonspecific active methods include use of interferons and interleukins (IL-2 and IL-12, for example), as well as bacillus (or bacilli) Calmette-Guérin (BCG), the organism that causes tuberculosis. It is a weakened form of a live tuberculosis bacterium that does not cause disease in humans. It was first used medically as a vaccine against tuberculosis. When inserted directly into the bladder with a catheter, BCG stimulates a general immune response that is directed not only against the foreign bacterium itself but also against bladder cancer cells.

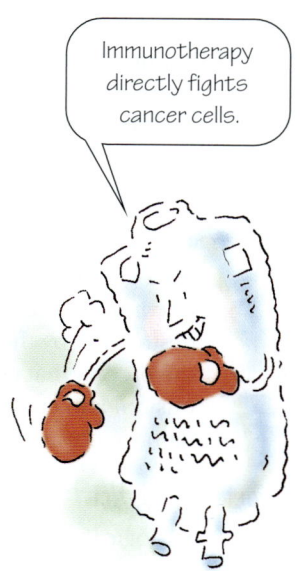

Immunotherapy directly fights cancer cells.

Passive immunotherapy, sometimes called adoptive immunotherapy, gives the patient antibodies and other agents so that the patient adopts an immune response that has been developed in a test tube. The passive approach can be specific or nonspecific. Specific treatments include monoclonal antibodies (mAbs), which can be designed to target certain cancer cells.

One nonspecific technique involves removing some of the patient's T cells, culturing the cells in the lab, and then injecting expanded populations of the treated cells into the patients. An alternative approach is to activate lymphocytes taken from a tumor to create yet another agent, called tumor-infiltrating lymphocytes (TILs), and returning these "stranger" cells to the patient where they can fight the cancer cells.

Cytotoxic therapy (tumor cell modulation)

Tumor cell modulation changes the cancer cell's biology so that they become weak and die. Some biologic agents in this approach are called cytotoxins. Perhaps the best-known cytotoxin is tumor necrosis factor (TNF), a toxin secreted by activated macrophages to selectively kill tumor cells, principally by interfering with their blood supply.

Certain agents make the antigens on cancer cells more recognizable to antibodies or make them stickier so that antibodies bind to them more easily. Other compounds interfere with the cell's ability to metastasize.

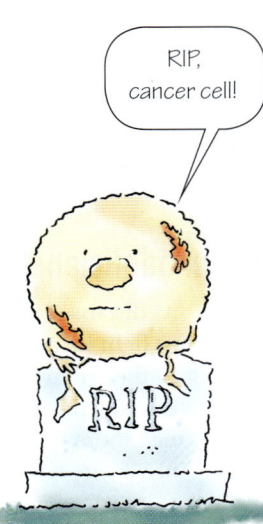

Autoimmune disorders

In a variety of autoimmune disorders involving numerous anatomical body systems, the immune system attacks healthy tissue. Causes are divided into genetic and environmental reasons; however, there are no clear answers yet to pinpoint the specific triggers or cause for each type of autoimmune disease.

Inflammation gone awry

Signs and symptoms of inflammation are the hallmark of autoimmune diseases. Inflammation is useful for fighting infection, but in autoimmune diseases, it damages normal tissues. Autoimmune diseases affect many anatomical structures, and there is no single medical specialty that treats patients with autoimmune disorders. Biologic agents are prescribed by rheumatologists, dermatologists, gastroenterologist, neurologists, oncologists, and others.

Examples of autoimmune diseases include:
- rheumatoid arthritis
- inflammatory bowel diseases, including ulcerative colitis and Crohn's disease
- multiple sclerosis
- psoriasis and psoriatic arthritis.

Immunosuppress to impress

Effectiveness of biologic agents against autoimmune diseases is thought to stem from their immunosuppressant properties. Biologic agents change the relationship between the body and the immune cells—in essence, restoring, augmenting, or modulating the immune system. They inhibit key factors such as interferon, tumor necrosis factor, and T lymphocytes known to cause inflammation.

Monoclonal antibodies are used with autoimmune diseases. Biological therapies can cool off this harmful inflammation by targeting immune cells or chemical messengers involved in inflammation.

Immunodeficiency diseases

As discussed above, antigens produce antibodies or immunoglobulins to fight invasion of infectious organisms and other types of invaders. In these patients, components of the immune system are missing or not functioning correctly. The World Health Organization has identified more than 185 primary immunodeficiency diseases with some being rare while others are very common.

No resistance

Both the innate and adaptive immune systems cause immunodeficiency disorders. Alteration in the production and function of antibodies is usually associated with the adaptive immune system, and the innate immune system indicates direct problems with natural killer cells, neutrophils, or complement proteins. The outcome is a patient with no resistance to infection. These infections can be severe or recurrent, along with increasing damage to the organs actually infected. For instance, recurring pneumonia could lead to lung damage. Additionally, patients with immune deficiencies may also develop an autoimmune disease such as inflammatory bowel disease or rheumatoid arthritis. They are also at risk for certain types of leukemia and lymphomas.

Immunoglobulins to the rescue

Immunoglobulin therapy (also known as Ig therapy) is given to replace missing antibodies or correct the nonfunctioning immune system. Examples of immunodeficiency disorders include common variable immune deficiency (CVID), hyper-IgM syndromes, and Wiskott-Aldrich syndrome, which may benefit from replacement therapy with immunoglobulins.

Types of biologic agents

Biological agents use living organisms, substances derived from living organisms, or laboratory-produced versions of these substances to treat disease. These agents are categorized as:
- interferons
- interleukins

- colony-stimulating factors
- monoclonal antibodies
- immunoglobulins.

The United States Adopted Names (USAN) Council, comprised of members from the U.S. Food and Drug Administration, U.S. Pharmacopeia, American Society of Health-System Pharmacists, and the American Medical Association, has established a nomenclature for generic names for all medications, including biological agents. Each group of agents is given a unique stem or addition to the chemical name. This identifies agents from the group with similar or common characteristics.

Natural but still potentially hazardous

Many people mistakenly believe that because biologic therapies work with the body's immune system, they are more "natural" and less toxic than other drugs. Although adverse effects of these drugs differ from those of antineoplastic and other drugs, all agents that interfere with the immune system can have unintended and generally undesirable effects. Two major concerns emerge with expansion of the lists of biologic agents — infusion-related reactions and the hazardous nature of these agents. Infusion-related reactions can be life threatening unless recognized and treated immediately. (See *Managing infusion reactions,* page 321.)

Many biologic agents are considered to be hazardous drugs, which require specialized training on preparation and administration, preparation in specialized biological safety cabinets, appropriate types and layers of personnel protective equipment, and special techniques for administration such as the use of closed system drug transfer devices. Biologic agents considered to be hazardous drugs include the following:
- ado-trastuzumab
- brentuximab vedotin
- panitumumab
- pertuzumab
- ziv-aflibercept.

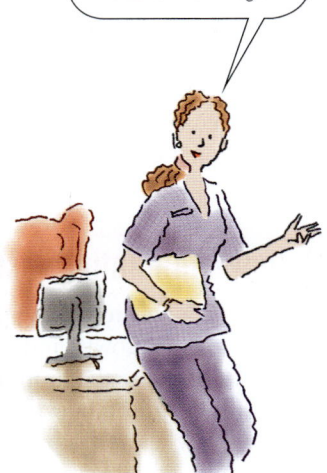

NIOSH, USP, and Material Safety Data Sheets have information about hazardous drugs.

Check your policies

Facilities should have current policies and procedures on handling all hazardous drugs. Resources for current information on hazardous drugs come from the following organizations:
- The National Institute for Occupational Safety and Health (NIOSH) continually gathers data on health risk related to all drugs and biologic agents, creating a list of drugs and agents considered to be hazardous.
- The U.S. Pharmacopeia has a new set of standards, USP <800>, for handling all hazardous drugs.

- Manufacturers create Material Safety Data Sheets and include complete drug information in each package of the agents. (See *Chapter 6, Antineoplastic Therapy* for more details on management of hazardous drugs, page 278.)

Interferons

Through recombinant DNA technology, various interferons have been genetically engineered for use in the medical treatment of disease including leukemia, melanoma, sarcoma, hepatitis B and C, AIDS-related Kaposi sarcoma, human papilloma virus genital warts, severe malignant osteoporosis, and multiple sclerosis.

Interferon classes

There are three known classes of interferons: alpha-, beta-, and gamma-interferons. Names for agents in this group begin with "interferon" followed by alpha, beta, or gamma and ending with a number and a letter to differentiate between subcategories and specific manufacturers. Most are administered by intramuscular (I.M.) or subcutaneous (S.C.) injection, although interferon alfa-2b (Intron A) is given by the intravenous (I.V.) route. This agent is indicated for treatment of metastatic melanoma and renal cell cancer.

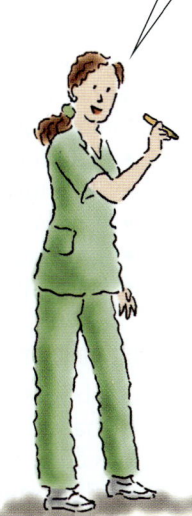

Interleukins end in -kin. That's pretty easy to remember!

Interleukins

Interleukins (IL) are used in the treatment of melanoma, renal cell carcinoma, and rheumatoid arthritis. Additionally, IL can be used to prevent severe thrombocytopenia in patients receiving antineoplastic agents. The generic name for this group of biologic agents ends with "-kin." Recombinant interleukin-2 (Proleukin, aldesleukin) is given by the I.V. route to treat metastatic melanoma and renal cell cancer.

Colony-stimulating factors

Colony-stimulating factors are hematopoietic growth factors promoting the growth and maturation of normal blood cells, which then stimulates the immune system. CSFs are used after cancer therapies to help grow a new population of red blood cells, white blood cells, and platelets and support the immune system to reduce the risk of infection and decrease anemia.

Colony-stimulating factors and other blood cell growth factors

Agent	Action	Indications
Filgrastim (Neupogen)	Stimulates proliferation, differentiation, and functional activity of neutrophils, causing a rapid rise in the WBC count	• Antineoplastic-induced neutropenia • Acute myeloid leukemia • Bone marrow transplant • Peripheral blood progenitor cell collection • Severe chronic neutropenia
Sargramostim (Leukine)	Stimulates progenitor cells to divide and differentiate; activates mature granulocytes and macrophages	• Bone marrow transplant failure and engraftment delay • Neutrophil recovery in acute myelogenous leukemia • Peripheral blood progenitor collection
Erythropoietin (Epogen, Procrit)	Induces maturation of red blood cells (RBCs); increases the release of reticulocytes from the bone marrow, which stimulates red blood cell production and might reduce the number of blood transfusions needed by the patient	• Anemia in chronic kidney disease • Antineoplastic-induced anemia • Postoperative anemia in some elective surgical patients
Darbepoetin alfa (Aranesp)	Stimulates RBC production by bone marrow	• Anemia in chronic kidney disease • Antineoplastic-induced anemia

Giving normal cells a boost

Bone marrow transplant patients receive CSFs to stimulate stem cell production for autologous stem cell transplant and white blood cell recovery after high-dose antineoplastic therapy. CSFs are given to bone marrow donors to stimulate their production of stem cells. They are also used for patients who develop anemia or low white blood cell counts because of cancer or cancer therapy. Names for agents in this group end with "-stim."

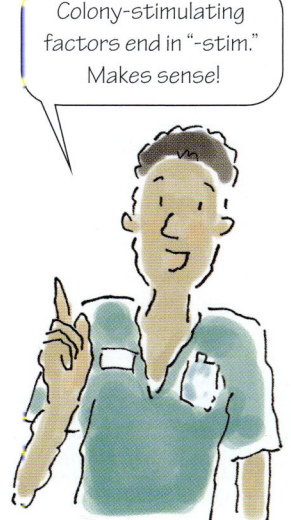

Colony-stimulating factors end in "-stim." Makes sense!

Monoclonal antibodies

Monoclonal antibodies are lab-engineered products derived from mouse (murine) antibodies, human antibodies, or a combination of both (chimeric). They target specific elements of the cell membrane surface, known as clusters of differentiation (CD). Mouse antibodies can elicit an immune response in humans; therefore, mouse antibodies are "humanized" by replacing 70% to 75% of the murine DNA with human DNA. This is done through genetic engineering and reduces the formation of antidrug antibodies (ASA), responsible for hypersensitivity reactions to these agents.

Combining for effectiveness

Monoclonal antibodies link to their target antigen but may not completely destroy the antigen. To improve their effectiveness for cancer treatment, monoclonal antibodies may be combined with antineoplastic drugs or radioactive substances. Immunoconjugates, conjugated monoclonal antibodies, or antibody–drug conjugates (ADC) are terms used to describe this group of agents.

Monoclonal antibodies have been approved to treat cancer, cardiovascular disease, rheumatoid arthritis, psoriasis and psoriatic arthritis, macular degeneration, Crohn's disease, multiple sclerosis, and viral infection. They are also used for prevention of organ rejection in transplant patients and skeletal events in patients with bone metastasis. Conjugated monoclonal antibodies are used for lymphoma, Crohn's disease, and moderate or severe active rheumatoid arthritis.

Generic names for monoclonal antibodies end in "-mab." Conjugated monoclonal antibodies have at least 2 words in the name, one for the monoclonal antibody and the other for the drug or agent attached to it.

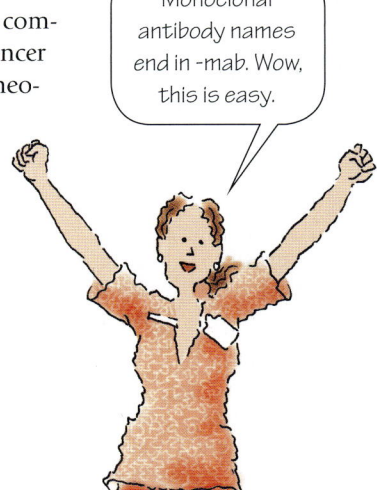

Monoclonal antibodies

Agents	Diseases treated
Abciximab (ReoPro)	Prevention of cardiac ischemia with percutaneous coronary intervention
Abatacept (Orencia)	Rheumatoid arthritis
Ado-trastuzumab emtansine (Kadcyla)	HER-2–expressing metastatic breast cancer cells
Alemtuzumab (Campath)	Chronic lymphocytic leukemia
Basiliximab (Simulect)	Immunosuppression in renal transplantation
Belimumab (Benlysta)	Systemic lupus erythematosus
Bevacizumab (Avastin)	Certain type of brain tumor and kidney, colon, rectal, lung, and breast cancers
Brentuximab vedotin (Adcetris)	Hodgkin's lymphoma
	Systemic large cell lymphoma
Cetuximab (Erbitux)	Colon and rectal cancers
	Head and neck cancer
Daclizumab (Zinbryta)	Relapsing-remitting multiple sclerosis
Eculizumab (Soliris)	Paroxysmal nocturnal hemoglobinuria
	Atypical hemolytic uremic syndrome
Ibritumomab tiuxetan (Zevalin)	B-cell non-Hodgkin's lymphoma

Monoclonal antibodies (continued)

Agents	Diseases treated
Infliximab (Remicade)	Crohn's disease Rheumatoid arthritis Psoriasis, psoriatic arthritis Ankylosing spondylitis
Ipilimumab (Yervoy)	Melanoma
Muromonab-CD3 (Orthoclone)	Acute allograft rejection in renal, heart, and liver transplant
Natalizumab (Tysabri)	Multiple sclerosis
	Crohn's disease
Ofatumumab (Arzerra)	Chronic lymphocytic leukemia
Panitumumab (Vectibix)	Metastatic colon and rectal cancers
Pertuzumab (Perjeta)	HER-2–positive metastatic breast cancer
Raxibacumab (ABthrax)	Inhalation of anthrax due to *Bacillus anthracis*
Rituximab (Rituxan)	Non-Hodgkin's lymphoma and chronic lymphocytic leukemia
	Rheumatoid arthritis not responding to other agents
Tocilizumab (Actemra)	Severely active rheumatoid arthritis
	Active juvenile idiopathic arthritis
Trastuzumab (Herceptin)	Breast cancer when the tumor expresses excess amounts of a protein called HER-2

Immunoglobulin

In the 1940s, immune globulins became available to prevent hepatitis, measles, and polio. Clinical use as a replacement therapy for immunodeficiency began in the early 1950s. Both of these uses required large amounts to be given by I.M. injection, resulting in painful sites and limiting their usefulness. In the 1980s, the first preparations for I.V. administration were introduced, and products for the subcutaneous route were available commercially in 2006.

Making immunoglobulins

To prepare immunoglobulins (Ig), human plasma from up to 60,000 units is pooled with the final product containing high amounts of IgG. Because immunoglobulins are derived from human blood, careful donor screening and testing are required. In addition, the FDA has mandated that all plasma used must be donated in the United States. Despite these precautions, transmission of an existing or emerging pathogen can happen.

Not interchangeable!

A variety of manufacturing processes are used resulting in different concentrations, sodium and sugar content, and osmolarity. The donated plasma contains a broad range of antibodies to many different bacteria and viruses. The immunoglobulin is first purified from the plasma resulting in about 96% IgG, along with very small amounts of IgM and IgA. The product is mixed with some type of sugar or amino acid to prevent aggregates. The final product contains highly purified IgG with a broad range of specific antibodies. Because these factors require careful consideration when prescribed, Ig preparations are not interchangeable. Patients with cardiac conditions require consideration of the total volume, while those with renal disease require careful assessment of sodium content. When these immunoglobulins are administered intravenously or subcutaneously, the body metabolizes them, and therefore, they must be constantly replenished (approximately every 3 to 4 weeks).

Ig products are available in either a liquid or a freeze-dried powder that requires reconstitution. Follow specific manufacturer instructions for preparation of each Ig product. All solution should be at room temperature before administration. Do not freeze or heat the product by any means such as a microwave, as this can alter the stability of the product. Generically, all products are "immune globulin intravenous"; however, there are numerous trade names. Dosages, frequency of administration, indications, preparation instructions, compatibility, and rate of administration will vary. Verify that the prescribed Ig product is what is being given and that you have read all information about the specific preparation.

Patient assessment prior to therapy

Prior to beginning biologic therapy, you will need to take a thorough medical history. Assess your patient's current status for:
- heart and vascular disease such as hypertension
- lung disease
- cancer
- nervous system diseases
- liver disease
- hematology disease
- diabetes.

Knowledge of recent bacterial, viral, or fungal infections must be included in this assessment, along with their outcome. When biologic agents that suppress tumor necrotic factor (TNF) are indicated, screening for tuberculosis is required. This may be performed with a skin test and/or a chest radiograph with results known before therapy starts. TNF is necessary to kill *Mycobacteria*; therefore, suppressing TNF activity could allow reactivation of latent tuberculosis.

Review all medications your patient is taking, carefully assessing for potential drug interactions. Obtain details about any previous drug reactions. Also confirm all allergies to drugs, food, and other substances.

Before administration of a biologic agent, confirm the necessary laboratory tests. Obtain the samples, send to the laboratory, and review results before giving the agent. This could include complete blood counts, platelet and reticulocyte counts, electrolytes, coagulation tests such as prothrombin time and partial thromboplastin time, liver and kidney function tests, and/or thyroid function tests. These tests will provide valuable information about the degree of myelosuppression present, along with the metabolism and excretion of the agent.

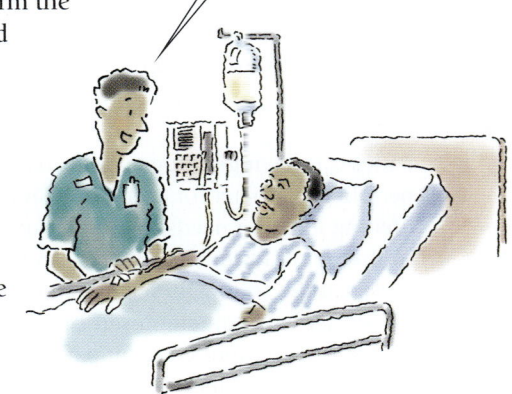

Patient assessment is crucial before beginning biologic therapy.

Obtain the patient's current weight and vital signs. Examine the skin for its appearance and integrity, and assess for hydration status.

Administration of biological therapies

Interferons, colony-stimulating factors, and some monoclonal antibodies (for example, adalimumab, etanercept) are given by subcutaneous injection. A clinician will show the patient how to prepare the needle and syringe for self-injection. A family member or other caregiver can learn the injection technique in case the patient feels too weak or ill to self-administer.

Some immunoglobulins are administered by subcutaneous infusion. After the first dose, the patient and/or family may be taught to self-administer these agents after a thorough assessment of their ability and willingness to learn the procedure. This procedure involves insertion of one or more subcutaneous infusion needles attached to an administration set that is bifurcated near its distal end. Each side of the administration set has a separate luer-locking hub that is attached to one S.C. infusion needle, allowing the total dose to be infused in smaller quantities into different S.C. sites.

IFN, IL-2, and other monoclonal antibodies are given intravenously in the medical office or an outpatient infusion center. Preparation of these agents should follow the standards established in the USP <797> chapter on compounding sterile preparations. For biologic agents considered to be hazardous drugs, USP <800> chapter on hazardous drug handling is the required standard. Both chapters indicate the need for preparation within a laminar airflow workbench. If the agent is classified as hazardous, this work area must meet the requirements of a biological safety cabinet, which has an appropriate number of air exchanges per hour, and it must be vented to the outside of the building. Appropriate attire such as gown, gloves, and face protection must be used. Transfer of all hazardous drugs should be done with a closed system drug transfer device to prevent exposure to the clinician and the environment. (See *Chapter 6, Antineoplastic Drug Administration*, page 269 for more details).

Tips for success

Patients receiving biologic agents usually require insertion of a short peripheral catheter for each dose. Since these are infrequent, but often lifelong infusion needs, the goal must be to preserve peripheral veins so that central venous catheters can be avoided. To accomplish vein preservation, follow these guidelines:

- Master your catheter insertion skills on healthy patients. Do NOT perform venipuncture on patients receiving a biologic agent unless you feel confident that you will be successful with one attempt. Multiple attempts cause vein damage, limiting their future use.
- Never make more than two venipuncture attempts; a second clinician may make two additional attempts. However, after a total of four unsuccessful attempts, another plan for vascular access should be created.
- Use strict attention to aseptic technique for hand hygiene, skin antisepsis, catheter insertion technique, and infusion methods.
- Ensure that the catheter and nearby joint (if those sites are unavoidable) are adequately stabilized.

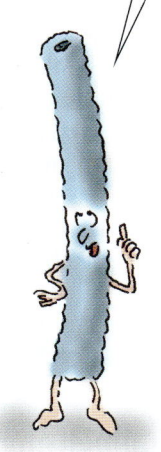

Preserve me when administering biologic agents!

Side effects of biologic agents

Biological therapies may cause side effects as do other medications. The type and severity of side effects depend on individual patient factors and their treatment plan, especially the type of biologic therapy that is used. Several agents have severe toxicities that require a "black box warning" in the package insert provided with the drug. Patient reactions may vary by the diagnosis being treated, with cancer patients having different types and rates of reactions than patients receiving the same agent for an autoimmune disease.

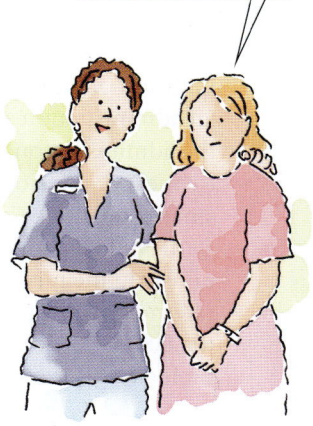

Side effects to biological therapies depend on the individual patient, their diagnosis, and their treatment plan.

Side effects by agent

The following are some common side effects caused by biological therapy drugs:

Interleukins

Side effects include flulike symptoms, including chills, fever, fatigue, headache, and muscle and joint pain and gastrointestinal side effects, such as nausea, vomiting, diarrhea, and decreased appetite. Other side effects include skin problems with or without a rash; hypotension and tachycardia; weight gain from fluid retention; and neurological problems such as confusion, disorientation, drowsiness, lethargy, anxiety, depression, and irritability.

Interferons

At the beginning of therapy, the patient will most likely experience flulike symptoms, such as chills and headaches, along with muscle and joint pain or discomfort. Chronic side effects tend to increase in intensity after several weeks on IFN therapy. Loss of appetite with weight loss and fatigue can be severe enough to limit the dose. Other side effects include lack of energy or ability to concentrate on a task, decreased blood counts, urinary protein, and low blood pressure.

Colony-stimulating factors

Colony-stimulating factor therapy is generally well tolerated. The side effects are usually minimal. Bone pain is one of the most commonly reported side effects.

Immunoglobulins

The most common side effects include chills and fever, irregular heartbeat, chest tightness and other respiratory problems, and unusual fatigue.

Monoclonal antibodies

Allergic reaction is a major concern and may occur with the first infusion or be delayed occurring after several doses. Rarely, the acute reaction can result in anaphylaxis, a severe, sometimes life-threatening, allergic reaction. Additional common side effects include fever, chills, nausea and vomiting, low blood pressure, and difficulty breathing. Flulike symptoms, fatigue, and digestive and renal problems may occur; however, the greatest concern is associated with infection, especially tuberculosis. Trouble concentrating, performing simple calculations, or remembering things may interfere with their normal daily activities and ability to work.

Managing infusion reactions

Successful prevention and management of the side effects caused by biologic therapies can be achieved by experienced clinicians with the cooperation of a well-informed patient. Close monitoring and prompt treatment are important components of coping with the side effects. Premedications are often ordered prior to the administration of these drugs and may include acetaminophen, diphenhydramine, dexamethasone, or methylprednisolone.

More serious reactions can occur during or shortly after infusion of a biologic agents. Types of infusion reactions may occur in patients receiving monoclonal antibodies including cytokine release syndrome and anaphylaxis. Be prepared to stop the infusion immediately and support the patient's airway, breathing, and circulation as necessary.

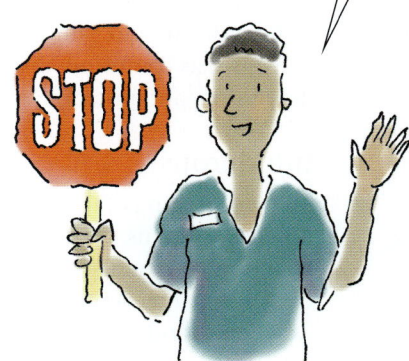

Stop the infusion if you suspect an infusion reaction.

Cytokine release syndrome

Cytokine release syndrome (CRS) is also known as cytokine storm; most nurses simply call it an "infusion reaction." CRS may happen more frequently in patients receiving monoclonal antibodies, but it is not limited to this group of biologic agents. CRS is a rapid, continuous release of cytokines. It may occur more frequently in women, older patients, those with a high tumor burden, and those with other drug sensitivities, although these risk factors do not predict their occurrence. It may occur with the first or subsequent infusions.

Clinical signs and symptoms may be mild including fever or chills, nausea, and vomiting. Problems that are more serious may include hypotension, headache, and dyspnea. Following symptomatic treatment with resolution of these problems, the infusion may be resumed, usually at a slower infusion rate. Premedicating patients with acetaminophen and diphenhydramine can minimize or prevent this reaction. CRS become less severe with subsequent infusions.

Anaphylaxis

Anaphylaxis is a severe allergic reaction to an agent, often beginning with sudden appearance of a rash and itching on the face, head, and hands. Progression includes hypotension, wheezing, and shortness of breath that can produce cardiovascular and or respiratory arrest. Treatment involves stopping the infusion, monitoring the patient's vital signs and airway, and giving epinephrine, corticosteroids, diphenhydramine, and oxygen as required. Continued monitoring for up to 6 hours is necessary. A patient who has had anaphylaxis should never receive that medication again.

Patient education

Prior to beginning therapy, the patient needs to know about their disease, purpose of therapy, potential side effects and how they will be managed, and the frequency of treatment. Many manufacturers provide patient teaching tools to support your efforts.

Cost and reimbursement for these agents can also be an issue that should be discussed as prior authorization from the insurance company may be required.

These agents require the nurse to remain with the patient during the infusion to monitor for adverse reactions and intervene appropriately in a timely manner. The patient should be knowledgeable about when to contact their LIP for any delayed reactions including:
- pain
- redness or swelling at the injection site
- a rash or hives
- light-headedness
- difficulty breathing
- a tight feeling in the throat
- fever, cough, or flulike symptoms
- first signs of depression (even if the patient thinks it might just be a passing case of the blues).

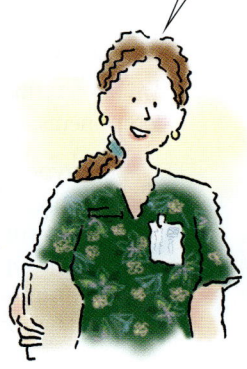

Educating your patient about when to notify you about a possible adverse reaction is key!

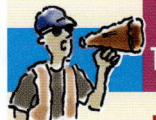

That's a wrap!

Biologic therapy review

Biologic agents
- Created from human blood or blood components, bacteria or viruses, and other types of biotechnology
- Processed much like other proteins in the body
- Interacted with the complex immune system to enhance or suppress human responses for cancer, autoimmune diseases, and immunodeficiency disorders

The immune system
- Two types of immunity include innate or nonspecific and adaptive or acquired immunity.
- White blood cells, especially lymphocytes, combat invading foreign substances to recognize and destroy them.

- Cytokines are small proteins that send signals between cells to cause a variety of actions from the immune system.
- Cytokines include interferons, interleukins, colony-stimulating factors, tumor necrosis factor, and chemokines.
- Immunoglobulins or antibodies, mainly IgG, are used for patients with immunodeficiency disorders.

Administration of biologic agents
- Some biologic agents are hazardous drugs requiring a high level of protection for any clinician preparing and administering these agents.
- Types of biologic agents are classified similarly to the cells of the immune system.

- Five categories of biologic agents include interferons, interleukins, colony-stimulating factors, monoclonal antibodies, and immunoglobulins.
- Prior to each administration, a thorough patient assessment is necessary.
- Assess laboratory values as needed for each agent.
- Side effects for each agent vary; know the specific ones for each agent and monitor the patient closely during infusion.
- Be prepared to stop the infusion and treat with appropriate medications to manage cytokine release syndrome or anaphylaxis.

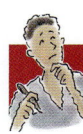

Quick quiz

1. Biologic agents are made from:
   A. beef protein.
   B. fish protein.
   C. human blood and blood components.
   D. plant components.

   Answer: C. Biologic agents are engineered from human blood and blood components, bacteria and viruses, and other forms of biotechnology.

2. The types of white blood cell most involved with the immune response are:
   A. eosinophils.
   B. basophils.
   C. monocytes.
   D. lymphocytes.

   Answer: D. Lymphocytes are concentrated in areas that frequently encounter hostile invaders and are divided into many different types of cells to modulate immune function.

3. Which immunoglobulin is found in the largest quantity in immunoglobulin products?
   A. IgG
   B. IgM
   C. IgA
   D. IgD

   Answer: A. Immunoglobulin products contain about 96% IgG.

4. Names of monoclonal antibodies end with:
   A. -mab.
   B. -kin.
   C. -beta or -alpha.
   D. -stim.

   Answer: A. Names of all monoclonal antibodies end in "-mab."

5. Cytokine release syndrome indicates the need to:
   A. slow the rate of the infusion of the biologic agent and continue patient monitoring.
   B. stop the infusion, treat the symptoms with appropriate medication, and restart the infusion if symptoms resolve.
   C. slow the infusion rate and provide other medications to treat the symptoms.
   D. stop the infusion permanently and treat the symptoms with appropriate medications.

   Answer: B. Temporarily stop the infusion, give other medications to treat the symptoms, and restart the biologic agent at a slower rate when the symptoms resolve.

Scoring

★★★ If you answered all five questions correctly, congratulations! Now treat yourself to some extra time in your resting phase.

★★ If you answered three or four questions correctly, not bad! You are getting into the flow of things.

★ If you answered fewer than three questions correctly, don't get discouraged! Sometimes, it takes a few learning cycles before the information starts taking effect.

Suggested References

AMA. (2016). *United States Adopted Names Council*. Chicago, IL: American Medical Association. Retrieved from http://www.ama-assn.org/ama/pub/physician-resources/medical-science/united-states-adopted-names-council/about-us.page?, on September 7, 2016.

Department of Health and Human Services Centers for Disease Control and Prevention National Institute for Occupational Safety and Health. (2014). *NIOSH list of antineoplastic and other hazardous drugs in healthcare settings 2014*. Retrieved from at http://www.cdc.gov/niosh/docs/2014-138/pdfs/2014-138_v3.pdf, on September 6, 2016.

IFD. (2013). *Immunoglobulin therapy and other medical therapies for antibody deficiencies*. Towson, MD: Immune Deficiency Foundation. Retrieved from at http://primaryimmune.org/treatment-information/immunoglobulin-therapy/, on May 20, 2016.

NCI. (2015). *Cancer vaccines*. Bethesda, MD: National Cancer Institute. Retrieved from http://www.cancer.gov/about-cancer/causes-prevention/vaccines-fact-sheet#q7

Younger, M. (Ed.) (2012). *Immunoglobulin therapy for primary immunodeficiency diseases*. Towson, MD: Immune Deficiency Foundation. Retrieved from http://primaryimmune.org/product/idf-guide-for-nurses-immunoglobulin-therapy-for-primary-immunodeficiency-diseases-3rd-edition/, on September 1, 2016.

Chapter 8

Parenteral nutrition

Just the facts

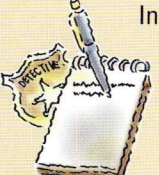

In this chapter, you'll learn:
- ♦ basic nutritional needs
- ♦ indications for parenteral nutrition
- ♦ nutritional solutions
- ♦ the proper way to perform a nutritional assessment
- ♦ the proper way to administer parenteral nutrition
- ♦ complications of parenteral nutrition.

Understanding parenteral nutrition

You may administer parenteral nutrition (PN) when illness or surgery prevents a patient from eating and metabolizing food. Common conditions that make PN necessary include:
- GI trauma
- pancreatitis
- ileus
- inflammatory bowel disease
- GI tract malignancy
- GI hemorrhage
- paralytic ileus
- GI obstruction
- short-bowel syndrome
- GI fistula
- severe malabsorption.

Critically ill patients may also receive PN if they're hemodynamically unstable or if GI tract blood flow is impaired.

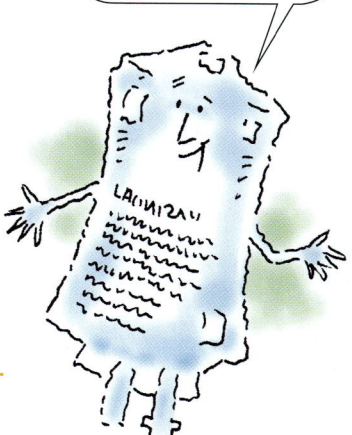

Is your patient unable to eat and metabolize food? Then, serve me up!

Nutritional needs

Essential nutrients found in food provide energy, maintain body tissues, and aid body processes, such as growth, cell activity, enzyme production, and temperature regulation. PN solution should

326

be used only when the gastrointestinal tract cannot be used. PN solutions are provided by the pharmacy in three ways:
- The solution is compounded to meet the specific nutritional needs of a patient, requiring a complex formula of all nutrients.
- The solution is a standard formula with fixed amounts of protein, carbohydrates, and fat.
- Premixed solutions are purchased from fluid manufacturers as a less costly alternative than custom compounded solutions and may be more commonly used in smaller facilities.

Nutrients in food are essential for me to remain active.

Turning food into fuel

When carbohydrates, fats, and proteins are metabolized by the body, they produce energy, which is measured in calories (also called *kilocalories*). A normal healthy adult generally requires 2,000 to 3,000 calories per day. Specific requirements depend on an individual's size, sex, age, and level of physical activity.

A nutritional solution: in more ways than one!

A parenteral nutrition solution will contain two or more of the following elements:
- dextrose
- proteins
- electrolytes
- vitamins
- trace elements including zinc, copper, chromium, manganese, and selenium
- water.

Intravenous fat emulsion (IVFE), commonly called lipids, may be added to the solution or given separately based on patient needs.

Minimize complications of parenteral nutrition by monitoring the catheter insertion site and patency, infusion rate, and laboratory test results.

It's a good thing…

PN solutions can provide all necessary nutrients when a patient is unable to absorb nutrients through the GI tract. It enables cells to function despite the patient's inability to take in or metabolize food.

…but risky

Like all invasive procedures, PN incurs certain risks, including:
- catheter infection
- hyperglycemia (high blood glucose)
- hypokalemia (low blood potassium).

Complications of PN can be minimized with careful monitoring of the catheter site, infusion rate, and laboratory test results.

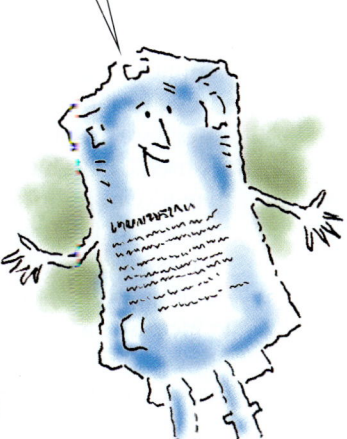

A matter of access

Another disadvantage of PN is the need for central vascular access device (CVAD), which is used because the hypertonic nature, primarily from high dextrose concentration, will cause sclerosis of peripheral veins. The rapid blood flow around the CVAD will allow for dilution of the PN solution by the blood.

Price is a premium

Parenteral nutrition is expensive — about 10 times as expensive as enteral nutrition for the solutions alone. Additionally, there are the costs of the electronic infusion pump, administration sets, CVAD insertion and management, and laboratory tests.

Parenteral nutrition infusion methods

Depending on the final osmolarity of the prescribed PN solution, nutritional support solutions are administered through either a CVAD or peripheral catheter. (See *Chapter 1* for discussion of osmolarity and tonicity, page 15.)

Central venous infusion

A patient needing PN will usually require a formula meeting complete nutritional needs. This solution was previously known as total parenteral nutrition (TPN), although that term is not used any longer. PN with a final dextrose concentration higher than 10% and a final osmolarity greater than 900 mOsm/L must be delivered through a CVAD with the catheter tip located in the superior vena cava near the junction with the right atrium. (See *Chapter 3, Infusion therapy requiring central venous access*, page 119.)

Peripheral infusion

Peripheral parenteral nutrition (PPN) is the delivery of nutrients through a catheter inserted into a peripheral vein. Generally, PPN provides fewer calories than PN because lower dextrose concentrations are used. The solution osmolarity must be less than 900 mOsm/L to reduce infusion site pain, phlebitis, and venous thrombosis. PPN formulas reduce the calories from protein and carbohydrates while increasing calories from fat, which could lead to excessively high levels of triglycerides and liver dysfunction. Another approach could be to increase the fluid volume to dilute the protein and carbohydrates; however, this could create fluid overload in many patients. PPN is also used to bridge the period between removal of a problematic CVAD and insertion of a new CVAD. Infusion of PPN through a midline catheter remains a controversial practice.

Indications for parenteral nutrition

The patient's condition determines whether PN or PPN is used.

Indications for PN

A patient may receive PN for:
- debilitating illness lasting longer than 2 weeks
- critical illness in an adult expected to remain in medical or surgical intensive care for 2 to 3 days or longer
- organ failure (liver, pulmonary, renal)
- deficient or absent oral intake for longer than 7 days, as in cases of multiple trauma, severe burns, or anorexia nervosa
- loss of at least 10% of preillness weight
- serum albumin level below 3.5 g/dL
- poor tolerance of long-term enteral feedings
- chronic vomiting or diarrhea
- inability to sustain adequate weight with oral or enteral feedings.
- GI disorders that prevent or severely reduce absorption, such as bowel obstruction, Crohn's disease, ulcerative colitis, short-bowel syndrome, cancer malabsorption syndrome, acute pancreatitis, and bowel fistulas
- inflammatory GI disorders, such as wound infection, fistulas, or abscesses such as after bariatric surgery.

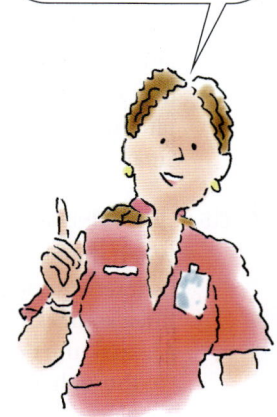

Use PN when lengthy or chronic illness leads to patient weight loss and decreased calorie and protein intake.

Indications for PPN

Patients who don't need to gain weight, yet need nutritional support, may receive PPN for as long as 3 weeks. It's used to help a patient meet minimal calorie and protein requirements. PPN therapy may also be used with oral or enteral feedings for a patient who needs to supplement low-calorie intake or who can't absorb enteral therapy.

Putting PPN on hold

PPN shouldn't be used for patients with moderate to severe malnutrition or fat metabolism disorders, such as pathologic hyperlipidemia, lipid nephrosis, and acute pancreatitis caused by hyperlipidemia. In patients with severe liver damage, coagulation disorders, anemia, and pulmonary disease as well as those at increased risk for fat embolism use parenteral nutrition cautiously.

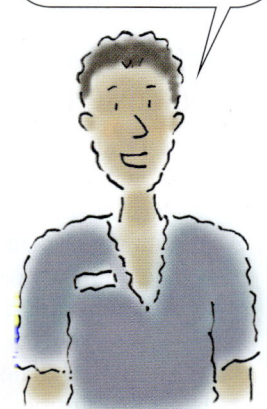

Use PPN to help the patient meet minimum calorie and protein requirements or to supplement oral or enteral feedings.

Nutritional deficiencies

The most common nutritional deficiencies involve protein and calories. Nutritional deficiencies may result from a nonfunctional GI tract, decreased food intake, increased metabolic need, or a combination of these factors.

Hunger strike

Food intake may be decreased because of illness, decreased physical ability, or injury. Decreased food intake can occur with GI disorders, such as paralytic ileus, surgery, or sepsis.

Metabolic activity up: need more calories!

An increase in metabolic activity requires an increase in calorie intake. Fever commonly increases metabolic activity. The metabolic rate may also increase in victims of burns, trauma, disease, or stress; patients may require up to twice the calories of their basal metabolic rate (the minimum energy needed to maintain respiration, circulation, and other basic body functions).

Effects of protein–calorie deficiencies

When the body detects protein-calorie deficiency, it turns to its reserve sources of energy. Reserve energy is drawn from three sources:
1. First, the body mobilizes and converts glycogen to glucose through a process called *glycogenolysis*.
2. Next, if necessary, the body draws energy from the fats stored in adipose tissue.
3. As a last resort, the body taps its store of essential visceral proteins (serum albumin and transferrin) and somatic body proteins (skeletal, smooth muscle, and tissue proteins). These proteins and their amino acids are converted to glucose for energy through a process called *gluconeogenesis*. When these essential body proteins break down, a negative nitrogen balance results (which means more protein is used by the body than is taken in). Starvation and disease-related stress contribute to this catabolic (destructive) state.

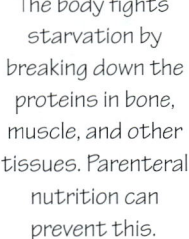

Fever, burns, trauma, disease, and stress all increase metabolic activity, causing an increased need for caloric intake.

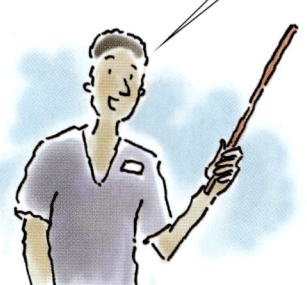

The body fights starvation by breaking down the proteins in bone, muscle, and other tissues. Parenteral nutrition can prevent this.

Nutrition disorders

Malnutrition is actually undernutrition, which results from not enough food intake or poor absorption of the nutrition from food consumed. With malnutrition, body composition changes, along with physical and mental capabilities. Clinical outcomes of illness and injury are complicated by the presence of malnutrition.

Malnutrition can be categorized as follows:
- disease-related malnutrition (DRM) with inflammation
- disease-related malnutrition without inflammation
- malnutrition without disease.

DRM with inflammation

An underlying disease produces the inflammatory response characterized by anorexia and tissue breakdown. The degree of metabolic changes depends upon the disease and its clinical course. Advanced age and inactivity produce more muscle breakdown. Diseases such as cancer, end-stage kidney disease, chronic obstructive pulmonary disease, and congestive heart failure can produce cachexia, a form of chronic DRM with inflammation characterized by muscle loss with or without fat loss. Stress from acute illness and injury such as burns or other trauma produces acute DRM with inflammation.

DRM without inflammation

In these conditions, inflammation is not the cause of the malnutrition. This group includes any condition that results in difficulty with eating including upper digestive obstruction, neurological conditions such as a stroke or Parkinson's disease, or many forms of dementia.

Malnutrition without disease

This group includes two situations. Natural disasters such as drought or flooding cause a lack of food and adequate nutrition. Socioeconomic conditions such as poverty, mourning, poor dental health, or self-neglect produces another cause of malnutrition.

Other nutrition-related conditions

Two societal trends influence nutrition — aging and obesity. Sarcopenia is the loss of skeletal muscle mass and strength, a condition often seen in older adults, and may be considered a precursor to frailty in older adults.

Overweight and obesity is overnutrition or abnormal fat buildup that affects health. This condition is commonly associated with a diet of high energy (that is, calories) but poor quality. Disease and injury can lead to malnutrition and greater clinical problems for the overweight/obese person. Sarcopenia may be combined with obesity in patients with cancer, type 2 diabetes, and post–organ transplantation. Another concern is the presence of central obesity in the intra-abdominal area. This condition is associated with insulin resistance, type 2 diabetes, hypertension, and high levels of cholesterol and triglycerides, producing greater cardiovascular risk to the patient.

Micronutrient deficiency is seen with osteoporosis from vitamin D deficiency or night blindness from vitamin A deficiency. Poor wound healing and a greater risk for infection are associated with micronutrient deficiency. On the other hand, excessive micronutrients can also produce clinical conditions such as skin rashes from excess niacin and peripheral neuropathy from too much vitamin B_6.

Refeeding syndrome is caused by overly aggressive provision of nutrition by oral, enteral, or parenteral routes. Fluid and electrolyte imbalances include peripheral edema and congestive heart failure from fluid retention, respiratory failure, delirium, and encephalopathy. The most common electrolyte disturbance is hypophosphatemia, but others such as low levels of potassium, calcium, and magnesium may also happen.

Malnutrition in hospitalized patients

Higher infection rates, poor or slow wound healing, greater lengths of hospital stays, and more frequent readmission are negative clinical outcomes associated with malnutrition in US hospitals. Data collection and analysis done by numerous methods have reported rates of malnutrition ranging from 21% of older adults to 24% of children and 54% of all hospitalized patients. A more recent study analyzed diagnostic codes on discharge from 1,051 hospitals in 45 states. Some form of malnutrition was diagnosed in 1.25 million patients, 3.2% of all discharges in 2010. Patients with a malnutrition diagnosis were older and had a longer length of hospital stay. Emergency or urgent reasons for admission were associated with more malnutrition diagnoses. Additionally, discharge for patients with these diagnoses were twice as likely to have home care and five times more likely to die.

Among this group of patients with diagnoses of malnutrition, infection represented three of the five most common diagnoses including septicemia, pneumonia, and aspiration pneumonitis. Acute renal failure and interstitial emphysema were the other two of the top five diagnoses. Only 8.9% of those with a malnutrition diagnosis received parenteral nutrition, while another 5% received enteral nutrition. Costs in this group were three times greater than patients without a malnutrition diagnosis.

This study of discharge diagnoses probably represents a very small portion of patients that actually have some type of malnutrition. Considering that older studies using other methods of data collection reported much higher rates, this could easily be significant under identification of malnutrition.

Nutritional assessment

When illness or surgery compromises a patient's intake or alters his metabolic requirements, you'll need to assess the relationship between nutrients consumed and energy expended. A nutritional assessment provides insight into how well the patient's physiologic need for nutrients is being met. Because poor nutritional status can affect most body systems, a thorough nutritional assessment helps you anticipate problems and intervene appropriately.

To assess nutritional status, follow these steps:
- Obtain a dietary history.
- Perform a physical assessment.
- Take anthropometric measurements.
- Review the results of pertinent diagnostic tests.

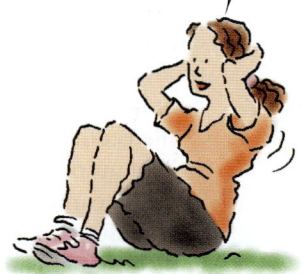

A nutritional assessment gives insight into how well the patient's need for nutrients is being met.

Dietary history

When obtaining a dietary history, check for signs of decreased food and fluid intake, increased metabolic requirements, or a combination of the two. Also, check dietary recall, using a 24-hour recall or diet diary. Note any factors that affect food intake and changes in appetite. Obtain a weight history.

Physical assessment

When performing a physical assessment, be sure to include:
- chief complaint
- present illness
- medical history, including previous major illnesses, injuries, hospitalizations, or surgeries
- allergies and history of intolerance to food and medications
- family history, including familial, genetic, or environmental illnesses
- social history, including environmental, psychological, and sociologic factors that may influence nutritional status, such as alcoholism, living alone, financial challenges, or lack of transportation.

Are you missing anything?

Also, be sure to observe for subtle signs of malnutrition. (See *Signs of poor nutrition*, page 333.)

Measuring up

Anthropometry compares the patient's measurements with established standards. (See *Taking anthropometric measurements*, page 334.) It's an objective, noninvasive method for measuring overall body size, composition, and specific body parts. Commonly used anthropometric measurements include:
- height
- weight
- ideal body weight
- body frame size.

Triceps skinfold thickness, midarm circumference, and midarm muscle circumference are less commonly used anthropometric measurements because they tend to vary by age and race. Using these measurements may be more meaningful for long-term PN, causing their use in the acute care hospital setting to be limited. Closely follow your facility's policy and procedure for taking these measurements as slight variations can produce inaccurate results.

Not up to 90%?

A finding of less than 90% of the standard measurement may indicate a need for nutritional support.

Signs of poor nutrition

When performing a physical assessment, note the patient's overall condition and inspect the skin, mouth, and teeth. Then, look for these subtle signs of poor nutrition:
- poor skin turgor
- bruising
- abnormal pigmentation
- darkening of the mouth lining
- protruding eyes (exophthalmos)
- neck swelling
- adventitious breath sounds
- dental caries or missing teeth
- ill-fitting dentures
- signs of infection or irritation in and around the mouth
- muscle wasting
- abdominal wasting, masses, and tenderness and an enlarged liver.

Taking anthropometric measurements

Follow the steps below to measure midarm circumference, triceps skinfold thickness, and midarm muscle circumference.

Midarm circumference
Locate the midpoint on the patient's upper arm using a nonstretching tape measure, and mark the midpoint with a marking pen.

Triceps skinfold thickness
Determine the triceps skinfold thickness by grasping the patient's skin between the thumb and forefinger approximately 1 cm above the midpoint. Place the calipers at the midpoint and squeeze the calipers for about 3 seconds. Record the measurement registered on the handle gauge to the nearest 0.5 mm. Take two more readings, and then, average all three to compensate for possible error.

Midarm muscle circumference
At the midpoint, measure the midarm circumference. Calculate midarm muscle circumference by multiplying the triceps skinfold thickness (in centimeters) by 3.143 and subtracting the result from the midarm circumference.

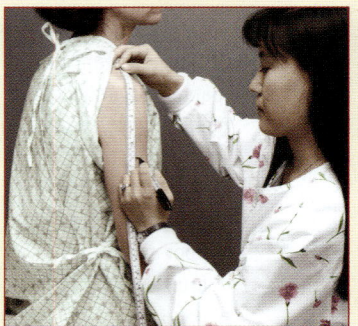
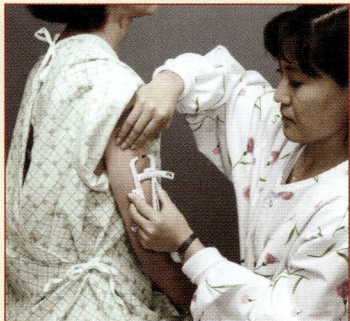
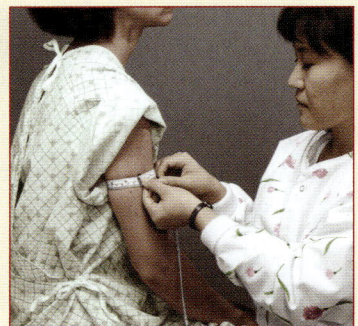

Interpreting your findings
Record all three measurements as percentages of the standard measurements using the following formula:

$$\frac{\text{Actual measurement}}{\text{Standard measurement}} \times 100.$$

Compare the patient's percentage measurements with the standard. A measurement less than 90% of the standard indicates calorie deprivation; a measurement over 90% of the standard indicates adequate or more than adequate energy reserves.

Measurement	Standard	90%
Midarm circumference	Men: 29.3 cm Women: 26.5 cm	Men: 26.4 cm Women: 23.9 cm
Triceps skinfold thickness	Men: 12.5 mm Women: 16.5 mm	Men: 11.3 mm Women: 14.9 mm
Midarm muscle circumference	Men: 25.3 cm Women: 23.2 cm	Men: 22.8 cm Women: 20.9 cm

Diagnostic studies

Evidence of a nutritional problem commonly appears in the results of a diagnostic test. Tests are used to evaluate:
- visceral protein status
- lean body mass
- vitamin and mineral balance.

Diagnostic studies are also used to evaluate the effectiveness of nutritional support. (See *Detecting deficiencies*, page 335.)

Detecting deficiencies

Laboratory studies help pinpoint nutritional deficiencies by aiding in the diagnosis of anemia, malnutrition, and other disorders. Check out this chart to learn about some commonly ordered diagnostic tests, their purposes, normal values, and implications. Albumin, prealbumin, transferrin, and triglyceride levels are the major indicators of nutritional deficiency.

Test and purpose	Normal values	
Creatinine height index Uses a 24-hour urine sample to determine adequacy of muscle mass	• Determined from a reference table of values based on a patient's height or weight	• Less than 80% of reference value: moderate depletion of muscle mass (protein reserves) • Less than 60% of reference value: severe depletion, with increased risk of compromised immune function
Hematocrit Diagnoses anemia and dehydration	• Male: 42%–50% • Female: 40%–48% • Child: 29%–41% • Neonate: 55%–68%	• Increased values: severe dehydration and polycythemia • Decreased values: iron deficiency anemia and excessive blood loss
Hemoglobin Assesses blood's oxygen-carrying capacity to aid in the diagnosis of anemia, protein deficiency, and hydration status	• Older adult: 10–17 g/dL • Adult male: 13–18 g/dL • Adult female: 12–16 g/dL • Child: 9–15.5 g/dL • Neonate: 14–20 g/dL	• Increased values: dehydration and polycythemia • Decreased values: protein deficiency, iron deficiency anemia, excessive blood loss, and overhydration
Serum albumin Helps assess visceral protein stores	• Adult: 3.5–5 g/dL • Child: same as adult • Neonate: 3.6–5.4 g/dL	• Decreased values: malnutrition, overhydration, liver or kidney disease, heart failure, and excessive blood protein losses such as from severe burns
Serum transferrin (similar to serum total iron-binding capacity [TIBC]) Helps assess visceral protein stores; has a shorter half-life than serum albumin and, thus, more accurately reflects current status	• Adult: 200–400 µg/dL • Child: 350–450 µg/dL • Neonate: 60–175 µg/dL	• Increased TIBC: iron deficiency, as in pregnancy, or iron deficiency anemia • Decreased TIBC: iron excess, as in chronic inflammatory states • Below 200 µg/dL: visceral protein depletion • Below 100 µg/dL: severe visceral protein depletion
Serum triglycerides Screens for hyperlipidemia	• 40–200 mg/dL	• Increased values combined with increased cholesterol levels: increased risk of atherosclerotic disease • Decreased values: protein-energy malnutrition (PEM) and steatorrhea

(continued)

Detecting deficiencies (continued)

Test and purpose	Normal values	
Total lymphocyte count Diagnoses PEM	• 1,500–3,000/µl	• Increased values: infection or inflammation, leukemia, and tissue necrosis • Decreased values: moderate to severe malnutrition if no other cause, such as influenza or measles, is identified
Total protein screen Detects hyperproteinemia or hypoproteinemia	• 6–8 g/dL	• Increased values: dehydration • Decreased values: malnutrition and protein loss
Transthyretin (prealbumin) Offers information regarding visceral protein stores; should be used in conjunction with albumin level. (Prealbumin has a shorter half-life [2–3 days] than albumin. This test is sensitive to nutritional repletion.)	• 16–40 mg/dL	• Increased values: renal insufficiency and patient on dialysis • Decreased values: PEM, acute catabolic states, postsurgery, and hyperthyroidism
Urine ketone bodies (acetone) Screens for ketonuria and detects carbohydrate deprivation	• Negative for ketones in urine	• Ketoacidosis: starvation

Parenteral nutrition solutions

The solution you administer depends on the type of parenteral nutrition and the patient's status. (See *Parenteral solutions*, page 337.)

Element roll call

Parenteral nutrition solutions may contain the following elements, each offering a particular benefit:
- *Dextrose* provides most of the calories that can help maintain nitrogen balance. The number of nonprotein calories needed to maintain nitrogen balance depends on the severity of the patient's illness.
- *Amino acids* supply enough protein to replace essential amino acids, maintain protein stores, and prevent protein loss from muscle tissues.
- *Fats,* supplied as lipid emulsions, are a concentrated source of energy that prevent or correct fatty acid deficiencies. These are available in several concentrations and can provide 30% to 50% of a patient's daily calorie requirement.

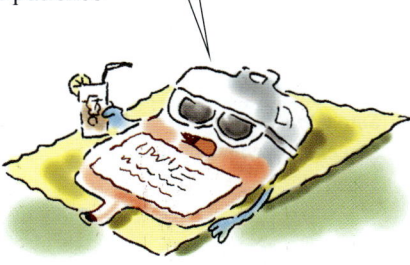

I'm not feeling very energetic today. Must be due to my solution's low dextrose content.

Parenteral nutrition solutions

Therapy and solution	Indications	Special considerations
Parenteral nutrition (PN) • Dextrose, 20%–70% (1 L dextrose 25% = 850 nonprotein calories) • Crystalline amino acids, 2.5%–15% • Electrolytes, vitamins, micronutrients, insulin, and heparin as ordered • Fat emulsion, 10% or 20% (can be given peripherally or centrally) • Water	Long-term therapy (2 weeks or more) is used to: • supply large quantities of nutrients and calories (2,000–3,000 calories/day or more) • provide needed calories, restore nitrogen balance, and replace essential vitamins, electrolytes, minerals, and trace elements • promote tissue synthesis, wound healing, and normal metabolic function • allow bowel rest and healing and reduce activity in the pancreas and small intestine • improve tolerance to surgery if severely malnourished.	• Is nutritionally complete • Requires percutaneous insertion of CVAD often at the patient's bedside. CVADs requiring surgical insertion (i.e., tunneled cuffed catheter and implanted ports) may be appropriate from some patients. • May result in metabolic complications (glucose intolerance or electrolyte imbalances) from hypertonic solution • May not be effective in severely stressed patients (such as those with sepsis or burns) • May interfere with immune mechanisms
Peripheral parenteral nutrition (PPN) • Dextrose, 5%–10% • Crystalline amino acids, 2.75%–4.25% • Electrolytes, minerals, micronutrients, and vitamins as ordered • Fat emulsion, 10% or 20% • Heparin or hydrocortisone as ordered • Water	Short-term therapy (3 weeks or less) is used to: • maintain nutritional state in patients who can tolerate relatively high fluid volume, who usually resume bowel function and oral feedings in a few days, and who aren't candidates for CV access devices • provide ~1,300–1,800 calories/day.	• Is nutritionally complete for short-term therapy • Shouldn't be used in nutritionally depleted patients • Can't be used in volume-restricted patients because it requires high volumes of solution • Avoids insertion and maintenance of CVAD, but the patient must have good peripheral veins. I.V. site should be changed at the first sign of any complication. • Delivers less hypertonic solutions • May cause phlebitis • Offers lower risk of metabolic complications *I.V. lipid emulsion* • Has increased risk of hyperlipidemia • Irritates vein in long-term use • May not be appropriate in patients with renal or liver failure

- *Electrolytes and minerals* are added to the parenteral nutrition solution based on an evaluation of the patient's serum chemistry profile and metabolic needs.
- *Vitamins* ensure normal body functions and optimal nutrient use for the patient. A commercially available mixture of fat- and

water-soluble vitamins, biotin, and folic acid may be added to the patient's parenteral nutrition solution.
- *Micronutrients,* also called *trace elements,* promote normal metabolism. Most commercial solutions contain zinc, copper, chromium, selenium, and manganese.
- *Water* is added to a parenteral nutrition solution based on the patient's fluid requirements and electrolyte balance.

Added features

Depending on the patient's condition, the practitioner may also order additives for the parenteral nutrition solution, such as insulin or heparin. (See *Understanding common additives*, page 338.)

PN solutions

Solutions for PN are hypertonic, with an osmolarity of 1,800 to 2,600 mOsm/L. Electrolytes, minerals, vitamins, micronutrients, and water are added to the base solution to satisfy daily requirements. Lipids may be given as a separate solution or as an admixture with dextrose and amino acids.

Understanding common additives

Common parenteral nutrition solutions include dextrose, amino acids, and any of the additives listed here, which are used to treat a patient's specific metabolic deficiencies:
- Acetate prevents metabolic acidosis.
- Amino acids provide protein necessary for tissue repair.
- Calcium promotes development of bones and teeth and aids in blood clotting.
- Chloride regulates the acid-base equilibrium and maintains osmotic pressure.
- $D_{50}W$ provides calories for metabolism.
- Folic acid is needed for deoxyribonucleic acid (DNA) formation and promotes growth and development.
- Magnesium aids carbohydrate and protein absorption.
- Micronutrients (such as zinc, manganese, and cobalt) help in wound healing and red blood cell synthesis.
- Phosphate minimizes the potential for developing peripheral paresthesia (numbness and tingling of the extremities).
- Potassium is needed for cellular activity and tissue synthesis.
- Sodium helps regulate water distribution and maintain normal fluid balance.
- Vitamin B complex aids the final absorption of carbohydrates and protein.
- Vitamin C helps in wound healing.
- Vitamin D is essential for bone metabolism and maintenance of serum calcium levels.
- Vitamin K helps prevent bleeding disorders.

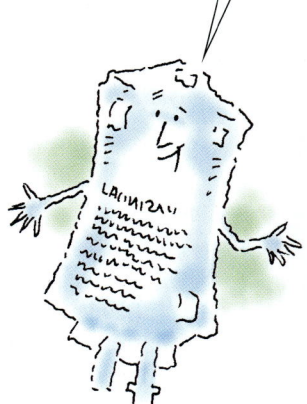

Some of these additives may be ordered for your patient's parenteral nutrition solution.

The 3:1 solution

Daily allotments of PN solution, including lipids and other parenteral solution components, are commonly given in a single 3-L bag, called a *total nutrient admixture (TNA)* or *3-in-1 solution*. (See *Understanding nutrient admixture*, page 339.)

Maintaining glucose balance without adding insulin

Glucose balance is extremely important in a patient receiving PN. Adults use 0.8 to 1 g of glucose per kilogram of body weight per hour. That means a patient can tolerate a constant I.V. infusion of hyperosmolar glucose without adding insulin to the solution. As the concentrated glucose solution infuses, a pancreatic beta-cell response causes serum insulin levels to increase.

To allow the pancreas to establish and maintain the necessary increased insulin production, start with a slow infusion rate and increase it gradually as ordered. Abruptly stopping the infusion may cause rebound hypoglycemia, which calls for an infusion of dextrose.

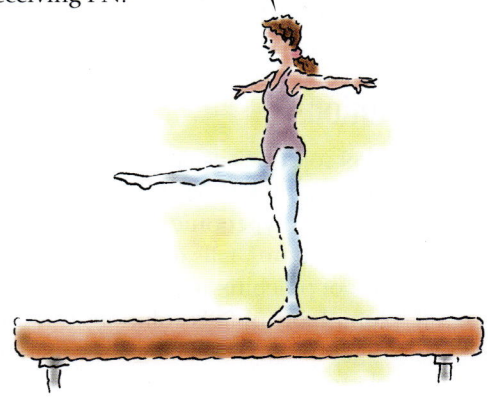

When administering PN, be sure to maintain the patient's glucose balance.

Understanding total nutrient admixture (TNA)

TNA is a white solution that delivers 1 day's worth of nutrients in a single 3-L bag. Also called *3-in-1 solution*, it combines lipids with other parenteral solution components.

Advantages
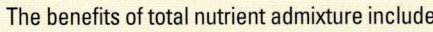
The benefits of total nutrient admixture include:
- less need to handle the bag (lower risk of contamination)
- less time required
- lower hospital costs
- increased patient mobility
- easier adjustment to home care.

Disadvantages
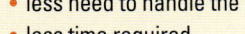
The disadvantages of total nutrient admixture include:
- the electronic infusion pump must be able to accommodate programming for larger volumes to be infused and to accurately deliver the needed flow rate
- 1.2-micron filter required (rather than a 0.22-micron filter) to allow lipid molecules through
- limited amount of calcium and phosphorus added because of the difficulty in detecting precipitate in the milky white solution.

Glucose balance may be further thrown off by:
- sepsis
- stress
- shock
- liver or kidney failure
- diabetes
- age
- pancreatic disease
- concurrent use of certain medications, including steroids.

PPN solutions

PPN solutions usually consist of dextrose 5% in water to 10% dextrose and 2.75% to 4.25% crystalline amino acids. PPN solutions are hypertonic or hyperosmolar — any solution greater than 350 mOsm/L falls into this category and is associated with a greater risk of phlebitis and thrombophlebitis. For this reason, the final osmolarity of PPN solutions is recommended by several professional organization to be no greater than 900 mOsm/L. Lipid emulsions, electrolytes, trace elements, and vitamins may be given as part of PPN to add calories and other needed nutrients.

Lipid emulsions

In an oral diet, lipids or fats are the major source of calories, usually providing about 40% of the total calorie intake. In parenteral nutrition solutions, lipids provide 9 kcal/g. I.V. lipid emulsions are oxidized for energy as needed. As a nearly isotonic emulsion, concentrations of 10% (1 kcal/mL) or 20% (2 kcal/mL) can be safely infused through peripheral or central veins. Lipid emulsions prevent and treat essential fatty acid deficiency and provide a major source of energy.

Administering parenteral nutrition

You may deliver parenteral nutrition in one of two ways:
1. continuously
2. cyclically.

Open for service 24 hours

With continuous delivery, the patient receives the infusion over a 24-hour period. The infusion begins at a slow rate and increases to the optimal rate as ordered. This type of delivery may prevent complications such as hyperglycemia caused by a high dextrose load.

Not-so-vicious cycle

A patient undergoing cyclic therapy receives the entire 24-hour volume of parenteral nutrition solution over a shorter period, perhaps 8, 10, 12, 14, or 16 hours. Home care parenteral nutrition programs have boosted the use of cyclic therapy. This type of therapy may be used to wean the patient from PN. (See *Switching from continuous to cyclic PN*, page 341.)

Administering PN

PN solutions must be infused through one of the following types of CVADs:
- peripherally inserted central catheter (PICC)
- nontunneled centrally inserted catheter
- tunneled cuffed catheter
- implanted port.

In it for the long haul

Long-term therapy requires the use of one of the following devices:
- tunneled cuffed catheter (for example, Hickman®, Broviac®)
- implanted port (for example, Infuse-A-Port® or Port-a-Cath®).

The dilution solution

Because PN solution has a solute concentration much greater than blood, peripheral I.V. administration can cause sclerosis and thrombosis. To ensure adequate dilution, the CVAD is inserted through the basilic vein of the upper extremity, the subclavian or internal jugular veins with the tip confirmed to be in the superior vena cava near its junction with the right atrium, a wide-bore, high-flow vein. For patients requiring insertion through the femoral vein, the tip should be confirmed to reside in the inferior vena cava near the right atrial junction above the diaphragm.

Preparing the patient

To increase compliance, make sure that the patient understands the purpose of treatment and enlist his help throughout the course of therapy.

Taking PN home

Understanding PN and its goals helps a home care patient assume a greater role in administering, monitoring, and maintaining therapy. When instructing a home care patient, focus your teaching on signs and symptoms of:
- fluid, electrolyte, and glucose imbalances
- vitamin and trace element deficiencies and toxicities
- catheter infection, such as fever, chills, discomfort on infusion, and redness or drainage at the catheter insertion site.

Switching from continuous to cyclic PN

When switching from continuous to cyclic parenteral nutrition (PN), adjust the flow rate so the patient's blood glucose level can adapt to the decreased nutrient load. Do this by reducing the flow rate by one-half for 1 hour before stopping the infusion. Draw a blood glucose sample 1 hour after the infusion ends, and observe the patient for signs of hypoglycemia, such as sweating, shakiness, and irritability.

To help prevent glucose imbalance, teach the home care patient receiving his first I.V. bag of PN how to regulate the flow rate so he maintains the rate prescribed by the licensed independent practitioner (LIP). Explain that a gradual increase in the flow rate allows the pancreas to establish and maintain the increased insulin production necessary to tolerate this treatment. When the goal rate of the PN infusion is met, there should be no reason to adjust the rate.

Finally, review the details of the administration schedule, the equipment the patient will use, and, to avoid incompatibilities, the prescribed and over-the-counter medications he takes and what to do in case of an emergency or treatment complication. Educate the patient and a caregiver regarding all above. Have the patient and caregiver practice each step of the procedure before hospital discharge when time allows. The patient and caregiver education will continue with the home care nurses until the patient or caregiver is competent to manage the infusion.

Be a compliance booster

To safely maintain this therapy, the prescribed regimen must be adhered to by the home care patient and his caregivers. Your teaching efforts and return demonstrations by the patient help boost compliance in all aspects of PN therapy.

Preparing the equipment

Before PN administration begins, a thorough assessment of vascular access needs should be performed to select the most appropriate CVAD. Following insertion, confirmation of tip location in the superior or inferior vena cava is required. This may be by a postprocedure chest X-ray or by electrocardiogram. (See *Chapter 3, Infusion therapy requiring central venous access*, page 146.)

Gather the PN solution, an electronic infusion pump, an administration set with the appropriate-sized filter, alcohol swabs, gloves, and an I.V. pole. Be sure to perform hand hygiene before preparing the PN solution for administration, and prepare the administration set in a clean area.

All PN solutions require filtration including lipids. For a PN solution with protein, carbohydrates and the other additives, use a 0.22-micron filter. Piggybacking lipid solutions must be done below this 0.22-micron filter, but a separate 1.2-micron filter is now required for all lipid infusion. For a TNA or 3-in-1 PN solution, a 1.2-micron filter is used. Using an administration set with an integral filter is preferred rather than adding a separate filter to the administration set; however, follow the policy and procedure in your facility.

60-minute warm-up

The infusion of a chilled solution can cause discomfort, hypothermia, venous spasm, and venous constriction. Plan to remove the bag or bottle of PN solution from the refrigerator about 60 minutes before hanging it to allow for warming.

Checking the order

Check the written order against the label on the bag or bottle. Make sure that the volumes, concentrations, and additives are included in the solution. Also, check the infusion rate.

Infusate inspection is imperative

Careful inspection of the infusate should be a habit. Check for clouding, floating debris, or a change in color. Any of these phenomena could indicate contamination, problems with the integrity of the solution, or a pH change. If you see anything suspicious, notify the pharmacy. Inform the LIP that there may be a delay in hanging the solution; he may want to order 5% or 10% dextrose in water until a new container of PN solution is available. Also, be prepared to return the solution to the pharmacy.

Handle with care

PN solutions may have lipid emulsions piggybacked at an injection port on the administration set or be compounded as a TNA solution. Either way, special precautions are required because of the potential for contamination. Additionally, the high dextrose solution supports the growth of microorganisms, so close attention to infection prevention is required. (See *Administering lipid emulsions*, page 344.)

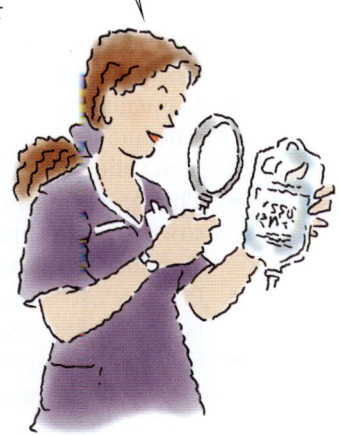

Check every solution for cloudiness, debris, or color changes.

Beginning the infusion

Before beginning the infusion, inspect the catheter insertion site for any signs or symptoms of any complication. Attach a saline-filled syringe and flush the CVAD to assess for resistance and aspirate to confirm a blood return. If there is no resistance to flushing, the presence of a blood return that is the color and consistency of whole blood, and an absence of any other signs or symptoms, begins the infusion as ordered. Watch for swelling at the catheter insertion site, neck, shoulder, or chest wall. Swelling may indicate extravasation of the PN solution, which can cause necrosis. If the patient reports discomfort at the start of or during the infusion, the catheter may be developing a complication. Contact the infusion nurse or vascular access specialist for a thorough assessment. Collaboration with the LIP is required to form the plan of care for diagnosing and managing the problem.

Administering lipid emulsions

To safely administer, follow these special precautions:
• Check the LIP orders for the rate of infusion. The first infusion is given at a slower rate to determine if adverse reactions will occur. The rate may be increased on the second day.
• Before the infusion, always check the lipid container or PN containing lipids for separation or an oily appearance. If either condition exists, the lipid may have come out of emulsion and cannot be used.
• Monitor the patient's vital signs and watch for adverse reactions, such as fever, a pressure sensation over the eyes, nausea, vomiting, headache, chest and back pain, tachycardia, dyspnea, cyanosis, and flushing, sweating, or chills. If the patient has no adverse reactions to the test dose, begin the infusion at the prescribed rate.
• Because lipid emulsions are at high risk for microbial growth, never rehang a partially empty bottle of emulsion.
• Lipid emulsion containers and separate administration set must be changed every 12 hours.

Maintaining the infusion

If the patient tolerates the solution well the first day, the practitioner usually increases intake to the goal rate by the second day. To maintain a PN infusion, follow these key steps:
- Check the order provided by the LIP against the label on the PN container.
- Check the label on the container for the expiration date, concentration of all solution components, rate, and total volume of solution. Add the time at which the solution was hung.
- Interruption in the infusion may come from a damaged fluid container or problems with the VAD. When this happens, hang a bag of 5% dextrose in water at the same infusion rate. Follow the standing orders or protocols from your facility. Some LIPs may prefer to use 10% dextrose in this situation, but it is now considered to be unwarranted.
- Maintain flow rates as prescribed, even if the flow falls behind schedule.
- Don't allow PN solutions to hang for more than 24 hours.
- Change the administration set and filter every 24 hours, using strict aseptic technique. Make sure that all junctions on the entire administration set are secured with luer-locked connections.
- Perform VAD site care and dressing changes according to your facility's policy and procedure.
- Check the infusion pump's volume meter and time tape to monitor for irregular flow rate. Gravity should never be used to administer PN.

- Record the patient's vital signs when you initiate therapy and every 4 to 8 hours thereafter (or more often, if necessary). Be alert for increased body temperature — one of the earliest signs of catheter-related bloodstream infection.
- Monitor your patient's glucose levels as ordered using glucose fingersticks or serum tests.
- Accurately record the patient's daily fluid intake and output, specifying the volume and type of each fluid. This record is a diagnostic tool that you can use to assure prompt, precise replacement of fluid and electrolyte deficits.
- Assess the patient's physical status daily. Weigh him at the same time each morning (after voiding), in similar clothing, using the same scale. Suspect fluid imbalance if the patient gains more than 1 lb (0.45 kg) per day. If ordered, obtain anthropometric measurements.
- Monitor the results of routine laboratory tests, such as serum electrolyte, blood urea nitrogen, and glucose levels, and report abnormal findings to the doctor so appropriate changes in the PN solution can be made.
- Check serum triglyceride levels, which should be in the normal range during continuous PN infusion. Typically, alanine aminotransferase, aspartate aminotransferase, alkaline phosphatase, cholesterol, triglyceride, plasma-free fatty acid, and coagulation tests are performed weekly.

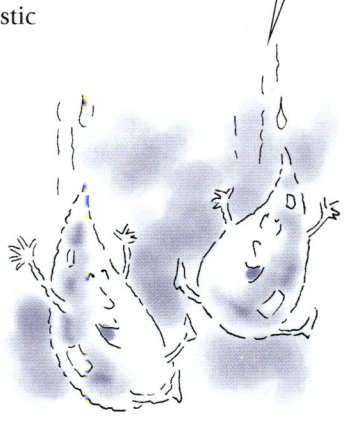

Gravity is great but not for controlling PN. Always use an electronic infusion pump.

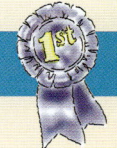

Best practice

Reducing the risk of infection

Because a parenteral nutrition (PN) solution serves as a medium for microbial growth and all types of vascular access devices provide systemic access to the bloodstream, the patient receiving PN risks infection. Maintaining strict aseptic technique when handling the equipment used to administer therapy has been shown to reduce the number of PN-related infections.

- Monitor the patient for signs and symptoms of nutritional aberrations, such as fluid and electrolyte imbalances and glucose metabolism disturbances. Some patients require supplementary insulin throughout PN therapy; the pharmacy may add regular insulin directly to the PN solution.
- Provide emotional support. Keep in mind that patients commonly associate eating with positive feelings and become disturbed when it's eliminated.
- Provide frequent mouth care for the patient.
- Document all assessment findings and nursing interventions.

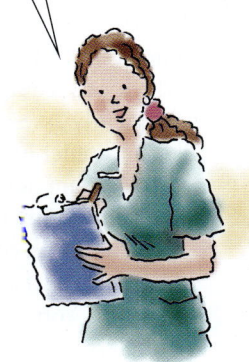

Don't forget to record your assessment findings and nursing interventions throughout treatment.

A port of last resort

Compatibility and stability of all solutions is a critical factor, thus using a PN infusion system for infusion of other medications or solutions should be avoided. When using a single-lumen CVAD, don't use the line to piggyback or infuse blood or blood products, give an I.V. push or piggyback medication, administer simultaneous I.V. solutions, measure CV pressure, or draw blood for laboratory tests. In unavoidable circumstances, the PN line may be used for electrolyte replacement or insulin drips because these infusions are common additives to the PN solution; however, checking with the pharmacy is necessary before attaching any other solution to the PN line. Remember, never add medication to a PN solution container.

Administering PPN

Using an amino acid, dextrose, and lipid emulsion solution, PPN fulfills a patient's basic calorie needs without the risks involved with a CVAD. PPN solutions have lower osmolarity and fewer calories than PN solutions; however, PPN may use a larger volume of total fluid. Administration of PPN through a peripheral vein requires use of all techniques to reduce the risk of phlebitis such as using the smallest gauge catheter, avoiding sites in areas of joint flexion, and adequate catheter stabilization. (See *Chapter 2, Infusion therapy through peripheral veins*, page 91.)

Preparing the patient

Make sure that the patient understands what to expect before, during, and after therapy.

Obtain the largest vein

Select the patient's largest available vein as the insertion site. Using a large vein enables the blood to adequately dilute the PPN solution, which can reduce risk of phlebitis. When using a peripheral catheter, frequently assess the site for signs and symptoms of all complications such as phlebitis, thrombophlebitis, and extravasation. Peripheral catheters are now changed based on the presence of these signs and symptoms rather than at a specific date or time. Any level of discomfort, change in color or temperature, swelling, leaking, or absence of a blood return indicates the need to remove the catheter and insert a new one. Your facility may still have a policy to change all peripheral catheters at a designated time interval (that is, 72 hours) and you will need to follow that policy; however, the catheter may require removal before this designated time.

Preparing the equipment

To administer PPN, gather the necessary equipment, including:
- ordered PPN solution (at room temperature)
- electronic infusion pump
- administration set with 0.22-micron filter
- alcohol swabs
- I.V. pole
- venipuncture equipment, if needed.

Checking the order

Check the written order against the written label on the bag. Make sure that the solution is for peripheral infusion and that the volumes, concentrations, and additives are included in the solution. Also, check the infusion rate.

A little lecture about lipids

In PPN therapy, lipid emulsions may be part of the solution. If given separately, piggyback the lipid emulsion below the 0.22-micron in-line filter close to the insertion site to avoid having lipids clog the filtration system. Ensure that the lipid administration set includes a 1.2-micron filter. When giving lipids, use an electronic infusion pump to ensure correct flow rate.

Beginning the infusion

Begin the PPN infusion as ordered. Watch for swelling at the peripheral insertion site. Swelling may indicate extravasation of the PPN solution, which can cause tissue damage.

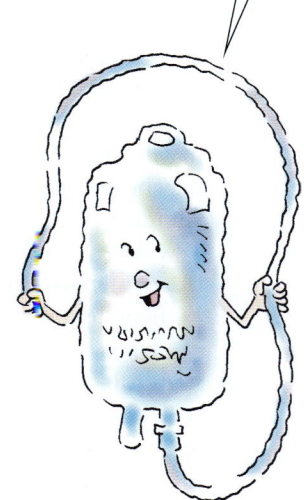

When giving lipid emulsions separately, add a 1.2-micron filter to the lipid administration set in addition to the 0.2-micron filter for the PN solution.

Maintaining the infusion

Caring for a patient receiving a PN infusion involves the same steps required for any patient receiving a peripheral I.V. infusion. You need to maintain the infusion rate and care for the administration set, dressings, infusion site, and vascular access device. In addition, monitor the patient for signs or symptoms of bloodstream infection, including:
- glucose in the urine (glycosuria)
- chills
- malaise
- increased white blood cells (leukocytosis)
- altered level of consciousness
- elevated glucose levels, measured by fingerstick or serum chemistry
- elevated temperature (usually higher than 100.4°F [38°C]).

Insulin insight

Because the synthesis of lipase (a fat-splitting enzyme) increases insulin requirements, the insulin dosage of a diabetic patient may need to be increased as ordered. Insulin is one of the additives that may be adjusted in the formulation of the PPN solution.

Patient reports

Patients receiving lipid emulsions commonly report a feeling of fullness or bloating; occasionally, they experience an unpleasant metallic or greasy taste. Some patients develop allergic reactions to the fat emulsion.

Lipid letdowns

Adverse reactions to lipid emulsion therapy include:
- headache
- flushing
- dizziness
- sweating
- drowsiness
- nausea
- vomiting.

More serious adverse reactions include:
- fever
- difficulty breathing
- cyanosis
- chest and/or back pain
- pain, redness, and swelling of the arms or legs.

Serious allergic reactions may occur, especially in patients reporting an allergy to eggs, safflower oil, soy, or peanuts as these may be ingredients in the lipid emulsion. A variety of liver diseases may be caused by long-term infusion of lipids, resulting in jaundice.

Changes in laboratory test results may also reveal problems when a patient receives lipid emulsions, including:
- hyperlipidemia
- hypercoagulability
- thrombocytopenia.

Considering clearance

The licensed independent practitioner (LIP) monitors the patient's lipid emulsion clearance rate. Lipid emulsion may clear from the blood at an accelerated rate in a patient with severe burns, multiple trauma, or a metabolic imbalance.

Precautions and complications

In this section, you'll find special considerations for administering PN to pediatric and elderly patients. You'll also find information about possible complications during therapy and pointers for discontinuing therapy safely.

Patients with special needs

Children and older adult patients are particularly susceptible to fluid overload and heart failure. With these patients, be particularly careful to administer the correct volume of PN solution at the correct infusion rate.

Pediatric patients

Parenteral nutrition for children serves a dual purpose:
1. It maintains a child's nutritional status.
2. It fuels a child's growth.

An extra helping

Children have a greater need than adults for certain nutrients, including:
- protein
- carbohydrates
- fat
- electrolytes
- trace elements
- vitamins
- fluids.

This greater need is an important consideration in accurately calculating solution components for pediatric patients.

Factor these in

As with adults, children receiving PN should be evaluated carefully by the nurse, LIP, and nutritional support team. Keep in mind the following factors when planning to meet children's nutritional needs:
- age
- weight
- activity level
- size
- development
- calorie needs.

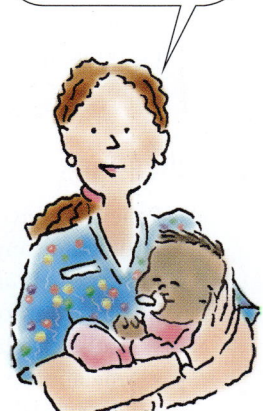

Because they're growing, children need more of some nutrients than adults do.

Lipid liabilities in little ones

Administering PN with lipid emulsions in a premature or low-birth-weight neonate may lead to lipid accumulation in the lungs. Thrombocytopenia (platelet deficiency) has also been reported in infants receiving 20% lipid emulsions.

Older adult patients

In older adults, overinfusion can produce serious adverse effects such as fluid overload, so always monitor flow rates carefully.

What lies underneath

An older patient may have underlying clinical problems that affect the outcome of treatment. For example, he may be taking medications that can interact with the components in the parenteral nutrition solution. For this reason, ask the pharmacist about possible interactions with any drug the patient is taking. Also, inquire about any alternative supplements such as vitamins and herbal products the patient may have been taking.

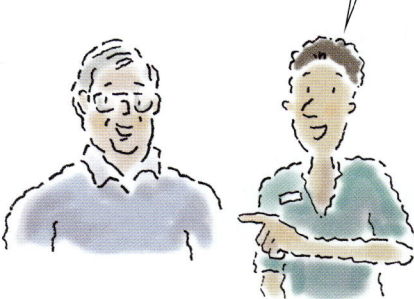

Older patients are prone to fluid overload and drug interactions, so watch carefully when administering PN solutions.

Complications

Patients receiving PN face many of the same complications as patients undergoing any type of peripheral or central infusion therapy. (See *Managing metabolic PN hazards*, page 351.) Complications of PN may be divided into two categories:
- catheter-related
- metabolic.

Peripheral catheter-related complications include local and systemic complications. Phlebitis, thrombophlebitis, and extravasation are local complications associated with PPN. (See *Chapter 2, Local complications of peripheral I.V. therapy*, page 107.) Systemic complications associated with peripheral catheters include bloodstream infection and fluid overload. (See *Chapter 2, Systemic complications of peripheral I.V. therapy*, page 111.)

Complications from CVADs associated with PN include the same insertion-related risks such as pneumothorax, along with complications occurring at any point in the life of the CVAD such as bloodstream infection, vein thrombosis, and venous air emboli. (See *Chapter 3, Risks of I.V. therapy via the central venous system*, page 164.)

Running smoothly

Managing metabolic PN hazards

Metabolic complications are primarily related to fluid and electrolyte imbalances. Prevention is associated with close monitoring of the patient for signs and symptoms along with laboratory test results. To help you treat these common complications, use this chart. (See *Chapter 1, Understanding electrolytes*, page 9.)

Complications	Interventions
Hyperglycemia	• Start insulin therapy or adjust the PN flow rate as ordered. • Carbohydrate intolerance or insulin resistance
Hypoglycemia	• Infuse dextrose as ordered. • May be related to sudden stop of PN infusion
Hyperosmolar hyperglycemic state	• Stop dextrose. • Rehydrate with the ordered infusate. • Maintain electrolyte balance.
Hypokalemia	• Increase potassium supplementation.
Hypomagnesemia	• Increase magnesium supplementation.
Hypophosphatemia	• Increase phosphate supplementation.
Hypocalcemia	• Increase calcium supplementation.
Metabolic acidosis	• Assess for contributing factors/diseases. • Adjust PN formula by replacing chloride with acetate. • Administer bicarbonate.
Metabolic alkalosis	• Assess for GI losses, diuretic, and steroid use. • Replace acetate for chloride solution.
Liver dysfunction	• Decrease carbohydrates and add I.V. lipids. • Consider cyclic infusions.
Hyperkalemia	• Decrease potassium supplementation.

Changing flow rate?

Suspect an occluded catheter lumen if the infusion flow rate becomes slower or pump occlusion alarms become more frequent. Lipids may accumulate on the intraluminal catheter wall leading to this type of lumen occlusion. This occlusion may be treated with instillation of 70% ethyl alcohol. The solution is prepared in the pharmacy. The amount equal to the internal volume of the CVAD is instilled into the lumen and allowed to reside there for up to 60 minutes. Avoid injecting the lumen contents into the bloodstream by aspirating the lumen contents and 3 to 5 mL of blood. Injection of ethyl alcohol may cause headache, dizziness, and nausea. Use this solution with extreme care in a CVAD made of polyurethane as damage may occur to the catheter from exposure to alcohol. Follow the catheter manufacturer instructions and your facility policies and procedures.

Metabolic complications

Metabolic complications include:
- hyperglycemia or hypoglycemia (high or low blood glucose level)
- hyperosmolar hyperglycemic state (HHS)
- hyperkalemia or hypokalemia (high or low blood potassium level)
- hypomagnesemia (low blood magnesium level)
- hypophosphatemia (low blood phosphate level)
- hypocalcemia (low blood calcium level)
- metabolic acidosis
- liver dysfunction.

Glucose: feast or famine

The patient may develop hyperglycemia if the formula's glucose concentration is excessive, the infusion rate is too rapid, or his glucose tolerance is compromised by diabetes, stress, or sepsis. Signs and symptoms of hyperglycemia include fatigue, restlessness, and weakness. The patient may become anxious, confused and, in some cases, delirious or even comatose. He'll be dehydrated and have polyuria and elevated blood and urine glucose levels.

Conversely, the patient may develop hypoglycemia if parenteral nutrition is interrupted suddenly or if he receives excessive insulin. Signs and symptoms may include sweating, shaking, confusion, and irritability.

S.O.S.! It's HHS!

An acute complication of hyperglycemic crisis, HHS is caused by hyperosmolar diuresis resulting from untreated hyperglycemia. A patient with HHS has a high serum osmolarity, is dehydrated, and has extremely high glucose levels. If untreated, he can develop glycosuria and electrolyte disturbances and even become comatose. Suspect HHS if your patient becomes confused or lethargic or experiences seizures.

Potassium: a plethora or pittance

Patients develop hyperkalemia because of too much potassium in the PN formula, renal disease, or hyponatremia. Look for skeletal muscle weakness, decreased heart rate, irregular pulse, and tall T waves on an electrocardiogram.

Patients develop hypokalemia because of too little potassium in the solution, excessive loss of potassium brought on by GI tract disturbances or diuretic use, or large doses of insulin. Look for muscle weakness, paralysis, paresthesia, and cardiac arrhythmias.

Magnesium mayhem

Hypomagnesemia results from insufficient magnesium in the solution. Suspect hypomagnesemia if your patient complains of tingling around the mouth or paresthesia in his fingers. He may also show signs of mental changes, hyperreflexia, tetany, and arrhythmias.

Phosphate funk

Hypophosphatemia results from insulin therapy, alcoholism, and the use of phosphate-binding antacids. Suspect hypophosphatemia if the patient shows irritability, weakness, and paresthesia. In extreme cases, coma and cardiac arrest can occur. Very rarely, a patient develops hyperphosphatemia. Patients with renal insufficiency are prone to hyperphosphatemia.

Calcium calamity

Hypocalcemia, a rare complication, results from too little calcium in the solution, vitamin D deficiency, or pancreatitis. The patient may develop numbing or tingling sensations, tetany, polyuria, dehydration, and arrhythmias.

Acid–base balance blues

Metabolic acidosis can occur if the patient develops an increased serum chloride level and a decreased serum bicarbonate level.

Last but not least, liver dysfunction

Increased serum alkaline phosphatase, lactate dehydrogenase, and bilirubin levels can indicate liver dysfunction.

The risk of rushing

If PN is infused too rapidly, the patient may feel nauseated, have a headache, and become lethargic. Heart failure is also a risk because of fluid overload.

Other complications

PN and lipid emulsion administration pose distinct risks.

Particular PPN problems

Significant complications of PPN therapy include phlebitis and extravasation.

Lipid low points

Prolonged administration of lipid emulsions can produce delayed complications, including an enlarged liver or spleen, blood dyscrasia (thrombocytopenia and leukopenia), and transient

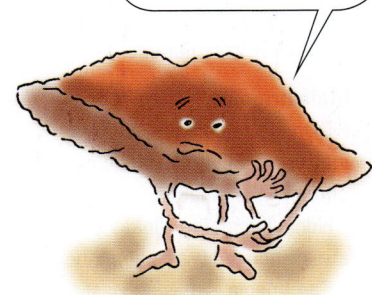

One of the delayed complications of prolonged administration of lipids is an enlarged liver or spleen. Oh, my!

increases in results of liver function studies. A small number of patients receiving 20% I.V. lipid emulsion develop brown pigmentation due to fat pigmentation.

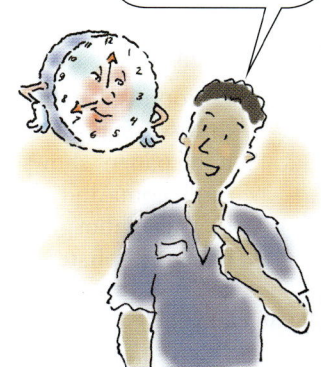

Patients should be weaned from PN therapy over 24 hours.

Discontinuing therapy

One major difference exists between the procedures for discontinuing PN and PPN therapy. A patient receiving PN should be weaned from therapy and should receive some other form of nutritional therapy such as enteral feedings.

When to wean and when not to wean

When the patient is receiving PPN, therapy can be discontinued without weaning because the dextrose concentration is lower than in PN. When discontinuing PN therapy, however, you should wean the patient over 24 hours to prevent rebound hypoglycemia.

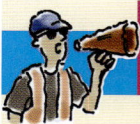 **That's a wrap!**

Parenteral nutrition review

Benefits
- Provides nutrition for patients who can't take nutrients through the GI tract because of illness or surgery
- Can be used when the patient is hemodynamically unstable or has impaired blood flow to the GI tract

Drawbacks
- Carries certain risks (catheter infection, hyperglycemia, hypokalemia)
- Requires vascular access

Malnutrition
- Disease-related malnutrition may be associated with acute and chronic inflammation.
- Noninflammatory illness and injury are associated with malnutrition.
- Sarcopenia is muscle wasting and is associated with aging.
- Overnutrition is found in overweight or obese patients.

Assessing nutritional status
Dietary history
- Check for decreased intake.
- Check for increased metabolic requirements.

Physical assessment
- Check for subtle signs of malnutrition.
- Obtain anthropometric measurements.

Diagnostic tests
- Major indicators of malnutrition are changes in the albumin, prealbumin, transferrin, and triglyceride levels.

PN vs. PPN
PN
- Dextrose 20% to 70%, amino acid, vitamins, trace elements diluted with water
- Administered through a central venous access device
- May be given in a 3-L bag with lipids daily, a 3-in-1 solution, or TNA
- Requires starting slow infusion with gradual increase

PPN
- Dextrose 5% to 10% with amino acids, vitamins, and trace elements
- Administered through a peripheral catheter
- Doesn't require starting with slow infusion rate

Potential complications
- Metabolic problems
- Catheter-related complications are the same as with other infusion therapy.

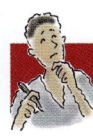

Quick quiz

1. What's the maximal amount of time that PN solutions are permitted to infuse before the bag must be replaced?
    A. 24 hours
    B. 48 hours
    C. 12 hours
    D. 72 hours

Answer: A. Don't allow PN solutions to hang for more than 24 hours.

2. Lipid residue on the intraluminal catheter walls is treated with:
    A. instilling a thrombolytic agent.
    B. removal of the catheter.
    C. stopping the infusion to reposition the CVAD.
    D. instilling ethyl alcohol.

Answer: D. Ethyl alcohol will dissolve the lipid residue on the internal CVAD wall.

3. A commonly used anthropometric measurement that helps determine nutritional status is:
    A. biceps skinfold.
    B. lean body mass.
    C. weight and height.
    D. head circumference.

Answer: C. Weight and height are anthropometric measurements that help to determine nutritional status.

4. Most of the calories in PN are contributed by which element?
    A. Fats
    B. Dextrose
    C. Amino acids
    D. Electrolytes

Answer: B. Most calories in PN solutions come from dextrose.

5. What type of solution is PN?
    A. Isotonic
    B. Hypotonic
    C. Hypertonic
    D. Emulsion

Answer: C. Solutions for PN are hypertonic with an osmolarity of 1,800 to 2,600 mOsm/L.

6. A common laboratory test that indicates protein status is:
   A. hemoglobin.
   B. albumin.
   C. total protein.
   D. triglycerides.

   Answer: B. Albumin, with a half-life of 21 days, is a good marker of nutritional status over time.

Scoring

★★★ If you answered all seven questions correctly, feel fulfilled! You've metabolized the chapter components and converted them to cerebral energy.

★★ If you answered five or six questions correctly, sit back and digest! Your mind has been well nourished.

★ If you answered fewer than five questions correctly, have a snack and review this book! There's nothing wrong with enhancing your diet of knowledge with a fact-filled supplement.

Suggested References

Ayers, P., Adams, S., Boullata, J., Gervasio, J., Holcombe, B., Kraft, M. D., …, Guenter, P. (2014). A.S.P.E.N. parenteral nutrition safety consensus recommendations: Translation into practice. *Nutrition in Clinical Practice, 29*(3), 277–282.

Cederholm, T., Barazzoni, R., Austin, P., Ballmer, P., Biolo, G., Bischoff, S. C., …, Singer, P. (2017). ESPEN guidelines on definitions and terminology of clinical nutrition. *Clinical Nutrition, 36*(1), 49–64. doi:http://dx.doi.org.ezproxyhost.library.tmc.edu/10.1016/j.clnu.2016.09.004

Corkins, M. R., Guenter, P., DiMaria-Ghalili, R. A., Jensen, G. L., Malone, A., Miller, S.,…, Resnick, H. E.; American Society for Parenteral and Enteral Nutrition. (2013). Malnutrition diagnoses in hospitalized patients United States, 2010. *Journal of Parenteral and Enteral Nutrition, 38*(2), 186–195.

Gorski, L., Hadaway, L., Hagle, M., McGoldrick, M., Orr, M, & Doellman, D. (2016). Infusion therapy standards of practice. *Journal of Infusion Nursing, 39*(1S), 159.

Gura, K. M. (2009). Is there still a role for peripheral parenteral nutrition? *Nutrition in Clinical Practice, 24*(6), 709–717.

O'Grady, N., Alexander, M., Burns, L., & Dellinger, E. (2011). Guideline for the prevention of intravascular catheter-related infections. Retrieved from http://www.cdc.gov/hicpac/BSI/BSI-guidelines-2011.html, on April 4, 2016.

Phillips, L., & Gorski, L. (2014). *Manual of I.V. therapeutics* (6th ed.). Philadelphia, PA: FA Davis.

Weinstein, S. M., & Hagle, M. (2014). *Plumer's principles and practice of infusion therapy* (9th ed.). Philadelphia, PA: Wolters Kluwer Health.

Chapter 9

Infusion therapy in pediatrics

Just the facts

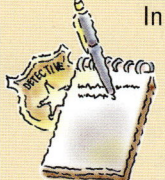

In this chapter, you'll learn:
- ◆ common uses of infusion therapy in pediatric patients
- ◆ how to calculate children's fluid needs
- ◆ how to select an appropriate I.V. site in infants and older children
- ◆ appropriate I.V. insertion techniques to use with pediatric patients
- ◆ monitoring techniques and complications to watch for
- ◆ alternative fluid delivery systems used with children.

Delivering infusion therapy to children

One of your most challenging experiences related to infusion therapy will occur when caring for an infant or child. It may also be a memorable event for the child because your skills and knowledge can have a lasting effect on his future hospitalizations and experiences with infusion therapy especially with venipuncture. In relating to children, it is helpful to understand developmental stages and nursing implications related to I.V. therapy at each stage.

(Text continues on page 359)

Growth and developmental stages of children

Age group	Developmental stage and characteristics	Nursing implications
Premature infant (born before 37 completed weeks of gestation) **Neonate** (birth to 1 month)	Basic trust vs. mistrust • Develops trust as basic needs are met. Separation anxiety and fear of strangers with infant >6 months	• Keep infants, especially premature infants, warm. • Use a pacifier for comfort. • Avoid feeding immediately before procedure (risk of vomiting and aspiration).

(continued)

357

Growth and developmental stages of children *(continued)*

Age group	Developmental stage and characteristics	Nursing implications
Infant (1 month to 1 year)	• Communicates by crying	• May wrap in blanket to restrain or use assistants other than family to restrain infant. • Encourage parental tactile contact and soothing verbal stimuli immediately after procedure and throughout duration of therapy. • Protect site from infant's reach.
Toddler (1–3 years)	Autonomy vs. shame • Has little understanding of cause and effect • Communicates by crying, pointing, basic words • May calm with security items • May regress in developmental milestones	• Prepare immediately before procedure. • Use simple and honest explanations. • Tell child of impending I.V. insertion immediately before procedure. • Use positioning for comfort techniques. • Transitional objects provide comfort (blanket, toy). • Likes rewards, that is, stickers. • *Note:* Secure stabilization of I.V. site is essential for this age group.
Preschool (4–6 years)	Initiative vs. guilt • Follows directions but has short attention span. • Needs support with invasive procedures and may perceive pain as punishment • Involve in decisions when possible	• Prepare just before procedure. • Use equipment for medical play (with dolls and stuffed animals). • Use short simple words (that is, "small straw") for catheter. • Positioning for comfort. • Explain that holding still is a big help and that it is OK to cry. • Curious about I.V. but able to keep from touching with frequent reminders or protective covering that allows visualization. • Never bribe or threaten ("If you don't drink, you'll get an I.V.") • Praise cooperation.
School age (6–12 years)	Sense of industry • Understands directions and likes to see cause and effect • Magical thinking exists • May try to delay procedure, likes sense of control, participation • Able to conceptualize the element of time	• Prepare several hours ahead of time. • Provide privacy and distraction during procedure. • Electronic tablets work well to distract. • Allow child to help and give tasks, such as ripping tape, holding still, and slow breathing. Explain each step. • Offer choices as much as possible. • Reassure that crying is OK.

Growth and developmental stages of children (continued)

Age group	Developmental stage and characteristics	Nursing implications
Adolescence (13–19 years)	Sense of identity • Vacillates between dependence and independence • Questions authority figures • Exaggerated response to pain; minor illness magnified • Fears altered body image	• Preparation several hours to days in advance is vital. • Show equipment, and explain function and allow time for questions. • Offer choices such as site location, if peers or family can be present. • Explain therapy as to an adult patient. • Provide privacy. • Teach adolescent to report observations about I.V.

Reprinted from Infusion Nurses Society. (2010). *Infusion nursing: An evidence-based approach* (3rd ed.). St. Louis, MO: Saunders/Elsevier, with permission.

Why infusion therapy is needed

The most common reasons for providing infusion therapy to a child include:
- replacement of body fluids and prevention or correction of electrolyte imbalances
- blood and blood product administration
- nutrition maintenance
- medication administration.

Maintaining fluid and electrolyte balance

Read the signs

Clinical symptoms of dehydration (such as decreased skin turgor, sunken eyes or fontanels, and dry mucous membranes) and symptoms of electrolyte imbalance (such as arrhythmias, altered respiratory effort, and muscle spasms) can give an estimation of the severity of the child's condition. To maintain fluid and electrolyte balance, remember that you'll need to adjust the maintenance fluid volume based on the child's condition, treatments, and ongoing losses (such as from vomiting, diarrhea, and insensible losses through respiration and sweating). Dehydration is described as mild, moderate, or severe based on history and physical examination.

Clinical signs and dehydration severity

Use the information below to help correlate the child's dehydration severity with his clinical status. This chart can also be used alone to help determine the severity of dehydration.

Sign	Severity		
	Mild (3%–5%)	**Moderate (6%–9%)**	**Severe (>10%)**
Physical appearance	Alert, restless, thirsty	Lethargic, postural dizziness	Limp, cold, unconscious, cyanotic extremities
Heart rate	Normal for age	Weak, rapid	Feeble
Blood pressure	Normal for age	Normal; possibly orthostatic hypotension	Hypotension
Pulse	Normal for age	Thready	Faint impalpable
Respirations	Normal for age	Slightly increased; deep	Deep rapid
Skin	Normal turgor; pinch retracts immediately	Decreased turgor; pinch retracts slowly	Tenting; pinch retracts very slowly (>2 seconds)
Extremities	Normal temperature and color; possible muscle fatigue and weakness	Cool temperature; normal color or mottling; extreme fatigue and muscle cramping	Cool to cold temperature; mottling or gray color; muscle spasms
Capillary refill	Normal (<2 seconds)	Slow (2–4 seconds)	>4 seconds
Mucous membranes	Slightly dry	Very dry	Parched or cracked
Eyes and tears	Normal eyes; presence of tears	Sunken eyes; decreased tears	Sunken eyes; absence of tears
Anterior fontanelle	Normal	Slightly depressed	Sunken
Urine	Slightly decreased output; dark yellow color	Moderately decreased output; very dark yellow color	Oliguria or anuria

Dehydration double check

Make sure you correlate your findings with the child's clinical symptoms. If you can't accurately determine the child's weights, estimate his dehydration severity by clinical signs alone. (See *Clinical signs and dehydration severity*, page 360.)

Calculating fluid needs

Calculating the fluid maintenance and replacement needs for a child is complex and requires the LIP to perform a thorough assessment and consider many factors when ordering the type and amount of fluid to be infused. As the nurse administering the fluids, you're responsible for double-checking the order for accuracy and ensuring that it meets the child's needs but doesn't put him at risk for fluid overload.

Daily fluid fill-up

After you've determined the percentage of fluid the child has lost, and before you calculate the amount of fluid replacement required, you first need to determine the child's daily maintenance fluid requirements. Check your facility's protocol because many facilities use charts listing the amount of maintenance fluid therapy required based on the child's weight. (To figure this amount yourself, see *Calculating maintenance and replacement fluid requirements*, page 361.) Once you've determined the maintenance fluid therapy the child requires, you can calculate the amount of replacement fluid needed.

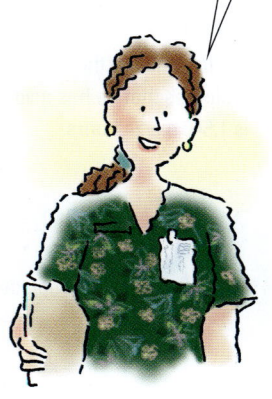

Double-checking the order for accuracy and determining whether it meets the child's fluid needs... Now that's one tall order!

Calculating maintenance and replacement fluid requirements

To calculate a pediatric patient's maintenance fluid requirements, use the appropriate formula based on the child's current status from the chart below.

Child's status	Formula
Neonate (0–72 hours)	60–100 mL/kg/24 hours
0–10 kg	100 mL/kg/24 hours
11–20 kg	1,000 mL for first 10 kg + 50 mL/kg/24 hours for each kilogram over 10 kg
21–30 kg	1,500 mL for first 20 kg + 25 mL/kg/24 hours for each kilogram over 20 kg

Example

A child is admitted to your facility after several days of vomiting and diarrhea. He has no signs of dehydration, is afebrile and, according to his mother, hasn't lost any weight. The vomiting and diarrhea have resolved, but his LIP has ordered that he receive maintenance I.V. fluids. His current weight is 22 kg.

The formula to calculate the 24-hour maintenance fluid requirements for this child is:

(1,500 mL for each of the first 20 kg) + (25 mL for each kg over 20)
1,500 mL + (2 × 25)
(1,500 mL) + (50 mL) =
1,550 mL/24 hours

Once you've determined the amount of replacement fluid needed and you know the child's severity of dehydration, you can calculate his replacement fluid requirements using the chart below.

(continued)

> **Calculating maintenance and replacement fluid requirements** *(continued)*
>
> | Fluid deficit (dehydration severity) | Formula for calculating amount of replacement fluid/24 hours |
> |---|---|
> | Mild | Maintenance + (maintenance × 0.5)/24 hours |
> | Moderate | Maintenance + (maintenance × 1.0)/24 hours |
> | Severe | Maintenance + (maintenance × 1.5)/24 hours |
>
> To continue the example from above, the child's clinical assessment indicates that he has mild dehydration. Therefore, his maintenance fluid need is 1,540 mL/24 hours.
>
> 1,540 mL + (1,540 mL × 0.5)/24 hours
> 1,540 mL + 770 mL/24 hours
> 2,310 mL/24 hours
>
> The child's total replacement fluid requirement is 2,310 mL/24 hours.

Replacement therapy

Generally, replacement therapy will be based on the child's stage of dehydration, which is measured as mild, moderate, or severe. The most accurate way to determine this is by obtaining the child's current and immediate preillness weights in kilograms, if known. (See *Formula for calculating percentage of fluid loss*, page 361.)

Tally those losses, too

When calculating replacement fluid needs, it's important to consider ongoing losses, such as those occurring from vomiting, diarrhea, diaphoresis, hyperthermia, and fluids collected from nasogastric tubes and drains. Ongoing fluid losses should be measured, if possible, and replaced with physiologic equivalents of the fluids.

A stickler for scheduling

Replacement fluids are given based on the child's condition. The LIP may order you to administer one or more bolus fluid infusions, followed by the remainder at a specified drip rate, or he may order all of the fluids to be administered over a specified time period.

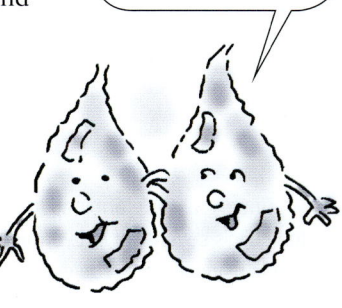

Don't forget to account for us ongoing losses when calculating a child's replacement fluid needs.

Formula for calculating percentage of fluid loss

To determine the child's percentage of fluid loss, or dehydration, first calculate his weight change, which will provide his fluid deficit in kilograms:

$$\text{Deficit} = \text{preillness weight (kg)} - \text{current weight (kg)}$$

Then, use the fluid deficit to determine the percent of dehydration:

$$\text{Dehydration percent} = (\text{deficit} \div \text{preillness weight [kg]}) \times 100$$

The percent of dehydration will then tell you if a child has mild, moderate, or severe dehydration:
- Mild dehydration—3%–5%
- Moderate dehydration—6%–9%
- Severe dehydration—>10%

Example
A child is admitted to your facility with signs of dehydration. His current weight is 30 lb (13.6 kg) and his mother tells you that his weight before he became ill (obtained 1 week earlier at the doctor's office) was 32 lb (14.5 kg).

First, determine the amount of the child's fluid deficit:
Deficit = 14.5 kg − 13.6 kg
Deficit = 0.9 kg

Then, determine the percentage of dehydration:
Dehydration percentage = (0.9 kg ÷ 14.5 kg) × 100
Dehydration percentage = (0.06) × 100
Dehydration percentage = 6

This child's dehydration percentage, 6%, places him within the range of moderate dehydration. *Remember:* Always correlate this finding with the child's clinical status.

Following a typical replacement schedule, you'll administer one-half of the deficit plus the maintenance amount over the first 8 hours of therapy and the remaining one-half of the deficit plus the maintenance amount over the next 16 hours. The child should be monitored at least every 2 hours for ongoing losses and fluid excess, which will necessitate adjustment of the replacement amounts.

Preventing or correcting electrolyte imbalances

Children can quickly become dehydrated and develop electrolyte imbalances — for example, when they have vomiting, diarrhea, fever, or other disorders that affect body fluid or electrolyte levels. (See *Common fluid and electrolyte imbalances in pediatric patients*, page 364.)

Common fluid and electrolyte imbalances in pediatric patients

Imbalance	Causes	Signs and symptoms	Treatment
Hypovolemia (fluid volume deficit)	Dehydration, vomiting, diarrhea, decreased oral intake, and excessive fluid loss	Thirst, oliguria or anuria, dry mucous membranes, weight loss, sunken eyes, decreased tears, depressed fontanelles (in infants), tachycardia, and altered level of consciousness	Oral rehydration (in mild to moderate dehydration), I.V. fluid administration (in severe dehydration), or electrolyte replacement
Hypernatremia (serum sodium > 145 mEq/L [>145 mmol/L])	Water loss in excess of sodium loss, diabetes insipidus (insufficient antidiuretic hormone [ADH] production or reduced response to ADH), insufficient water intake, diarrhea, vomiting, fever, renal disease, and hyperglycemia	Decreased skin turgor; tachycardia; flushed skin; intense thirst; dry, sticky mucous membranes; hoarseness; nausea; vomiting; decreased blood pressure; confusion; and seizures	Gradual replacement of water (in excess of sodium) or ADH replacement or vasopressin administration (for patients with diabetes insipidus); frequent neurologic assessments
Hyponatremia (serum sodium < 130–135 mEq/L [<130–135 mmol/L])	Syndrome of inappropriate antidiuretic hormone (SIADH), edema (from cardiac failure), hypotonic fluid replacement (for diarrhea), DKA, burns, cystic fibrosis, malnutrition, fever, and excess sweating	Dehydration, dizziness, nausea, abdominal cramps, and apprehension, disorientation, seizures, coma, increased ICP	Sodium replacement, water restriction, diuretic administration, or fluid replacement (with ongoing fluid loss, such as with diarrhea); frequent neurologic assessment
Hyperkalemia (serum potassium >5 mEq/L [>5 mmol/L])	Acute acidosis, hemolysis or rhabdomyolysis, renal failure, excessive administration of I.V. potassium supplement, and Addison's disease	Arrhythmias, weakness, paresthesia, electrocardiogram (ECG) changes (tall, tented T waves; ST segment depression; prolonged PR interval and QRS complex; and absent P waves), nausea, vomiting, hoarseness, flushed skin, intense thirst, and dry, sticky mucous membranes	Dialysis (for renal failure), sodium polystyrene (Kayexalate) (to remove potassium via the GI tract), I.V. calcium gluconate (antagonizes cardiac abnormalities), I.V. insulin or hypertonic dextrose solution (shifts potassium into the cells), bicarbonate (for acidosis), or restricted potassium intake
Hypokalemia (serum potassium < 2.5–3 mEq/L [<2.5–3 mmol/L])	Vomiting, diarrhea, nasogastric suctioning, diuretic use, acute alkalosis, kidney disease, starvation, and malabsorption	Fatigue, muscle weakness, muscle cramping, paralysis, hyporeflexia, hypotension, tachycardia or bradycardia, apathy, drowsiness, irritability, decreased bowel motility, and ECG changes (flattened or inverted T waves, presence of U waves, and ST segment depression)	Oral or I.V. potassium administration (I.V. infusions must be diluted and given slowly)

Other electrolyte disorders not included in the table above include imbalances of calcium, magnesium, and phosphorous.

Dehydration demands diligence

When you assess the child receiving infusion therapy for dehydration, be sure to compare your results with the child's baseline findings. Monitor the child's pulse rate and volume, blood pressure, temperature, capillary refill, urine output, and laboratory test results. Also assess the child's peripheral pulses, skin color, and the temperature of his extremities.

Timely weights and measures

All children receiving infusion therapy should be weighed before the fluid administration is started and once per shift throughout the course of treatment. Blood tests should include serum electrolytes and glucose levels, depending on the type of fluid being infused.

Count on calculating

When you're monitoring a child receiving I.V. therapy, calculate the amount of fluid that has been infused to ensure that the child is receiving the ordered amount. Also verify that the flow rate corresponds with the most recent LIP orders.

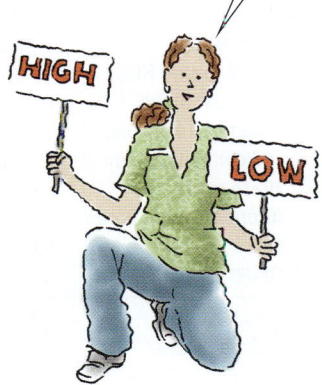

Pay attention to signs of dehydration and electrolyte imbalances, and adjust the fluid volume accordingly.

Administering blood or blood products

Expect to administer blood or blood products to a child who has:
- bone marrow failure due to disease process or therapy
- severe anemia
- a sudden loss of blood
- a low hemoglobin level before, during, or after surgery.

A whole lot o' blood...and O_2

Whole blood transfusion replenishes both the volume and the oxygen-carrying capacity of the circulatory system by increasing the mass of circulating red cells. Transfusion of packed red blood cells, from which 80% of the plasma has been removed, restores only the oxygen-carrying capacity. Both types of transfusion treat decreased hemoglobin levels and hematocrit.

Portioned-out products

Other blood transfusion products that you may give to a neonate or child include albumin, fresh frozen plasma, platelets, and factor VIII concentrate. (See *Blood administration guidelines*, page 366.) as well as other clotting factors, depending on the specific deficiency, granulocytes, and cryoprecipitate.

Blood administration guidelines

This chart lists some of the common blood products you may give to a child.

Component	Indications	Rate	Administration guidelines
Whole blood *5–10 mL/kg* Single-donor anticoagulated blood	• Massive blood loss • Exchange transfusion • Special procedures (extracorporeal membrane oxygenation [ECMO] to prime the circuit, apheresis)	• As rapidly as necessary to re-establish blood volume • 45–60 minutes (longer if hemodynamically unstable)	• Always administer ABO group and Rh type specific.
Packed red blood cells (RBCs) Concentrated RBCs with most of the plasma, leukocytes, and platelets removed *10–15 mL/kg* **Acute massive blood loss** *10–20 mL/kg*	• Severe anemia • Surgical blood loss • Suppression of erythropoiesis (such as thalassemia or sickle cell anemia) • ECMO — blood loss from bleeding or multiple sampling for laboratory analysis	• 5 mL/kg/hour	• Administer ABO group and Rh type specific if possible. If not, compatible group and type can be transfused safely. • O-negative uncrossmatched blood may be used for infants up to age 4 months.
Albumin Plasma protein available in 5% and 25% solutions	• 5% solution: hypoproteinemia, volume deficits • 25% solution: severe burns, cerebral edema	• 5%: 1–2 mL/minute (60–120 mL/hour); can be administered as fast as possible to correct shock • 5%: Do not exceed 2–4 mL/minute in patients with normal plasma volume; 5–10 mL/minute in patients with hypoproteinemia • 25%: 0.2–0.4 mL/minute (12–24 mL/hour). Do not exceed 1 mL/minute in patients with normal plasma volume; 2–3 mL/minute in patients with hypoproteinemia	• Some products may require a filter; refer to product labeling. • Infusion rate depends on indication and clinical situation. In emergencies, may administer as rapidly as necessary to improve clinical condition after initial volume replacement. • 25% albumin rapidly mobilizes large volumes of fluid into circulation. Watch for pulmonary edema or other symptoms of fluid overload. • Product is stored at room temperature and has a very long shelf life.
Fresh frozen plasma Contains all the clotting factors and some fibrinogen *10–15 mL/kg*	• Massive hemorrhage • Hypovolemic shock • Multiple clotting deficiencies	• Hemorrhage: as indicated by patient's condition • Clotting deficiency: over 2–3 hours	• Donor's plasma should be ABO compatible with recipient's RBCs. • Rh compatibility isn't required because product doesn't contain RBCs. • Administer within 6 hours of thawing to preserve clotting factor activity.

Blood administration guidelines *(continued)*

Component	Indications	Rate	Administration guidelines
Platelets Platelets suspended in a small amount of plasma ***Random donor*** 1–8 units per transfusion ***Single-donor unit from pheresis*** May be split for neonates and infants	• Severe thrombocytopenia (platelet count <20,000/mm³) • Platelet count <50,000–100,000/mm³ in a child who requires surgery or in a child with hemorrhage or imminent bleeding • Cardiac surgery with massive blood replacement • Platelet count <80,000–100,000 in a child undergoing ECMO	• May be given by I.V. push (5–10 minutes/unit); if volume overload is a concern, transfuse the total dose over 2–3 hours using an electronic infusion pump	• Rh compatibility is required; ABO plasma compatibility is preferred. • Platelets may be irradiated to inactivate donor lymphocytes that cause graft-versus-host disease in immunocompromised patients • If single-donor or HLA platelets are ordered, obtain 1-hour and 24-hour platelet counts after the transfusion to determine adequate platelet response. • Gently agitate every hour because platelets tend to clump.
Factor VIII concentrate Sterile lyophilized powder containing blood coagulation factor VIII, which is prepared from pooled human plasma *10–50 units/kg*	• Hemophilia A	• I.V. push over about 5 minutes (2 mL/minute maximum) • If patient complains of headache: slow the rate because product is high in protein	• Dose is ordered in units. • No compatibility testing is required. • Administer within 1 hour of reconstitution.

Maintaining nutrition

When a child is unable to obtain adequate nutritional requirements orally or through a gastrostomy tube, you'll need to administer parenteral nutrition. The goal of parenteral nutrition (PN) is to meet anabolic needs and allow normal growth and development. Conditions that may require PN include prematurity, and congenital or acquired anomalies of the digestive tract.

A formula for success

Nutritional formulas containing water, glucose, amino acids, lipids, electrolytes, vitamins, and minerals are delivered by an electronic infusion pump and filtered during infusion.

Main components of parenteral nutrition (PN) intravenous solutions

Component	Composition	Purpose
Protein	Crystalline amino acids; infants younger than 6 months require a special amino acid mixture that mimics breast milk components	For growth
Carbohydrates	Dextrose (PN solutions with dextrose concentration >10% or other additives resulting in an osmolarity of >900 mOsm/L should be administered via a central venous access device.)	Provides energy so the body does not break down protein or fat to meet calorie needs
Fat	Fat emulsions or lipids (filtered with a 1.2-micron filter, hang no longer than 12 hours)	Provide a high-calorie content per volume, making them ideal sources of calories for children; vein buffer

In addition to the above: Electrolytes, vitamins, trace elements minerals, and other additives may be needed. (See *Chapter 8, Parenteral nutrition*, page 326.)

For children receiving long-term PN, continued growth can change the nutritional requirements, so careful monitoring is essential. Continuous monitoring is required to ensure safe infusion of PN that meets the changing needs and growth of the child. This includes monitoring the infusion itself and assessing laboratory and nutritional measurements on a scheduled basis. A multidisciplinary team approach can result in the successful clinical application and monitoring of PN, with a minimal number of complications.

Administering medications

An I.V. medication may be prescribed for a child when:
- the child can't take medications orally
- the oral route changes the drug or interferes with its ability to be absorbed by the GI tract
- the drug isn't available in another form or is too irritating for I.M. administration
- rapid therapeutic action is needed, such as during an emergency.

Quick and highly efficient

Compared with other routes of administration, the I.V. route is the fastest, most efficient way to deliver medications throughout the body. The most commonly used calculations for medication administration in neonatal and pediatric patients are those based on body weight and body surface area (calculated by nomogram). Dosing of pediatric medications is usually ordered as milligrams (mg) per kilogram or, in the case of antineoplastic agents, mg per meter squared.

I.V. medications may be administered by three different methods:

1. I.V. push is the slow injection of a concentrated dose of medication; usually for a small volume of medication contained in a syringe that is manually injected into the venous access device (VAD).
2. I.V. secondary piggyback or intermittent dose is a medication diluted in a small quantity of fluid (for example, 10 to 100 mL, depending upon child's age) and infused over a short period (for example, 30 minutes) at specific intervals (for example, every 8 or 12 hours); syringe pumps are commonly used for this method of delivery in children.
3. I.V. continuous infusion with the medication mixed in a larger fluid volume and given by a constant infusion; flow rate is controlled by an electronic infusion pump.

Antibiotics are the most common medications given by intermittent infusion, while most antineoplastic drugs will be given by I.V. push or as a continuous infusion. Vasoactive drugs, such as those given to neonates and children in intensive care settings, are often given by continuous infusion and titrated according to the response of the patient.

Venous access to administer infusion therapy

A child requires special care during I.V. catheter insertion and throughout therapy. Although your venipuncture technique will be basically the same for most pediatric patients, your approach, restraint method, and manner of securing the I.V. catheter will depend on the child's age and medical condition. You'll need to monitor the child closely during therapy to determine whether the fluid is infusing correctly to prevent fluid overload, infiltration, and other complications.

Selecting a peripheral I.V. catheter site

Perhaps your greatest challenge in providing I.V. therapy to a child will be choosing an appropriate vein. The veins of infants and toddlers are usually difficult to visualize or palpate, especially when the child is dehydrated or hypovolemic from another medical condition. In addition, toddlers and prepubescent children have more subcutaneous tissue covering their veins than adults, which makes finding a suitable vein more difficult. Vascular visualization technology can greatly enhance vein location, particularly in patients with difficult venous access. (See *Chapter 2, Vascular visualization technologies*, page 82.)

Chill! It's simply a child challenge...

In children, I.V. therapy is typically prescribed to administer medications or to correct a fluid deficit, improve serum electrolyte balance, or provide nourishment. Your first concern related to pediatric I.V. therapy includes correlating the I.V. site and equipment with the reason for therapy and the patient's age, size, and activity level. For example, a scalp vein is a typical I.V. site for an infant, whereas a peripheral hand, wrist, or foot vein may suit older children.

...or is it?

When you know a child's vein anatomy, it will make palpating for veins and documenting the location of an I.V. site easier.

Only the best will do

When you're choosing the best I.V. site for a child, first consider his age, activity level, and the reason for the I.V. therapy. An ideal vein for a 10-year-old child may not be the best choice for an 8-month-old child. Other factors to consider include how difficult the venipuncture will be for you and the patient and which site carries the lowest risk of device-related local and bloodstream infection. You should always avoid previously used or sclerotic veins. For children who have had chronic I.V. therapy or frequent hospitalizations, veins may be difficult to locate. Vein location is greatly improved by using a visible light or near-infrared light or ultrasound device. Blindly making venipunctures when veins cannot be seen or palpated is no longer an acceptable practice.

Neonates and infants

Until a child is about 12 months old, the scalp veins are readily accessible for a short peripheral catheter because they have no valves and are easy to stabilize for catheter insertion. However, they're best reserved for neonates and infants younger than 6 months old because the child's hands can easily dislodge them. To locate an appropriate scalp vein, carefully palpate the site for arterial pulsations. If you feel these pulsations, select another site. (See *Identifying scalp veins*, page 371.) However, in hypotensive or premature infants, the pulse may be more difficult to detect.

Other veins can be gold mines, too

The large saphenous vein in front of the malleolus on the inner aspect of the foot and the small saphenous vein on the outer lateral aspect of the foot are also good I.V. sites for infants and young children under walking age. Dorsal veins of the foot, even though they can be seen easily, tend to have a high rate of skin sloughing should an infiltration occur.

Children over age 1

Palpate for a suitable vein in the hands, forearms, or upper arms when selecting an I.V. site in a child or adolescent, and always try to select the most distal site available. Start with the child's nondominant side to avoid interference with self-care or other activities, and move to the dominant side if necessary. Also keep in mind whether the child is young and sucks his thumb; if so, make sure to use the opposite side. For sites in the hand or wrist, plan to use a handboard for joint stabilization as complications are more frequent in areas of joint flexion.

Antiantecubital

Although antecubital veins are appropriate for children of all ages and are usually easy to view and palpate, you should try to avoid their use for peripheral I.V. therapy. Antecubital sites can be uncomfortable for the child, and they must be securely supported at all times.

For the mobile guitar hero

For a mobile patient, select an I.V. site on the upper extremity so that he can still get out of bed. Also avoid starting the I.V. in the same arm as the patient's identification band. Remove the band and replace it on the other arm, to prevent potential circulatory impairment.

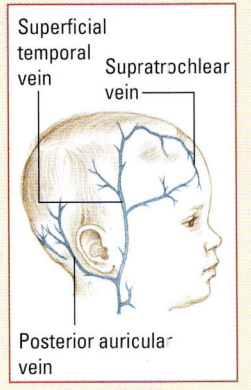

Identifying scalp veins

This illustration shows the scalp veins most commonly used for venipuncture in infants.

- Superficial temporal vein
- Supratrochlear vein
- Posterior auricular vein

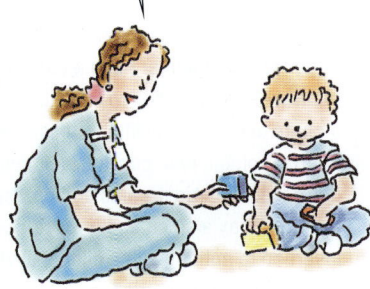

Always consider the child's age and activity level when choosing an I.V. site, especially if he's young and still sucks his thumb.

Preparing for insertion

The preferred venous access device for infants and young children, no matter which vein you are using, is a small 24- or 22-gauge safety catheter with or without wings. This device is less likely to cause traumatic injury to the vein.

Tailored to size and need

Choose the needle and catheter that you'll use to obtain I.V. access based on the size of the child's veins and the type of fluid he'll be receiving. Use the smallest gauge catheter in the shortest length possible to allow blood to flow around the catheter while I.V. fluids are infusing. Blood products can also be administered through a small gauge catheter, even 24 gauge catheters.

Forewarned and forearmed

Explain to the child's parents what you'll be doing when inserting the I.V. catheter and why it's necessary. Forewarn them if you'll be using a scalp vein, and tell them that you may have to clip the hair from a small section of the infant's head. Give an age-appropriate explanation to the child when the time is right.

Restrain for safety's sake

At times, you may have to restrain the child to ensure that you obtain I.V. access and for the child's safety. If possible, enlist the aid of a coworker, or show the parents how to use positioning for comfort techniques to assist with restraint. Encourage them to talk to the child and comfort him by holding his hand or stroking his arm instead of involving them directly in what may be a frightening experience. Provide the child with a favorite toy or blanket for comfort;

Best practice

Easing the pain of venipuncture

For most children, receiving a needlestick — especially during venipuncture — can be a traumatic experience. In neonates, painful procedures have been shown to cause increase in need for oxygen and vital sign changes. You can lessen your neonatal and pediatric patient's anxiety, increase comfort, reduce pain, and improve compliance during the procedure by employing nonpharmacologic as well as pharmacologic pain control measures prior to venipuncture.

In neonates and infants, small amounts of oral glucose dripped either into the cheek or on a pacifier have a calming effect. In older infants and children, multiple measures can be used to decrease the trauma of I.V. insertion. These measures include use of a child life professional for distraction and medical play and usage of pharmacologic pain control, including application of a local anesthetic such as transdermal anesthetic creams and pressure-accelerated lidocaine before the venipuncture. You may also consider placing warm packs on the site for 10 minutes prior to insertion to enhance vein dilation. When using an anesthetic agent, be sure to assess for allergies, age restrictions according to the manufacturer, and other contraindications for the agent you are administering.

utilize child life therapist for preparation prior to and distraction during the procedure.

If the child is an infant, wrap him in a blanket with the site exposed. Utilize positioning for comfort measures for older infants, toddlers, preschool, and school-age children when appropriate. If he's a toddler or school-age child, seat him across from you or in your assistant's lap. You can also have him lie down on the bed or a treatment table. Ask your assistant to hold the extremity chosen for the I.V. in one hand while restraining the other extremities. The assistant's hand can be also be used as a tourniquet while restraining the child.

Provide an age-appropriate explanation about the venipuncture when the time is right. Oops…I think I might have jumped the gun a bit with this one.

Inserting the catheter

If you need to use a tourniquet to dilate a vein, make sure it's appropriately sized for that particular child, and tie the tourniquet over a sleeve or gauze to avoid pinching the extremity with the tourniquet.

Check for the child's pulse to make sure that you haven't overtightened the tourniquet. When accessing a scalp vein, use a special latex-free rubber band with a tape tab and place it above the child's eyes and ears.

Having a flashback to childhood

Insert the I.V. needle and catheter into the vein, and watch for blood to flow backward through the catheter or attached extension set, which confirms that the needle is in the vein. In children, blood return in the flashback chamber may be minimal. Several peripheral I.V. catheters are designed so you can see blood return inside the plastic catheter before it reaches the flashback chamber. When you see a blood return, advance the needle about ⅛" (0.3 cm) and slowly thread the catheter into the vein. If you feel resistance, allow the child to relax for a few seconds and try again. Loosen the tourniquet, and attach a small preflushed microbore luer-locking tubing with a needleless connector to the hub of the catheter. You can either flush the I.V. with saline to maintain patency or begin the infusion.

Securing the site

Stabilizing the I.V. site can be a little tricky with pediatric patients. Always begin by applying an engineered stabilization device and then taping the site as you would for an adult so the skin over the access site is easily visible.

Finger-proof and protect

In addition to securing the I.V. catheter with a catheter stabilization device and tape, you must take care to make sure the I.V. insertion site is inaccessible to the child's prying fingers and that the administration set is safely secured. Several types of protective devices to place over the I.V. site are available commercially, including plastic covers, fabric wraps, and elastic netting. (See *Protecting an I.V. site*, page 374.)

To safeguard the catheter, loop the administration set and tape it so that if it's pulled, the strain will be exerted on the taped set and not the catheter. If possible, thread the administration set through the child's shirt to exit out the back, where it can't be reached, and to help prevent an accidental strangulation with the tubing.

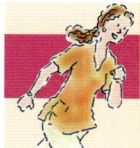

Running smoothly

Protecting an I.V. site

Protecting a child's I.V. site can be a challenge. An active child can easily dislodge an I.V. catheter, which will necessitate you reinserting it — thus causing him further discomfort. A child may also injure himself by dislodging the I.V. catheter.

To prevent a child from dislodging an I.V. catheter, first secure the catheter carefully. Stabilize the catheter and dress the I.V. site as you would for an adult, so that the insertion site and surrounding area are easily visible. However, avoid over taping the site because doing so makes it harder to inspect the site and the surrounding tissue. Protect the skin from injury from the I.V. device by putting a small gauze pad under the hub of the I.V. catheter and connector tubing. Also use skin barrier solution to prevent medical adhesive-related skin injury (MARSI).

If the child is old enough to understand, warn him not to play with or jostle the equipment, and teach him how to walk with an I.V. pole to minimize tension on the line. If necessary, you can restrain the extremity.

You should also create a protective barrier between the I.V. site and the environment using one of the following methods. Site protection is useful to prevent accidental dislodgement; however, the insertion site and vascular pathway must remain visible. Other concerns for site protection include compromising the blood flow through the extremity or the fluid flow through the attached set and catheter and skin damage from tight application. Follow manufacturers' instructions to ensure correct application of the devices chosen.

Stretch netting
Cut a piece of 4" (10.2-cm) stretch netting the same length as the patient's arm. Slip the netting over the patient's arm, and lay the arm on an arm board. Then grasp the netting at both sides of the arm, and stretch it under the arm board. Securely tape the stretch netting beneath the arm board.

Note: You may also protect a scalp site by placing netting on the patient's head, leaving a hole to allow access to the site.

Protecting an I.V. site *(continued)*

I.V. Site Protectors
These are plastic rounded dome device with smooth edges, with or without attached fabric for securing the dome over the I.V. site; usually vented to prevent trapping moisture and heat near the I.V. site. These devices eliminate the need to cut or modify other items used in patient care to adapt for site protection.

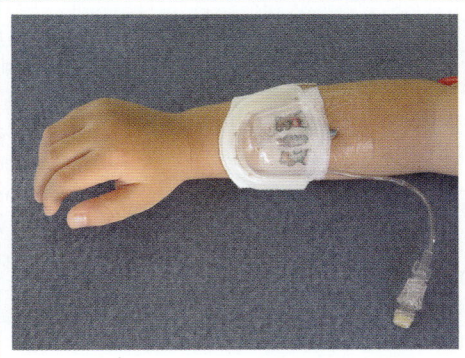

Example of a pediatric I.V. site protector device. (Reprinted from I.V. House, Inc., St. Louis, MO, with permission.)

Handboard
Improvements in handboards include attached straps with Velcro closures; rounded edges with a shape that contours to the shape of the hand and wrist, and openings on the palm side to allow for assessment of both sides of the extremity. (See example in *Chapter 2*, page 93.)

Still stuck on stickers

After inserting the I.V. catheter, remember to reward your preschool or school-age patient. Colorful stickers to wear on clothes or on the I.V. dressing are always popular with this age group.

Assessment and management

The frequency of monitoring will depend on the child's condition, age, and the reason for I.V. therapy. For instance, a child who's receiving replacement fluids for dehydration will require continuous monitoring, whereas a child with an I.V. access site for medication administration will require less frequent monitoring. You'll need to assess the I.V. site of an infant or toddler frequently because he's more likely to dislodge the catheter than the adolescent who understands the necessity of the I.V. and the discomfort associated with having it reinserted.

Around-the-clock assessments

Assess the child's infusing I.V. site at least hourly, or more frequently, depending on the nature of the infusion, and compare extremities. Observe for redness, streaking, edema, and soiled dressings. Palpate for swelling, skin tenseness, or cordlike feel of the accessed blood vessel and note the temperature of the surrounding skin. Make sure that you also assess the areas above and below the insertion site. Check that the dressing and I.V. administration set are secure to prevent the child from dislodging the device or becoming tangled in the set. Don't reinforce wet or soiled dressings, tapes, or protective devices. Change them if they become loose or dislodged or if there's blood or fluid leakage.

Check that pain!

Use a standardized assessment tool or a face rating scale, where the child points to the face that describes how he feels, to determine whether the child is experiencing pain at the I.V. site. Observe closely for facial or body language reactions when you assess the site. Ask the child if the access site hurts and give him permission to tell you that it does. Some children may be reluctant to admit that they're having pain. You should constantly be aware of the amount of discomfort that I.V. therapy can cause and work to minimize the pain as quickly as possible.

Flushed and duly noted

Flush the VAD after each medication delivery to maintain patency and prevent complications. Make sure that if saline flushes are ordered, you use preservative-free normal saline solution.

Be sure to document all of your findings and interventions, according to facility policy, on flow sheets and in the nurses' notes.

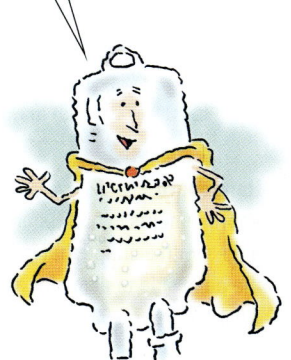

Use a standardized pain assessment tool to rate your patient's pain, and do whatever it takes to ease his discomfort. Even if it means drawing faces or wearing a corny cape, it is worth it, right?

Dealing with I.V. complications

The potential complications associated with I.V. therapy are similar in children and adults. However, some aren't as common in children as they are in adults and others occur more frequently. The most common complications associated with I.V. therapy in children include infiltration, occlusion, dislodgment, and phlebitis. Allergic reactions, emboli, and infection occur less often in children than adults.

Infiltration and extravasation

Infiltration can occur when the I.V. fluid or medication infuses into the tissue surrounding the vein, instead of entering the venous circulation. Extravasation occurs when the infiltrated fluid is extensive or the fluid infusing is a vesicant capable of causing tissue damage to the skin and subcutaneous tissue. It typically occurs as a result of an accidental vein puncture from the catheter, dislodgment of the catheter from the vein, or leakage between the catheter and the wall of the vein. Infiltration involves a substance that's nonvesicant, whereas extravasation involves a vesicant substance.

Give it a grade

Signs of infiltration include localized swelling, pain, and coolness to the touch. It is important to consider the size of an infiltration in relationship to the size of the affected extremity using a validated pediatric I.V. assessment tool. Infiltrations can be graded from 0 (no symptoms) to 4 (severe symptoms) based on appearance as well as percentage of the extremity affected. The following infiltration scale has been tested for reliability and validity in the pediatric population.

Infiltration scale

Grade	Characteristics
0	No symptoms Flushes with ease
1	Localized swelling (1%–10% of extremity) Flushes with difficulty Pain at site
2	Slight swelling at site (up to ¼ of the extremity above or below site, or 10%–25% of the extremity above or below site) Presence of redness Pain at the site
3	Moderate swelling at site (¼ to ½ of extremity above or below site, or 25%–50% of the extremity above or below site) Pain at site Skin cool to touch Blanching Diminished pulse below site
4	Moderate swelling at site (¼ to ½ of extremity above or below site, or more than 50% of the extremity above or below site) Infiltration of blood products, irritants, and/or vesicants (any amount of swelling) Skin cool to touch Blanching Skin breakdown/necrosis Blistering Diminished or absent pulse Pain at site Capillary refill >4 seconds

Reprinted from Pop, R. S. (2012). A pediatric peripheral intravenous infiltration assessment tool. *Journal of Infusion Nursing, 35*(4), 243–248. doi:10.1097/NAN.0b013e31825at323, with permission.

Cease and desist

When you identify an infiltrated I.V., you should immediately stop the infusion. Check your policies to see if an antidote might be recommended. Detach the administration set from the catheter hub, attach a syringe, and attempt to aspirate. The volume of fluid aspirated will probably be very small, but you might be able to retrieve the volume inside the catheter lumen. Then remove the catheter. Treatment depends on the severity of the infiltration and whether the substance is a vesicant or nonvesicant. The first step is always elevation of the extremity to aide in fluid reabsorption by the lymphatic system.

Heat or cold: Which one to use?

The choice for applying warm or cold compresses is based on the medication that has entered the tissue. Cold compresses cause vasoconstriction and reduces the exposure of additional tissue to the extravasated fluid. However, cold compresses cannot be used with vasoocclusive diseases such as sickle cell anemia. Application of cold compresses is indicated for most fluids and medications. This is usually applied for 20 to 30 minutes four to six times per day.

Heat application in an infant or child poses greater risk for burns, but it is indicated for certain antineoplastic agents (See *Chapter 6, Extravasation management guidelines,* page 293.) and vasopressors. Heat causes vasodilation, allowing the extravasated fluid to spread to additional tissue possibly extending the size of the damaged area. The method for applying heat must be one that can be controlled and monitored. Towels or other devices should not be heated in microwave ovens or under hot running water because the actual temperature cannot be measured.

The highest temperature that is safe for children is 42°C (107.6°F). Place a dry towel between the patient and the heat source. Application is usually for 15 to 30 minutes. Follow your facilities policies and procedures for application of both heat and cold in all pediatric patients.

Fluid overload

Fluid overload occurs when fluids are given at a higher rate or in a larger volume than the child's system can absorb or excrete. It can potentially be a severe complication of pediatric I.V. therapy because it can occur in a very short time and can be life threatening.

Beware the ominous signs!

Signs of fluid overload include edema, dyspnea, hypertension, weight increase, a third heart sound, and crackles. Careful monitoring of the child and rapid notification of the LIP when the child's status changes can help prevent the infusion of too much fluid in too short of a time. Consequently, you should check the I.V. flow rate at least hourly, even when you're using an electronic infusion pump.

Infection

Infection can occur at the I.V. insertion site for several reasons, including:
- inadequate hand hygiene
- improper skin antisepsis before the venipuncture
- contaminated equipment
- disruption of the occlusive dressing, which allows bacteria to enter the area
- moist or wet dressings that encourage bacteria colonization
- improper management of the administration set and all injection sites.

Taking the local or septic route

Infection of I.V. sites is usually local, resulting in redness, warmth, and swelling of the area. The child may also develop a fever. Bloodstream infection, though rare, can also occur if bacteria enter the bloodstream, especially in children who have compromised immune systems.

Strictly aseptic

You can usually prevent I.V. site infection if you use strict aseptic technique during I.V. insertion, provide safeguards to prevent the child from playing with or removing the dressing, and frequently monitor the integrity of the dressings and change them as soon as they become moist. I.V. sites are not routinely changed in pediatric patients so close monitoring is essential. Instead, pediatric peripheral catheters are removed based on signs and symptoms of any complication, also known as clinical indications.

Allergic reactions

Skin antiseptics and medications and their preservatives may cause allergic reactions. Some children are also allergic to the materials used in the manufacturing or packaging of the catheters. Latex may be used in the manufacture of some products and their packaging. Be sure to assess your patient for all allergies including latex and to read all product labels for the presence of latex.

While adhesive dressings and tape applied to cover the site and secure the catheter may cause skin damage, this is usually not a true allergic reaction. Most often, skin irritation from adhesive devices occurs because they were applied before solutions were thoroughly dry or were stretched during application causing tension on the skin. Follow the manufacturer instructions for correct application of all adhesive products and use skin barrier solutions to promote skin integrity.

Redness and, possibly, a rash are the first signs of local inflammation. If the child has been previously exposed to the allergen, anaphylactic shock is possible, though rare.

Preventing and predicting occurrences

You can't always prevent an allergic reaction or accurately predict which child will experience one. Make sure that you ask the parents whether the child has any known allergies or has ever had a previous reaction. Make sure that gloves and other supplies are latex-free, especially in patients with a known latex allergy.

Severe I.V. therapy complications can be prevented through diligent monitoring and thorough assessments. Early identification of problems and prompt interventions to correct them can prevent minor complications from becoming serious ones.

Other vascular access methods

In some instances, it may not be possible or in the child's best interest to insert a peripheral I.V. catheter. In these situations, other types of fluid delivery systems, such as central vascular access devices (CVADs), intraosseous infusion, or an umbilical vessel catheter, may be used.

Central vascular access devices

Central catheters are recommended when an infant or child needs therapy for a week or longer and for the administration of solutions or medications that are hyperosmolar or considered vesicants.

A CVAD is a device whose tip is located in the superior vena cava near the cavoatrial junction for insertions sites in the arms, scalp, or neck. For insertion sites from the lower extremities, the tip should be located in the inferior vena cava above the diaphragm and near the cavoatrial junction. In children with long-term needs for a CVAD, growth will cause changes in the tip location and will require periodic assessment and possible removal and insertion of a new catheter with a correct tip location. Intracardiac tip location in infants should be avoided as this can result in the CVAD tip eroding through the cardiac wall, producing cardiac tamponade.

CVAD options include peripherally inserted central catheters (PICCs), nontunneled catheters, tunneled cuffed catheters, and implanted ports. (See *Chapter 3, Infusion therapy requiring central venous access*, page 382.) The type of CVAD chosen for a pediatric patient should be based on the:
- age and size of the child
- cognitive and compliance ability
- type and duration of the therapy
- infusate characteristics
- vein quality and ability to access
- body image considerations and
- location where therapy will be provided, such as hospital, alternative care, or homecare.

Care of CVADs varies by device but includes site assessment, flushing or infusion to maintain patency, and periodic dressing changes, depending on type of catheter dressing and device securement. An insertion "bundle" of specific practices is strongly recommended to prevent complications of CVADs, particularly blood stream infections, which can be costly. Essential components of assessing a CVAD include noting the security of the catheter, change in external length if applicable, intactness of dressing, and lack of visible complications at the exit/insertion site. The most common complications of CVADs in children include catheter lumen occlusion, partial or complete dislodgment, and infection, which may lead to early catheter removal.

Nontunneled CVADs

Nontunneled CVADs are single or multiple lumens and are generally made of polyurethane that is originally stiff but softens as it reaches body temperature. Nontunneled CVADs are placed directly into the superior vena cava by way of the right or left subclavian, the internal or external jugular veins, or the inferior vena cava via the femoral veins at the groin. Nontunneled catheters are inserted by physicians, advanced practice nurses, physician's assistants, and vascular access specialist and are used for short-term access in critical care patients. These catheters are often inserted in emergency situations and dwell only several days due to high risk of infection. Site preferences in children — in order of preference, safety, and accessibility — are the:
- femoral vein with a short subcutaneous tunnel to avoid the diaper area
- internal jugular veins
- subclavian vein.

Tunneled cuffed CVADs

Surgically placed tunneled cuffed catheters (that is, Broviac) are single-lumen or multilumen silicone or polyurethane catheters with one or two Dacron polyester cuffs to anchor the catheter in the subcutaneous tunnel under the skin. This technique helps hold the catheter in place for long-term use and protects against infection from the skin; however, bloodstream infection remains likely from introduction of organisms through the catheter hub and lumen. These catheters are surgically tunneled under the skin of the chest with the catheter entering the internal jugular or subclavian vein and tip located in the superior vena cava. The catheter exits the skin on the chest wall or may be tunneled to the upper back to prevent the child from reaching it. An alternative site is the inferior vena cava, with the catheter tunneled to the abdomen, thigh, or back. Tunneled catheters are used for longer-term indications such as long-term parenteral nutrition or cancer treatment.

Implanted ports

An implantable port is a surgically placed CVAD that is made up of a catheter attached to an implanted metal or plastic dome containing a self-sealing injection port. An implanted port is sutured to the surgically created pocket and the catheter tip located in the superior or inferior vena cava. Ports are indicated for long-term intravascular access, particularly when intermittent I.V. therapy is needed, such as in children with cancer or cystic fibrosis. Although the port is implanted under the skin and not visible, the downside is that the port has to be accessed periodically by inserting a special noncoring needle through the skin and into the self-sealing septum so that blood samples can be obtained, the port flushed to maintain patency, or therapy administered. Using a topical numbing agent prior to access can lessen pain of port accessed.

Peripherally inserted central catheter

A PICC is a catheter that's inserted percutaneously into a peripheral vein. The catheter tip resides in the lower one-third of the superior vena cava, at the junction of the superior vena cava and right atrium. Available sizes for premature neonates, infants and children include one to five French and are available in single or multiple lumen configurations.

PICC a peck of reasons

PICC placement is indicated for intermediate to long-term I.V. access for the administration of antibiotics, pain medications, antineoplastic agents, noncytotoxic vesicants, parenteral nutrition or other hyperosmolar solutions, or blood products. The early use of PICCs may also spare peripheral veins and limit the pain of repeated needlesticks, which can be traumatic to children. Another reason to use a PICC is that PICCs are also associated with fewer complications in infants and children.

Generally, good to go

In general, to maintain good blood flow around the catheter, children are encouraged to use the arm with the PICC as usual, rather than guard it. However, very active children are at a greater risk for breaking or dislodging a PICC; immobilization of the extremity may be necessary in these children.

Intraosseous infusion

Usually performed in an emergency, an intraosseous infusion (IO) may be necessary to provide resuscitative fluids, medication, and blood until a vein can be accessed for I.V. administration. When a successful I.V. catheter insertion is not possible within 1 to 2 minutes, the IO route should be used. An intraosseous needle with a battery-powered drill is commonly used. If one isn't available, a 16G or 19G straight needle may be used; however, excessive force is needed to drive the needle through bone. For children, this means the need for analgesic medications as this is a painful procedure. The needle is placed in the medullary cavity of a bone, usually in the distal end of the femur or the proximal or distal ends of the tibia. In an infant or child, the thigh may have additional subcutaneous tissue making the femur a difficult site to enter and maintain. The sternum is not appropriate for use in children due to its thinner dimension. The solution is then infused directly into the cavity, which is rich in blood. (See *Understanding intraosseous infusion*, page 383.) While the IO route in now the first choice in emergent life-threatening situations, once the patient is stable, another plan for vascular access is needed as the IO device must be removed within 24 hours.

Umbilical vessel catheter

An umbilical catheter may be inserted into the neonate's umbilical artery or vein for I.V. therapy, when necessary.

Arterial access

An umbilical artery catheter is commonly inserted for:
- taking frequent blood samples
- providing direct arterial blood pressure measurement.

> **Understanding intraosseous infusion**
>
> During intraosseous infusion, the bone marrow serves as a noncollapsible vein; thus, fluid infused into the marrow cavity rapidly enters the circulation by way of an extensive network of venous sinusoids.

This type of catheter is contraindicated in neonates older than 7 days and in those who have abdominal wall defects, necrotizing enterocolitis, peritonitis, or vascular compromise in the buttocks or lower limbs.

Vote for venous

An umbilical venous catheter may be inserted to administer fluids and medications and to provide venous access for exchange transfusions. It's also typically the first choice of intravascular access in neonatal resuscitation.

Specialized equipment

Administration sets

Keeping it just right

The administration set for infants and children is different from that of adults in that the flow rates requirements are much slower. Precise infusion rates are required to prevent the possibility of medication overdose or fluid volume overload.

Make sure that the I.V. administration set is connected to a syringe and correctly placed in a syringe pump or an electronic infusion pump with an anti–free flow feature to reduce the risk of fluid overload. Infusion by gravity is no longer a common practice in pediatrics; however, for some situations (for example, conscious sedation for invasive procedures), a microdrip administration set with or without a volume control set may be used. Administration sets should be free of Di[2-ethylhexyl] phthalate (DEHP).

Electronic infusion devices

Electronic infusion devices or pumps that regulate fluid delivery are used in neonates, infants, and children and should demonstrate ±5% accuracy, guard against free flow, and have occlusion alarm ratings that fall within safety limits. Infusion pumps are necessary in infants and children who require arterial lines and highly accurate infusions, such as PN, antineoplastic agents, blood products, and vasoactive and other rate-dependent medications that must be delivered accurately to achieve desired effect. A popular volumetric pump often used for children is the syringe pump. This highly portable pump incorporates a syringe as the volume chamber to deliver the infusate. The syringe pump is indicated in children for infusion of intermittent doses of medications, such as antibiotics, low volume therapy, and need to infuse at very low flow rates.

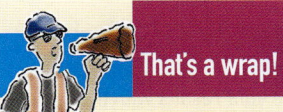

That's a wrap!

Pediatric I.V. therapy review

Reasons for I.V. therapy in children
- Replacement of body fluids
- Prevention or correction of electrolyte imbalances
- Blood and blood product administration
- Nutrition maintenance
- Medication administration

Calculating fluid needs
- Amount of fluid replacement is based on child's stage of dehydration.
- If available, obtain the child's current and immediate preillness weights in kilograms.
- Determine the child's dehydration percentage.
- Correlate the results with the child's clinical symptoms.
   - If precise weights aren't available, estimate the dehydration severity by clinical signs alone and adjust percentage based on whether the child weighs more or less than 10 kg.
   - Determine the child's daily maintenance fluid requirements.
   - Adjust the maintenance fluid amounts based on the child's condition, activity level, treatments, and insensible fluid losses.
- Add the child's replacement amounts to his maintenance amounts to determine daily fluid needs.
- Consider ongoing losses, such as those occurring from vomiting, diarrhea, diaphoresis, and hyperthermia and fluids collected from nasogastric tubes and drains, when determining fluid replacement needs.
- Typical replacement schedule is to administer one-half of the deficit plus the maintenance amount over the first 8 hours of therapy and the remaining one-half of the deficit plus maintenance over the next 16 hours.
- Monitor the child at least every 2 hours for ongoing losses and fluid excess, to determine if adjustment of the replacement amounts is necessary.

Site selection
- Consider the child's age, activity level, and the reason for the I.V. therapy when choosing the best I.V. site.
- Avoid previously used or sclerotic veins.

Scalp veins
- Reserve use for infants younger than 6 months old.
- Be aware that they have no valves and are easy to stabilize for catheter insertion.
- Palpate the site for arterial pulsations; if you feel these pulsations, select another site.

Hand, forearm, and upper arm veins
- Choose the most distal site available.
- Start with the child's nondominant side and move to the dominant side if necessary.
- Make sure that you use the opposite hand if the patient is a young child who sucks his thumb.
- Avoid starting the I.V. in the same arm as the patient's identification band.
- Keep in mind that hand veins are ideal sites for long-term therapy.
- Immobilize the arm with an arm board if you insert the catheter near the wrist or elbow.
- Avoid using antecubital, wrist, knee, and axillary veins.

Foot and leg veins
- Use the dorsal surface of the foot and the lower leg for children prior to walking age.
- Immobilize an I.V. site on the hand, wrist, and foot with a padded board and place padding under the foot.
- Remember that femoral veins can be used for children of all ages.

I.V. catheter insertion
- Choose the catheter based on the size of the child's veins and the type of fluid he'll be receiving.
- Use the smallest gauge catheter in the shortest length that will allow blood to flow around the catheter while the I.V. fluid is infusing.
- Regulate flow rate with a syringe pump or electronic infusion pump with an anti-free flow feature.

(continued)

Pediatric I.V. therapy review *(continued)*

- Give an age-appropriate explanation to the child when the time is right.
- Apply a transdermal anesthesia cream before the venipuncture to lessen the child's anxiety, reduce his pain, and improve compliance, if he's older than 1 month.
- Place warm packs on the site for 10 minutes to enhance vein dilation.
- Restrain the child, as necessary.
- In children, the blood return in the flashback chamber may be minimal after inserting the I.V. needle and catheter into the vein.
- Using an engineered stabilization device and sterile tape, secure the catheter.
- Cover the insertion site and external VAD with a transparent semipermeable dressing.
- Place a protective device over the VAD site to prevent dislodgment by the child.
- Loop the set and tape it so that, if it's pulled, the strain will be exerted on the tubing and not the catheter.

Assessment and management
- Frequency of monitoring depends on the child's condition, age, and the reason for I.V. therapy.
- Monitor the child's pulse rate and volume, blood pressure, temperature, capillary refill, urine output, peripheral pulses, skin color, extremities temperature, and laboratory test results.
- Compare your results with the child's baseline findings.
- Weigh the child before fluid administration is started and once per shift throughout the course of treatment.
- Monitor the amount of fluid infused and confirm flow rates.
- Assess the child's VAD site and entire infusion system at least hourly for signs of complications.
- Determine if the child is having pain.
- Document all findings and interventions according to facility policy, on flow sheets and in the nurses' notes.

Complications
- Infection
- Infiltration or extravasation
- Fluid overload
- Allergic reactions
- Phlebitis and emboli (uncommon)

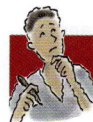

Quick quiz

1. A child with moderate dehydration will have:
    A. normal skin turgor.
    B. a rapid, weak pulse.
    C. extreme fatigue and muscle cramping.
    D. normal capillary refill.

Answer: C. A child with moderate dehydration has cool extremities and experiences extreme fatigue and muscle cramping.

2. A child's preillness weight was 12 kg and his current weight is 11 kg. What is his percent of dehydration?
    A. 1%
    B. 8%
    C. 20%
    D. 25%

Answer: B. To determine the child's percent of dehydration, subtract his current weight (11 kg) from his preillness weight (12), divide your answer (1 kg) by the child's preillness weight (12 kg), and then multiply that number (0.08) by 100 to arrive at 8%.

3. When you're providing maintenance I.V. fluids to a child, it's important to:
    A. use the child's current weight as the basis for determining the child's fluid needs.
    B. determine the child's percent of dehydration.
    C. administer bolus injections, followed by the remaining amount of fluid.
    D. adjust the amounts based on the child's activity level, treatments, and insensible fluid losses.

Answer: D. The child's activity level, treatments, and insensible fluid losses affect the amount of maintenance fluids required.

4. A scalp vein is usually an ideal I.V. site for the:
    A. neonate.
    B. 10-month-old child.
    C. 2-year-old child.
    D. adolescent.

Answer: A. Scalp veins are best reserved for infants younger than 6 months old because they can easily be dislodged by the child's hands.

5. The most common complications associated with I.V. therapy in children include:
    A. infiltration/extravasation, lumen occlusion, dislodgment, and phlebitis.
    B. infection, infiltration/extravasation, phlebitis, and allergic reactions.
    C. infection, emboli, fluid overload, and allergic reactions.
    D. infiltration/extravasation, fluid overload, and deep vein thrombosis.

Answer: A. Infiltration/extravasation, lumen occlusion, dislodgment, and phlebitis are the complications of I.V. therapy that are most often seen in children.

Scoring

☆☆☆ If you answered all five questions correctly, two toddler thumbs up! You're practically a pediatric parenteral pro!

☆☆ If you answered four or five questions right, great goin'. You earned yourself an I.V. bagful of M & Ms!

☆ If you answered fewer than four questions correctly, no worries. Have a little snack, then begin your chapter infusion over again. You'll do better next time!

Suggested References

Centers for Disease Control and Prevention. (2011). *Guidelines for the prevention of intravascular catheter-related infections* (p. 10, 26, 28). Retrieved from http://www.cdc.gov/hicpac/pdf/guidelines/bsi-guidelines-2011.pdf, on September 25, 2016.

Ebbinghaus, S., & Kobayashi, H. (2010). Safe heat application for pediatric patients: A hot item. *Journal of Nursing Care Quality, 25*(2), 168–175.

Frey, A. M., & Pettit, J. (2010). Intravenous therapy in children. In M. Alexander, A. Corrigan, L. Gorski, J. Hankins, & R. Perucca (Eds.), *Infusion nursing: An evidence based approach* (3rd ed.). St. Louis, MO: Saunders.

Gorski, L. A., Hadaway, L., Hagle, M. E., Mcgoldrick, M., Orr, M., & Doellman, D.; Infusion Nurses Society (INS). (2016). Infusion therapy standards of practice. *Journal of Infusion Nursing, 39*(Suppl 1), S1–S159.

Gorski, L. A., Hallock, D., Kuehn, S. C., Morris, P., Russell, J. M., & Skala, L. C. (2012). Recommendations for frequency of assessment of the short peripheral catheter site. *Journal of Infusion Nursing, 35*(5), 290–292. doi:10.1097/NAN.0b013e318267f636.

Harrison, D., Beggs, S., & Stevens, B. (2012). Sucrose for procedural pain management in infants. *Pediatrics, 130*(5), 918–925. doi: 10.1542/peds.2011-3848.

Hockenberry, M. J., & Wilson, D. (2010). *Wong's nursing care of infants and children* (9th ed.). St. Louis, MO: Mosby.

Pop, R. S. (2012). A pediatric peripheral intravenous infiltration assessment tool. *Journal of Infusion Nursing, 35*(4), 243–248.

Chapter 10

Infusion therapy in older adults

Just the facts

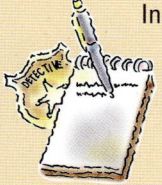

In this chapter, you'll learn:
- ◆ physiologic changes associated with aging
- ◆ considerations for administering infusion therapy to older adults
- ◆ potential complications of infusion therapy in older adult patients
- ◆ teaching considerations and techniques to use with older adult patients
- ◆ what to document when providing infusion therapy.

The older adult

In 2014, the average life expectancy at birth for Americans was 78.8 years. Over the 35 years from 1980 to 2014, life expectancy has risen for both white and black Americans and both sexes with the white female having the longest life expectancy at 81.2 years. Although there is no consensus on age groupings, rates for death, disease, and disability are examined by some type of grouping. A commonly used example of age groups of the older adult is:
- the young old — age 65 to 74
- the middle old — age 75 to 84
- the old-old — 85 years and older.

The old-old group has the fastest rate of increase with those over age 85 comprising 14% of all older adults. By 2050, projections estimate that 21% of all older adults will be 85 years or more. While those 85 years and more account for only 2% of the total US population, they represent 9% of hospital discharges and 11% of days of hospital care, rates that are much higher than other age groups.

Another concern for adults over age 65 is the overall burden of disease, especially the presence of multiple chronic conditions (MCC), sometimes known as multimorbidity. MCC is having two or more chronic conditions, adding a heightened level of complexity to their care. About half of all Americans have no chronic medical condition while about 25% have MCC and older adults have greater proportion than younger adults. Those with MCC have more hospitalizations and emergency department visits. Of those 85 years or more, transfer from hospital to a skilled nursing facility was more common than discharge to their personal home.

From 2000 to 2010, the rates of hospitalization for congestive heart failure, pneumonia, stroke, and hip fracture saw a decline for those 85 and older, with congestive heart failure listed as the most frequent medical diagnosis. For MCC in all older adults, the most common combination for diagnoses is ischemic heart disease, hypertension, and hyperlipidemia.

These facts add up to more older adults needing infusion therapy. This population group is growing, and it is important to recognize that the older adult has special needs and physiologic changes, which affect the clinician's approach to infusion therapy for this population.

Modify your technique

When caring for older adult patients, you must make certain modifications to the techniques you normally use for other adults. You need to take into account the physiologic changes that normally occur during aging and understand how these changes affect infusion therapy.

Aging and inflammation

Aging involves a series of structural and functional changes affecting all organs in the human body. Oxidative stress plus chronic low-grade inflammation work together to produce changes throughout the body. Levels of C-reactive protein, tumor necrotic factor alpha, and interleukins, all components of the immune system, measure this proinflammatory condition. Many researchers apply the name "inflammaging" to this process that involves all systems in the human body. Vascular endothelium, the lining of all blood vessels, is the site of inflammation-induced chemical and structural changes that produce disease with aging. Remember the most common diagnoses in this age group listed above involve the vascular system.

The most effective ways to reduce the impact of inflammaging is to maintain activity including exercise, avoid a sedentary lifestyle, eat a healthy diet with high amounts of antioxidants, and reduce calories eaten.

Another concept in the older adult population is frailty. Its presence is characterized by at least three of these conditions:
- Weakness, especially grip strength
- Decreased physical activity
- Reduced motor function, usually measured by walking speed
- Exhaustion
- Unintentional weight loss

Frailty is seen in up to 10% of all older adults; however, it is seen in about one-third of those over age 80. A major cause of frailty is abnormal regulation of the immune system leading to an increase in chronic inflammation.

Innate immunity comes from mechanical barriers of skin and mucous membranes, while acquired immunity comes from many different types of cells creating a specific response to a foreign substance known as an antigen. (See *Chapter 7, The immune system*, page 306.) Alterations in the immune system put older adults at increased risk for infection, reduced protection from vaccines, and the chronic inflammatory state.

Physiologic changes of aging

With aging come the loss of some body cells, reduced metabolism of others, altered intercellular communication, loss of the ability to regenerate new cells, and the accumulation of genetic damage from our entire life. These changes lead to altered body composition and reductions in certain body functions. Consequently, the older adult patient is more susceptible to complications with infusion therapy.

Skin and connective tissue

Perhaps some of the most obvious signs of aging occur with changes to the integumentary system.

The skinny on skin changes

Subcutaneous fat loss, dermal thinning, and decreasing collagen lead to the development of facial lines around the eyes, mouth, and nose. Mucous membranes become drier, and sweat gland output reduces as the number of active sweat glands decrease.

Skin also loses elasticity with age, to the point where it may seem almost translucent. As the thickness and amount of connective tissue in the dermal layer decrease, veins become more fragile. Typically, veins will appear tortuous because of the increased transparency and decreased elasticity of the skin. (See *Aging and its effect on skin*, page 392.)

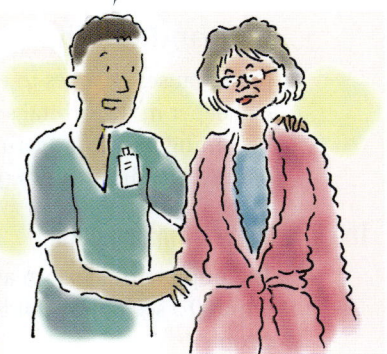

Aging alters the body composition and reduces certain bodily functions, so it makes sense that you'll need to modify your technique.

Aging and its effect on skin

Although the effects of aging vary with the specific tissue or organ, all older adults eventually become more susceptible to fatigue and disease. Some of the physiologic changes that occur in skin with aging include:
- gradual loss of subcutaneous fat and elastin, which causes the skin to wrinkle and sag
- decreased dermal thickness, which can lead to skin tears and other skin damage from adhesive devices.

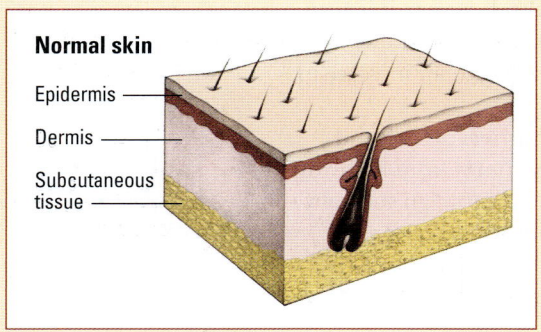

Normal skin
- Epidermis
- Dermis
- Subcutaneous tissue

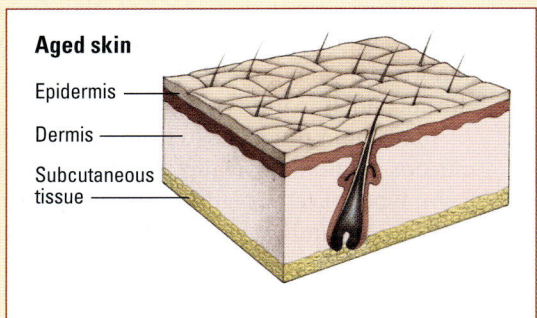

Aged skin
- Epidermis
- Dermis
- Subcutaneous tissue

Hair pigment decreases with age as the number of melanocytes decreases, so the hair may turn gray or white. Hair also thins as the patient ages. Nail growth slows and longitudinal ridges, thickening, brittleness, and malformations may increase.

Slow to heal

Besides wounds taking longer to heal, other common skin conditions in elderly people include:
- senile keratosis — overgrowth and thickening of the horny epithelium
- acrochordon — benign skin tags
- senile angiomas — benign tumors made up of blood vessels or lymph vessels.

Eyes and vision

Aging causes changes to eye structure and visual acuity. The eyes sit deeper in the orbital socket and the eyelids lose their elasticity, becoming baggy and wrinkled. As the lacrimal apparatus loses fatty tissue, tears diminish in quantity.

The incredible shrinking pupil

The pupil shrinks, decreasing the amount of light that reaches the retina. To see objects, older adults need more light than younger people.

Who dimmed the lights?

Aging also diminishes night vision and depth perception. Many older adults develop presbyopia, a vision defect in which objects very close to the eye can't be seen clearly without corrective lenses.

Ears and hearing

Many elderly persons lose some degree of hearing. By age 60, most adults have difficulty hearing about 4,000 Hz. (The normal range for speech recognition is 500 to 2,000 Hz.) Many older adults have trouble distinguishing higher-pitched consonants, such as *s*, *sh*, *f*, *ph*, *ch*, *z*, *t*, and *g*.

Some people may not be immediately aware of the onset or progression of a hearing defect. Others may recognize it but view it as a natural part of aging. Both vision changes and hearing changes need to be taken into account when preparing and teaching an older adult patient about infusion therapy. These limitations must be considered when infusion therapy will continue after hospitalization. An ambulatory infusion center or a skilled nursing facility may be a better option than home care due to these changes.

Respiratory system

Age-related changes occur in all areas of the respiratory system. In the upper airway, the nose enlarges from continued cartilage growth and the tonsils atrophy. Many patients also experience some degree of tracheal deviation. In the thorax, the anteroposterior chest diameter increases, which may result in decreased chest wall mobility. Respiratory muscle degeneration or atrophy may also occur, reducing pulmonary function.

Airway closed

Aging also results in the closing of some airways, which impairs ventilation of the basal areas of the lungs and reduces the maximum breathing capacity, forced vital capacity, and inspiratory reserve. This decreases the elderly patient's tolerance of excess fluid and increases the risk for complications due to fluid overload.

Cardiovascular system

The heart usually decreases slightly with age. The heart muscle becomes less efficient and loses contractile strength, and fibrotic and sclerotic changes thicken the heart valves and reduce their flexibility. The aorta grows more rigid, causing systolic blood pressure to rise proportionately more than diastolic blood pressure.

> Impaired ventilation of the lungs' basal areas causes an older adult patient to have less tolerance for excess fluid. This puts her at increased risk for fluid load complications with infusion therapy.

Fluid-shifting sensitivity

By age 70, many people experience a decrease in cardiac output at rest, making the older adult more sensitive to fluid shifts that may occur with infusion therapy.

Gastrointestinal system

Normal age-related changes in the GI system include diminished mucosal elasticity and reduced GI secretions, which in turn may alter digestion and absorption. GI tract motility, esophageal sphincter

---

Preventing dehydration in older patients

To maintain adequate hydration, an older patient needs 1,000 to 3,000 mL of fluid daily. Less than 1,000 mL daily may lead to constipation, which can contribute to urinary incontinence. It may also result in more concentrated urine, which predisposes the patient to urinary tract infections. Follow these guidelines to make sure the patient is adequately hydrated.

Monitoring
- Monitor intake and output. Ensure an intake of at least 1,500 mL of oral fluids and urine output of 1,000 to 1,500 mL per 24 hours.
- Check skin turgor and mucous membranes.
- Monitor vital signs, especially pulse rate, respiratory rate, and blood pressure. An increase in pulse and respiratory rates with decreased blood pressure may indicate dehydration.
- Monitor laboratory test results, such as serum electrolyte, blood urea nitrogen, and creatinine levels, hematocrit, and urine and serum osmolarity. Check for signs of acidosis.
- Weigh the patient at the same time daily, using the same scale and with the patient wearing the same type of clothes.
- Listen to bowel sounds for any increase in activity. Monitor stools for character: hard stools may indicate dehydration; loose, watery stools indicate loss of water.
- Be aware of diagnostic tests that affect intake and output (for example, laxative or enema use, which causes fluid loss), and replace any lost fluids.

Providing fluids
- Provide oral fluids often throughout the day, for example, every hour and with a bedtime snack.
- Provide modified cups that the patient can handle; help those who have difficulty.
- Offer fluids other than water; find out the types of beverages the patient likes and the preferred temperatures (for example, ice cold or room temperature drinks).
- Monitor coffee intake; coffee acts as a diuretic and may cause excessive fluid loss.
- If the patient is unable to take oral fluids, request an order for I.V. or subcutaneous hydration.

tone, and abdominal muscle strength may also decrease with age. These changes may result in appetite loss, esophageal reflux, constipation, and an increased risk of dehydration. (See *Preventing dehydration in elderly patients*, page 394.)

Hematology and immune system

The older adult's immune system produces greater levels of interleukin-6 (IL-6), a proinflammatory cytokine associated with atherosclerosis, and osteoporosis, which in turn produces an overall decline in function. C-reactive protein (CRP) is a marker for cardiovascular disease and is usually elevated in frail older adults. White blood cell (WBC) counts on the high side of the normal range in the older adult may be associated with cardiovascular, cerebrovascular event, and cancer mortality. The ability of WBCs to trap and kill invading organisms is diminished with age and is likely the cause of increased infections in the older adult.

The adaptive or acquired immune system increases autoimmune antibody production and changes in cytokine production. Cytokines are cellular proteins responsible for communication and interaction between other cells. Age-related failure in the function of the innate immune system may lead to failure to activate the adaptive immune system, which in turn leads to more chronic diseases in the older adult.

Fluid balance and aging

As the body ages, its fluid reserves become limited and the total amount of body water is decreased. This places the older adult at higher risk for developing a fluid volume deficit.

Further fluid factors

Other contributing factors for fluid volume deficit in an older adult include:
- decreased saliva
- decreased thirst mechanism
- electrolyte imbalances (See *Common fluid and electrolyte imbalances in elderly patients*, page 396.)
- increased urination.

Mind your elders!

When caring for an older adult patient, especially one who is receiving infusion therapy, remain mindful of his fluid volume status. (See *Assessing fluid volume status*, page 397.)

(Text continues on page 398.)

Common fluid and electrolyte imbalances in older patients

The following chart lists some of the common fluid and electrolyte imbalances you may encounter while caring for older patients.

Imbalance	Causes	Signs and symptoms	Treatment
Hypervolemia Fluid volume excess	• Renal failure • Heart failure • Cirrhosis • Increased oral or I.V. sodium intake • Mental confusion • Seizures • Coma	• Edema • Weight gain • Jugular vein distention • Lung crackles • Shortness of breath • Bounding pulse • Elevated blood pressure • Increased central venous pressure	• Diuretics • Fluid restriction (<1 qt [1 L]/day) • Sodium restriction • Hemodialysis for patients with renal failure
Hypovolemia Fluid volume deficit	• Dehydration • Vomiting • Diarrhea • Fever • Polyuria • Chronic kidney disease • Diabetes mellitus • Diuretic use • Hot weather • Decreased oral intake secondary to anorexia or nausea • Diminished thirst mechanism and inadequate water intake (common in nursing home patients)	• Dry mucous membranes • Oliguria or concentrated urine and anuria • Orthostatic hypotension • Dizziness • Weakness • Confusion or altered mental status • Possible severe hypotension • Increased hemoglobin, hematocrit, blood urea nitrogen, and serum creatinine levels	• Fluid administration (may be oral or I.V. or S.C.) depending on degree of deficit and patient's response • Urine output of 30–50 mL/hour usually signals adequate renal perfusion.
Hypernatremia Serum sodium >145 mEq/L (145 mmol/L)	• Water deprivation hypertonic tube feedings without adequate water replacement • Diarrhea • Low body weight	• Dry mucous membranes • Restlessness • Irritability • Weakness • Lethargy • Hyperreflexia • Seizures • Hallucinations • Coma	• Gradual infusion of hypotonic electrolyte solution or isotonic saline solution
Hyponatremia Serum sodium <138 mEq/L (138 mmol/L)	• Diuretics • Loss of GI fluids • Kidney disease • Excessive water intake • Excessive I.V. fluids or parenteral feedings	• Nausea and vomiting • Lethargy • Confusion • Muscle cramps • Diarrhea • Delirium • Weakness • Seizures • Coma	• Gradual sodium replacement, water restriction (1–1.5 L/day), or discontinuation of diuretic therapy (if ordered)

Common fluid and electrolyte imbalances in older patients *(continued)*

Imbalance	Causes	Signs and symptoms	Treatment
Hyperkalemia Serum potassium >5 mEq/L (5 mmol/L)	• Renal failure • Impaired tubular function • Potassium-conserving diuretic use (in patients with renal insufficiency) • Rapid I.V. potassium administration • Metabolic acidosis • Diabetic ketoacidosis	• Arrhythmias • Weakness • Paresthesia • Electrocardiogram (ECG) changes (tall, tented T waves, ST segment depression, prolonged PR interval and QRS complex, shortened QT interval, absent P waves)	• Dialysis (for renal failure) • Sodium polystyrene (Kayexalate) (to remove potassium) • I.V. calcium gluconate (antagonizes cardiac abnormalities) • I.V. insulin or hypertonic dextrose solution (shifts potassium into the cells) • Bicarbonate (for patients with acidosis) • Potassium intake restriction
Hypokalemia Serum potassium <3.5 mEq/L (3.5 mmol/L)	• Vomiting • Diarrhea • Nasogastric suction • Diuretic use • Digoxin toxicity • Decreased potassium intake	• Fatigue • Weakness • Confusion • Muscle cramps • ECG changes (flattened T waves, presence of U waves, ST segment depression, prolonged PR interval) and ventricular tachycardia or fibrillation	• Oral or I.V. potassium administration (I.V. infusions must be diluted and given slowly)

Assessing fluid volume status

Your usual assessments of fluid volume status need to be adjusted when caring for an older patient because of the normal changes associated with aging. For example, instead of testing skin turgor on the forearm, you should test skin turgor on the patient's forehead or sternum. The normal decrease in skin elasticity is diminished in these areas compared to the forearm. Other assessments used to assess fluid volume status include:

- temperature — an elevation in temperature may indicate a decrease in fluid volume
- decreased filling of veins in hands
- intake and output
- weight (daily)
- tongue — should be moist, midline, and pink
- blood pressure — normal for patient without orthostatic hypotension
- mental assessment — fluid volume deficit may result in confusion.

Preserving skin integrity

Skin, the largest organ in the human body and a significant component of the innate immune system, serves as a mechanical barrier to invasion by foreign substances especially microorganisms. It is imperative that skin integrity be given a high priority when managing infusion therapy. Skin punctures are required to insert venous access devices (VADs) and adhesive devices are required to secure, stabilize, and protect those VADs, with both factors presenting significant challenges to keep the skin surrounding VAD insertion sites as healthy as possible.

Medical adhesive products used for infusion therapy include tape, dressings, and engineered stabilization devices. Basically, these devices include a layer of fabric or plastic with an adhesive coating on one side. The adhesive can be made from acrylates, silicones, hydrogels, or hydrocolloids, although the purpose of the adhesive devices directs which type of adhesive is used. For example, transparent semipermeable dressings use either acrylates or silicone in the adhesive.

The amount of all adhesive devices used should be the minimum to secure the VAD effectively while at the same time reducing the risk of skin injury. Pressure applied to adhesive devices increases the adhesion to the skin. Increasing the contact time between the adhesive and the skin increases its adhesiveness because skin temperature warms the adhesive allowing it to fill in the spaces between the skin and the adhesive device.

There are multiple types of tape available for different needs and level of securement, although tape is not recommended to secure any type of VAD. Plastic-perforated tape may hold securely but can be hard to remove the adhesive if left in place for several days. Paper tape is a gentle alternative for the skin, but it does not easily mold to skin surfaces and may require more tape to hold the device securely. Silicone tapes and dressings are very gentle to the skin and attach and release easily. However, they have a weak adherence to plastic or other silicone device such as the VAD external segment and hub. Additionally, rolls of tape are easily contaminated with disease-producing organisms.

Medical Adhesive–Related Skin Injury (MARSI)

Medical adhesive–related skin injury (MARSI) is the result of adhesive attaching more strongly to the skin surface than the surface skin cells are attached to each other. MARSI is seen in a variety of clinical presentations, mainly at the time of adhesive device removal.

- Skin stripping or pulling apart of the epidermal layers of skin; skin appears shiny over an irregular area of the surface; may also include redness and blisters.
- Skin tear or complete separation of the epidermis from the dermis causing an open wound.
- Irritant contact dermatitis caused by chemical irritation to the skin; redness and swelling is seen where the device was in contact with the skin; usually a short duration.
- Allergic dermatitis is an immune response to the adhesive; a watery layer may appear along with redness and itching in the area where the adhesive was in contact with the skin; may last for several days or up to a week.
- Skin maceration appears when moisture is trapped under the dressing for extended periods; skin is gray or white and wrinkled in appearance.
- Folliculitis appears as small elevated areas around the hair follicle; associated with shaving or organisms trapped in the follicle.

Every time a dressing is removed from the skin, the surface skin cells are pulled off with the dressing. In older adults with thin, fragile skin, adhesive-related skin injury will result. Frequent dressing changes mean continual skin damage and reduce ability for healing. The use of special skin barrier solution before applying the dressing and the use of special adhesive remover are recommended to reduce these types of injuries.

Moisture under the dressing increases the risk of infection and MARSI. Skin antiseptic and skin barrier solutions applied to the skin must be thoroughly dry before applying the adhesive device. Moisture can also come from the puncture site in the form of bleeding or from excessive sweating. Transparent membrane dressings allow the passage of oxygen and moisture through the dressing; however, there are no recommendations for moisture vapor transmission rate (MVTR) for reducing local or bloodstream infection from the VAD.

Administering infusion therapy

Infusion therapy in older adults can be given by two routes — intravenous and subcutaneous. Because of the age-related skin changes and often fragile condition of older adults, administering infusion therapy to older adult patients by either route can be particularly challenging. The clinician must pay close attention to the mechanical aspects of accessing a vein or choosing the subcutaneous site and administering the fluids but also to the patient's tolerance of the fluids and medications and the therapy's overall ensuing physiologic effects.

The loss of subcutaneous tissue surrounding veins makes adequate stabilization very difficult while any type of adhesive device for stabilization and dressing can lead to greater skin damage. These factors may support the use of subcutaneous infusion over intravenous infusion, especially in long-term or palliative care. But remember that all medications cannot be given subcutaneously due to the potential for tissue damage. Subcutaneous infusion is easier to learn and administer and is less expensive than the I.V. route.

Keen on assessment

Ongoing assessment plays a crucial role when administering infusion therapy to the older adult. After you complete your initial assessment, you'll need to check the LIP orders to ensure that they don't conflict with your assessment findings or any advance directives the patient may have. Throughout therapy, you'll need to assess the patient frequently for signs of intolerance or complications.

Subtle signals

Remember that older adults have a decreased tolerance for too much or too little fluid, but their bodies tend to manifest symptoms slowly in response to such extremes. Therefore, you are responsible for monitoring for subtle changes that could signal a potential problem and alerting the LIP before they escalate to a more serious condition.

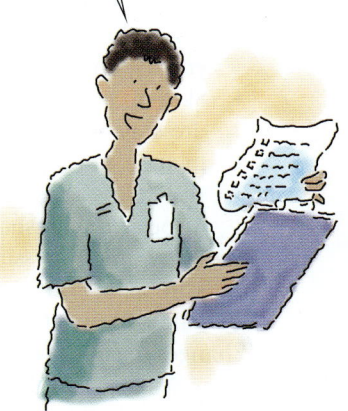

Monitor the patient often during therapy for subtle changes that can signal intolerance or impending complications.

Subcutaneous infusion

Subcutaneous infusion is limited to isotonic fluids for prevention or treatment of dehydration or fluid volume deficits. Dextrose 5% in water or 0.9% sodium chloride is most common, but other solutions such as lactated Ringer's may be infused by this route. Hyaluronidase, an enzyme to enhance the absorption of the fluids, may be added to subcutaneous infusions. The volume and rate of infusion for subcutaneous infusion is similar to those for the I.V. route. A single subcutaneous site may be able to tolerate 1,500 mL over a 24-hour period and manual regulation of the flow rate is preferred over electronic infusion pumps.

Medications that may be given by the subcutaneous route include insulin, opioids, corticosteroids, antiemetics, deferoxamine mesylate, and sedatives such as midazolam and haloperidol. Immunoglobulins are also given by the subcutaneous route. An infusion pump such as a syringe pump or an ambulatory infusion pump may be necessary to control the flow rate when medication is infusing.

Subcutaneous device and site selection

A subcutaneous infusion set will usually have a short needle extending at a right angle from an adhesive platform. Small gauge needles are used, usually 24- to 27-gauge size. Some designs have two small needles on one device to facilitate infusion into a larger subcutaneous area. An extension set is part of this infusion set to make it easier to attach the administration set. These devices are inserted at a right angle into the skin with the adhesive platform pressed against the skin to stabilize and secure it.

A 24-gauge short peripheral catheter may be used for subcutaneous infusion, but straight or winged needles are not recommended. The peripheral catheter is inserted using a 45- to 60-degree angle. The length of the needle or catheter should be relatively short to avoid placement into the muscle tissue as this can cause pain with infusion. Also, aspirate for the lack of a blood return on this site. If blood can be aspirated, immediately remove the device and find another site as this could mean a nearby vein or artery has been entered.

Sites for placement of the subcutaneous infusion set includes the back side of the upper arm, the upper chest area below the clavicle (but avoid breast tissue), the front or sides of the thigh, and the abdomen at least 2 inches away from the navel. Always avoid areas near a joint when an extremity is used.

Site selection requires assessment of skin integrity. Inspect the skin and avoid areas of redness or any type of discoloration, swelling, cuts or abrasions, or any type of pain or discomfort. Assess the amount of subcutaneous tissue in the area to ensure that it is adequate to avoid reaching the muscle tissue.

Site preparation

Skin antisepsis is equally as important for insertion of a subcutaneous device. Antiseptic agents may cause excessive skin drying, especially those with alcohol; however, alcoholic chlorhexidine gluconate solution is the preferred agent. Povidone-iodine, alcohol, and tincture of iodine may be used if there is a contraindication for chlorhexidine. Apply the antiseptic with a gentle back and forth scrubbing motion, and allow the area to dry completely before inserting the device.

Maintaining skin integrity at this site is a critical element requiring use of skin barrier solutions. Apply this solution to the area where any adhesive will be placed.

Make sure all solutions are thoroughly dry before adding the adhesive dressing. Usually, the transparent membrane dressing provides adequate securement for a subcutaneous device.

Site assessment and rotation

The site must be assessed frequently to ensure the absence of redness, hardness, pain, bruising, or leaking. A small amount of edema is to be expected, but it should not be excessive since fluid absorption should easily be occurring.

When used for hydration, each site may only be able to tolerate 1.5 to 2 L of fluid. This could indicate the need for rotating the site every 24 to 48 hours depending on the rate of infusion. When signs and symptoms indicate a problem, the site should be changed immediately. This also indicates the need for an evaluation of the flow rate and volume being infused. Adjustments may be necessary to allow for better fluid absorption. Addition of hyaluronidase to the infusion could speed up absorption and reduce these problems.

When used only for medication administration, the subcutaneous site is changed every 7 days or when signs and symptoms indicate the need to change it.

Intravenous infusion

Selecting an I.V. site

The basic steps for inserting a peripheral I.V. catheter are the same for the older adult as for a younger patient. (See *Chapter 2, Infusion therapy using peripheral veins*, page 53.) However, the approach, assessment, site and device selection, and stabilization are all unique to the older adult. The older the patient, the more critical these elements become in determining the appropriate techniques for peripheral I.V. access.

It is important to avoid sites that are already bruised and show signs of repeated venipuncture attempts or widespread subcutaneous bruising. Also avoid areas of flexion in the hands, wrists, and antecubital fossa as these sites have higher rates of complications such as infiltration, extravasation, and phlebitis. Evaluate both arms, and take into consideration the patient's need of his dominant hand for activities of daily living. Also, note any mobility restrictions or needs to use special devices (cane, wheelchair, crutches, etc.). The older adult may have other diseases, which limit use of their extremities for peripheral I.V. sites. Assess the medical history for all types of arthritis (for example, osteoarthritis, rheumatoid or psoriatic arthritis) and diseases that alter peripheral circulation such as lupus, Raynaud's syndrome, and diabetes.

Integral site integrity

Vein preservation in the older adult patient is difficult, but it's almost always necessary to accomplish successful treatment. Review the length and type of needed infusion therapy along with the number of potential peripheral venous access sites. Blindly making venipuncture attempts is never an appropriate way to insert a peripheral catheter. One clinician should never make more than two venipuncture attempts and no more than two clinicians should try, for a total of four attempts. Even four attempts may be too much for some older adults. When visible and palpable sites are not found or not anticipated to last for the entire course of therapy, another plan for vascular access is required. An alternative approach includes an ultrasound-guided peripheral catheter or a midline catheter inserted into deeper veins of the upper extremity. Characteristics of the fluid or medication (for example, osmolarity, pH, vesicant/irritant nature) may indicate the need for a central vascular access device; however, this choice requires assessment of the insertion risk in the older patient. A peripherally inserted central catheter (PICC) may have the greatest safety profile as the insertion site is in the upper extremity. A subclavian or jugular CVAD insertion in a frail older adult could increase insertion complications such as pneumothorax. A surgically inserted catheter such as a tunneled cuffed catheter or implanted port may present challenges with anesthesia. Subclavian and jugular sites require a Trendelenburg position that could be difficult or impossible for older adults with spinal problems or respiratory diseases.

Palpating the vein

Evaluate both arms carefully and palpate the veins completely along the vein tract. In the older adult, the vein may not have the bounce and distention as the vessels in a younger patient. The veins may readily pop up when a restrictive tourniquet is applied, but when palpated, they feel firm, corded, hard or ropelike. If possible, avoid veins that are thick and ropelike; this indicates thick, occluded vein walls and inserting and threading a catheter into them may be difficult.

Although a tourniquet may be necessary for some patients, you may find that many older adult patients have easily visible veins. It may be possible to gently access these visible veins without a tourniquet. If using a tourniquet is required, do not tie it tightly. Use the tourniquet as a gentle restrictive band. Another alternative would be to use a blood pressure cuff and only inflate it to a low pressure to restrict venous flow. The width of the blood pressure cuff helps to spread the inflation pressure over a wide area, so a lower pressure will still distend the vein for visualization.

Many types of medications can affect the clotting or bleeding times or the integrity of the vein wall of the older adult including anticoagulants, steroids, certain antibiotics, or antineoplastic agents. In these patients, the use of a tourniquet may cause bleeding, bruising, or hematoma formation.

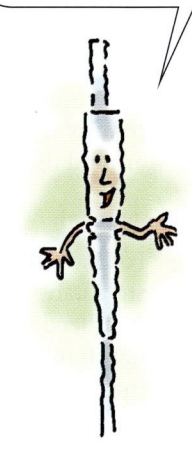

Avoid thick, ropelike veins. They're too thick-walled and occluded, making it hard for me to thread my way through them. Hey…thanks for listening!

Preparing the site

Site preparation is an important aspect with older adults. Their skin is typically dry and loose and may not tolerate some of the skin antiseptics. Alcoholic chlorhexidine gluconate is the preferred agent; however, povidone-iodine, alcohol, and tincture of iodine may be used if there is a contraindication for chlorhexidine. Apply the antiseptic with a careful back and forth motion, and allow the area to dry completely before inserting the catheter.

Inserting the device

Because the older adult has looser tissue, you may find stabilizing the vein difficult. These are sometimes referred to as "rolling veins." There are no rolling veins, but only veins that were not well stabilized prior to the insertion attempt. To help stabilize a vein for insertion, stretch the skin below the insertion site and anchor it firmly with your nondominant hand. Once you have the vein securely stabilized, then the insertion attempt can be made using either the direct or indirect approach.

Direct approach

With the vein stabilized, make the approach directly over the top of the vein with the smallest gauge catheter, shortest length needed to provide the ordered I.V. therapy. A smaller gauge catheter, such as 24 gauge ¾ inch length, may be more appropriate and easier to insert. The point of insertion should be 4 to 6 inches below the tourniquet, if one is used. Insertion into the vein too close to the point of the restrictive pressure may cause extreme back pressure inside the vein. When the vein is then punctured, it is like a pin exploding a balloon and the vein ruptures, causing subcutaneous bleeding and bruising at the site and a hematoma formation if not adequately controlled. Veins in the older adult are more fragile, so the venipuncture needs to be performed quickly and efficiently. Once the site is selected, and prepped, the insertion action should be a sure, quick motion into the vein to reduce the chance of excessive bruising. If a tourniquet or blood pressure cuff was used for restrictive pressure, remove it promptly to prevent bleeding back through the vein wall around the point where the needle penetrated the vein.

Indirect approach

For the older adult patient with very thin, delicate skin, where the subcutaneous tissue has deteriorated to the point that the vein is not stabilized with the tissue structure, the vein is very difficult to stabilize. It may be easier to use a two-step indirect approach to entering the vein. The goal is to penetrate the skin first, and then, once the catheter has entered the skin, the catheter angle can be lowered even more, so the angle of insertion into the vein is almost parallel to but not touching the skin. This will reduce the potential of going through the vein with a direct stick approach or injuring the back wall of the vein with the tip of the bevel of the needle.

First, determine the best place where you can secure the skin taut, close to the vein to be accessed, but not too close to accidently nick the vein or contaminate the catheter with your fingers. Using a steady direct motion, penetrate the skin. Once through the skin, lower the catheter angle and turn the tip toward the vein along a parallel line of the vessel. With a steady motion, move the catheter tip into the vein. Once the vein is accessed, open the tourniquet or release the BP cuff. It is important to reduce the restriction on the venous flow to avoid any leakage back out through the puncture site. After the vein is accessed, securement and stabilization can proceed.

Securing the VAD

VAD stabilization and securement should be based on the type of VAD, its location, the condition of the skin, and the potential activity level of the patient.

When securing the catheter, pay special attention to the patient's skin. Do not use more adhesive materials than is necessary, especially on the skin of frail older adults. The use of an engineered catheter stabilization device should be considered to reduce the risk of accidental dislodgement and local complications. Tape does not adhere well to the catheter and has been found to be contaminated with pathogenic microorganisms. Use a skin barrier solution to protect the skin from the adhesive and dressing materials.

Skin barrier solution

The use of a skin barrier solution as a protective coating on the skin will place a barrier between the epidermis and the adhesive/dressing materials. These solutions are manufactured in many forms, although wipes or applicators allow the solution to be directed to the area under the adhesive device. The composition of these barrier solutions can be acrylates, polymers of organic and inorganic substances, or silicone. Solutions without alcohol may be preferred since alcohol can be irritating or cause pain with existing skin breaks or irritation. After the skin barrier solution is applied, it must be allowed to air-dry by evaporation. The liquid part of the barrier evaporates leaving a transparent, breathable, and protective barrier on the skin surface. This will reduce the possibility for skin irritation, dermatitis, itching, or skin tears.

Applying the dressing

The TSM dressing should be applied to the skin without stretching it. Place it flat against the skin, smoothing it down on all sides to eliminate gaps.

Visualize the site

The insertion site must remain visible at all times. Neither the method of stabilization nor the dressing should prevent you from seeing the puncture site, the vein pathway, and the surrounding area. For the fragile skin of older adults, folded gauze padding under the catheter hub may be helpful to protect the skin from rigid plastic areas. It's also more comfortable for the patient.

Rolled bandage material, with or without elastic properties, should not be used around a VAD site. These bandages prevent adequately seeing the site and can easily restrict blood flow through the extremity and/or fluid flow into the vein. For severe skin conditions requiring reduction of adhesives, a tubular gauze mesh is better than rolled bandages.

Administration

When administering I.V. fluids and medications to the older adult, there are several special considerations that the clinician needs to evaluate. The older adult may have several physiologic conditions or comorbidities, which may affect the volume or rate at which I.V. fluids may be administered. Patients with chronic diseases such as diabetes, kidney disease, liver disease, heart disease, hypertension, or congestive heart failure are at greater risk for complications from I.V. fluid or medication administration.

Too-rapid administration of I.V. fluids can result in the older adult experiencing fluid overload or speed shock. Fluid overload results from infusing more fluid volume than the body can assimilate while maintaining cardiac function. Speed shock results when I.V. medication is given too fast. (See *Chapter 2, Systemic complications of peripheral I.V. therapy,* page 111.)

The older adult may also develop different tolerances for I.V. medications based on multiple chronic conditions. Drug dosages and dosing intervals may need to be adjusted to accommodate the older adult's tolerances. The older adult has a lowered metabolism rate along with changing liver and kidney functioning. All these elements must be taken into account when providing I.V. therapy for the older adult.

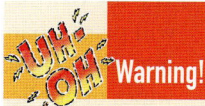

Don't go too fast with fluids

Older adult patients can develop heart failure if I.V. fluids are infused too rapidly. Therefore, use caution when administering I.V. fluids to replace fluid losses in these patients.

Controlling the flow

When administering I.V. therapy to the older adult patient, be sensitive to rapid variations of fluid volume and their effect on the patient. Keep in mind that the infusion of too much fluid at a too-rapid rate can trigger severe and often irreversible complications. (See *Don't go too fast with fluids,* page 406.)

Better safe than sorry

Regulation of fluid flow requires accuracy for the older adult. This can be achieved with an electronic infusion pump or other mechanical flow control devices such as elastomeric balloon pumps. (See *Chapter 1, Infusion flow rates*, page 32.) The specific care setting, type of medication, and patient risk factors must be considered when choosing a means of flow rate control. For instance, electronic infusion pumps are commonly used for all fluids and medications in an acute care setting. The administration set used in this pump would have an automatic device to stop the flow of fluids when the set is removed from the pump. For small volume intermittent medications given in the home, elastomeric balloon pumps may be sufficient to control the flow rate simply by the size of the opening where the set joins the fluid container. Make sure the administration set is long enough to provide adequate range of movement for the patient, but not so long that it drags on the floor and creates a fall hazard.

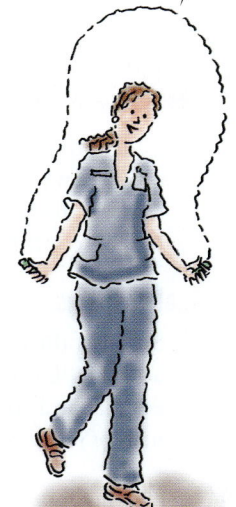

Use an electronic or mechanical flow device to control the flow rate of I.V. solution, and keep the administration set at a reasonable length to allow movement but prevent falls. Safety first!

Removing the catheter
It ain't over till it's over

Remove the peripheral catheter as soon as I.V. therapy is complete and the patient no longer needs I.V. access for their plan of care. This helps decrease the risk of all complications especially in the older adult patients. The current standard of practice is to change all short peripheral catheters based on clinical indications rather than a set time intervals, although some facilities may still have policies to change the catheter at 72 or 96 hours. Clinical indications include any sign or symptom of any complication. When a patient complains of pain or tenderness at the site, it is time for that catheter to be removed, regardless of how long it has been in place.

A little TLC won't hurt

Catheter removal can be difficult, especially when the skin is very thin. Follow the manufacturer's directions for removal of all stabilization devices and dressings.

Removing a TSM dressing can be done in several ways. Always pay close attention to holding the VAD while removing the TSM dressing to prevent dislodgment.
- Peel the dressing off by pulling parallel to the skin rather than pulling straight up from the edge at a 90-degree angle.
- Grasp one side of the TSM and pull outward to release the adhesive.
- Use an adhesive remover, gently working from one corner to peel the TSM dressing away from the skin.

Adhesive Removers

There are three categories of adhesive removers: alcohol-organic based, oil based, or silicone based. Alcohol-organic removers contain some hydrocarbon element or a petroleum distillate. Both of these have some types of toxicities. Oil-based removers may be made of mineral oil, petroleum, or citrus components. These solutions are very useful in removing adhesive residue; however, once they have been used at a site, another dressing cannot be placed in the same location immediately as the oil will prevent any adhesion. Consequently, this type cannot be used at sites where a dressing change is performed weekly (that is, PICC). Finally, silicone-based removers work to loosen the adhesion of the dressing or stabilization device; it evaporates readily and does not leave a residue.

Checking for complications

Older adults are extremely sensitive to the complications of I.V. therapy. Changes in metabolic systems, fluid and electrolyte imbalances, chronic disease, malnutrition, and changes to the integumentary system all contribute to this sensitivity.

The usual suspects

Some of the complications that are more likely to occur in an older adult patient include phlebitis, infiltration, extravasation, pulmonary edema, and speed shock. (See *Chapter 2, Local and systemic complications of peripheral I.V. therapy*, page 107.)

Can't feel the pain

Be aware that older patients may have a diminished pain sensation, especially in their hands and extremities. As a result, they may be unable to feel the pain caused by phlebitis and infiltration/extravasation of I.V. fluid. Frequency of site assessment of the peripheral I.V. infusion depends on many factors. Follow these recommendations to enhance patient safety:
- every 4 hours when nonvesicant fluid and medications are infusing in an alert and oriented patient
- every 1 to 2 hours in patients with cognitive deficits and sensory changes in the extremity, those receiving any sedative medication, or when the catheter must be placed in an area of joint flexion.
- every 5 to 10 minutes when a vesicant medication is infusing through a peripheral vein.

Assess the integrity and functionality of the entire infusion system to ensure adequate connections and correct flow rate.

Assess the entire patient for signs and symptoms of systemic complications such as fluid overload, hypersensitivities, and adverse drug reactions on a frequent basis.

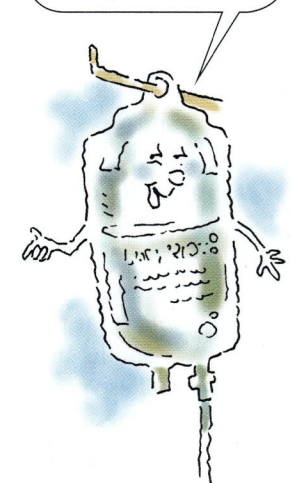

Older adults are more prone to phlebitis, but they can develop any of the usual complications of I.V. therapy, so assess for signs and symptoms often.

Patient teaching

When teaching an older adult about I.V. therapy, you need to tailor your approach to account for their different learning styles, abilities, and needs. To help ensure successful sessions, keep in mind how the aging process may affect their mental capacity, sensory perception, psychomotor function, hearing, and vision.

Mental capacity changes

A person's intellectual ability changes with age. Some factors of intelligence, such as those associated with experience and learning over time, increase with age. However, as degenerative processes occur, other mental processes decline, causing such changes as slowed processing time and slowed response time.

Have a chat

Talk to the patient and determine his previous experiences with I.V. therapy. Use this existing knowledge as a beginning for your teaching.

Older adults may need more time to process and react to information, especially when learning something new and complex. Modify your teaching sessions accordingly by:
- avoiding long explanations — keep it simple and short
- dividing your teaching into short segments of information
- providing plenty of time for the patient to review what you have said (allow extra time to answer your questions)
- repeating information if the patient seems confused or hesitant to answer questions.

Sensory losses

The ability to discriminate high-frequency sounds begins to diminish around age 60. Severe impairment can make the older adult feel isolated, suspicious, or even paranoid. The older adult may nod his head and agree with everything you say when you look like you're expecting a response.

Can you hear me now?

If the older adult speaks loudly or tilts his head when listening, assess for deafness. If he has a hearing aid, make sure he's wearing it and that it's turned on and functioning. Speak slowly, clearly, and in a normal tone while facing the individual. Do not raise your voice. Select a quiet room for teaching sessions.

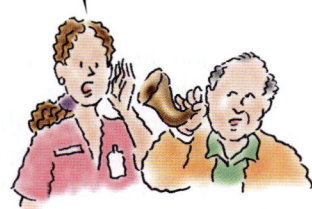

I said, "I think we'd better postpone the patient-teaching session until I can assess what's up with your hearing aid."

A bright idea

Impaired vision may prevent the patient from being able to read any patient-teaching handouts you give him, so take time to read the information with him if necessary. If possible, provide large-print handouts. Make sure that reading lights are properly placed and that they supply bright but diffused light.

More info, please!

Whenever possible, use the opportunity to teach the older adult patient about his infusion therapy and to answer any questions he may have. Being informed and receiving regular updates about his treatment will help foster his sense of control over his environment and situation.

End-of-life issues

Infusion therapy at the end of life raises many questions that have not been adequately addressed by clinical studies. This could involve starting infusions to prevent or treat fluid volume deficits or stopping infusions when it appears necessary. The entire health care team must carefully consider the patient's wishes, working collaboratively with the patient and/or legal surrogates. Comfort of the patient is the paramount concern. Fluid volume deficits may cause discomfort from dry oral mucous membranes, although this may be managed by local oral hygiene or other means. Administration of fluids may promote discomfort through accumulation of excess fluid in lungs, abdomen, or extremities. Additionally, the need for medications to control pain must be considered. If pain cannot be controlled by oral, transcutaneous, or other routes, the I.V. route may be the best option. The decision for each older adult should be based on their desires while promoting the greatest amount of comfort and the least risk of adverse reactions.

Documentation

Documentation of I.V. therapy for older adult is the same as for younger ones. In your nurse's notes or on the appropriate I.V. sheets, record the date and time of the venipuncture; the type, gauge, and length of the cannula; the specific anatomic location of the insertion site; the length of the catheter; and, if applicable, the reason the infusion site was changed. Also document the number of attempts at venipuncture (if you made more than one), the type and flow rate of the infusion solution, the name and amount of medication in the solution (if any), any adverse reactions and actions taken to correct them, patient teaching and evidence of patient understanding, and your initials.

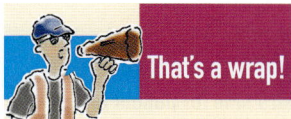

That's a wrap!

I.V. therapy for the older adult review

Physiologic changes associated with aging
Loss of some body cells, reduced metabolism, and other changes including:

Skin, hair, and nails
- Subcutaneous fat loss, dermal thinning, and decreased collagen
- Dry mucous membranes
- Decreased number and output of sweat glands
- Decreased elasticity
- Decreased vein thickness
- Decreased hair pigment, causing hair to turn gray or white; hair thinning
- Slowed nail growth, formation of longitudinal ridges; nails may also become thicker, brittle, and malformed
- Slowed wound healing
- Other possible skin conditions: senile keratosis, acrochordon, and senile angiomas

Eyes and vision
- Eyes sit deeper in the orbital socket.
- Eyelids lose their elasticity, becoming baggy and wrinkled.
- Tears diminish in quantity.
- Pupil shrinks and decreased light reaches the retina.
- Night vision and depth perception diminish.

Ears and hearing
- By age 60, most adults have difficulty hearing about 4,000 Hz. (Normal range for speech recognition is 500 to 2,000 Hz.)
- Many older adults have trouble distinguishing higher-pitched consonants (*s, sh, f, ph, ch, z, t,* and *g*).
- Vision and hearing changes should be considered when preparing patient teaching.

Respiratory system
- In the upper airway, the nose enlarges from continued cartilage growth, tonsils atrophy, and the trachea may be deviated.
- Anteroposterior chest diameter increases (may decrease chest wall mobility). Respiratory muscle degeneration and closing of some airways occur.
- Patient may have decreased maximum breathing capacity, forced vital capacity, and inspiratory reserve.

Cardiovascular system
- Heart size decreases.
- Heart muscle loses efficiency and contractile strength; fibrotic and sclerotic changes thicken heart valves, reducing their flexibility.
- Aorta grows more rigid, causing systolic blood pressure to rise proportionately more than diastolic blood pressure.
- By age 70, many people experience a 35% decrease in cardiac output at rest.

GI system
- Diminished mucosal elasticity and reduced GI secretions alter digestion and absorption.
- GI tract motility, lower esophageal sphincter tone, and abdominal muscle strength may decrease.

Hematologic and immune systems
- Less responsive to foreign antigens
- Increased risk for health care–acquired infections and time needed for healing

Fluid balance
- Fluid reserves become limited and the total amount of body water is decreased by 6%.
- Other factors contributing to fluid volume deficit: decreased saliva, decreased thirst mechanism, electrolyte imbalances, and increased urination.
- Patient requires frequent assessments for alterations in fluid volume.

Administering I.V. therapy
- Use same principles in selecting a site as for younger patients.
- Avoid using bruised areas and areas of flexion (particularly the hands).
- Review the length and type of treatment needed, and assess whether alternative access is required.
- Carefully palpate the patient's veins.

(continued)

I.V. therapy for the older adult review *(continued)*

- Tourniquet may not be necessary in many patients.
- Avoid veins that are thick and ropelike.
- Recommended skin antiseptic agents include disinfectants for cleaning the access site: alcoholic chlorhexidine gluconate, povidone-iodine, alcohol, and 2% tincture of iodine; apply antiseptic carefully and allow the area to dry completely before inserting the catheter.
- To stabilize the vein for insertion, stretch the skin below the insertion site and anchor it firmly with your nondominant hand.
- Perform venipunctures quickly and efficiently to avoid excessive bruising.
- A smaller gauge needle, such as 24-gauge ¾" needle, may be more appropriate and easier to insert.
- If a tourniquet is used, remove it promptly to prevent bleeding through the vein wall around the infusion device.
- Secure the catheter using an engineered stabilization device and transparent semipermeable dressing. Use a skin barrier solution and allow it to dry before securing the catheter.
- Keep the insertion site visible at all times, and insert gauze padding under the catheter to help protect skin and promote comfort.

Removing the catheter
- The same catheter can be left in place as long as no signs or symptoms of any complication are present, but it should be removed as soon as possible when treatment is completed.
- Removal can be difficult, especially when the skin is very thin.
- Be careful and use an adhesive remover to help reduce skin tearing.

Complications
- Most common complications include:
  - phlebitis
  - infiltration
  - extravasation
  - pulmonary edema
  - speed shock.
- Carefully assess I.V. insertion site with frequency determined by the characteristics of the fluid and the patient's ability to perceive and report discomfort.
- Assess for signs and symptoms of fluid overload, hypersensitivities, adverse drug reactions, and other complications on a frequent basis.

Patient teaching
- Keep in mind that older people may need more time to process and react to information, especially when learning something new and complex.
- Avoid giving long explanations, and divide sessions into short segments of information.
- Allow extra time for patient to comprehend what's been said and to answer questions; repeat information as necessary.
- If the patient speaks loudly or tilts his head when listening, assess for deafness.
- If the patient has a hearing aid, make sure he's wearing it and that it's turned on and functioning.
- Speak slowly, clearly, and in a normal tone; don't raise your voice.
- Hold teaching sessions in a quiet room.
- Read any patient-teaching handouts with the patient; if possible, provide large-print handouts.
- Make sure that reading lights are properly placed and supply bright, diffused light.

Documentation
Document the following:
- date and time of the venipuncture
- type, gauge, and length of the catheter
- anatomic location of the insertion site
- number of attempts at venipuncture
- type and flow rate of the I.V. solution
- name and amount of medication in the solution (if any)
- any adverse reactions and actions taken to correct them
- patient teaching and evidence of patient understanding
- your initials.

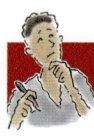

Quick quiz

1. Where should you measure skin turgor in an elderly patient?
    A. Forehead
    B. Forearm
    C. Abdomen
    D. Lower leg

Answer: A. Use the skin on the patient's forehead to test his skin turgor. This skin is less likely to have decreased elasticity.

2. The total body water in an older adult is decreased by:
    A. 3%.
    B. 6%.
    C. 9%.
    D. 12%.

Answer: B. As the body ages, its fluid reserves become limited and the total amount of body water is decreased by 6%.

3. Which skin change is characteristic of an elderly patient?
    A. Decreased amount of subcutaneous fat
    B. Thicker skin
    C. Increased elasticity
    D. Increased perspiration

Answer: A. As a person ages, his subcutaneous fat decreases and his skin tends to become thinner and less elastic. Perspiration usually decreases as well.

4. When teaching an older adult patient about I.V. therapy, which of the following considerations should you keep in mind?
    A. The patient probably won't want to know about his treatment.
    B. Patient teaching only needs to be done once.
    C. It's best to use only patient-teaching handouts.
    D. It's helpful to talk slowly and be prepared to repeat information.

Answer: D. Because of the potential for sensory losses associated with aging, it's best to talk slowly and clearly to the patient and repeat information as needed.

5. The physiological basis for disease in the older adult is:
    A. cardiac disease.
    B. chronic renal failure.
    C. chronic inflammation.
    D. pulmonary disease.

Answer: C. Chronic low-grade inflammation is thought to be the physiological cause of diseases in the older adult.

Scoring

⭐⭐⭐ If you answered all five questions correctly, brag all you want to your grandma! You're a first-generation older adult I.V. therapy whiz!

⭐⭐ If you answered three questions correctly, not too bad. Put on your reading glasses, brush up on your age-related physiological facts, and modify your study technique. You'll do fine next time.

⭐ If you answered fewer than three questions right, give yourself a break. You've only hit a few tiny wrinkles…nothing a little reviewing, tea, and retinol can't cure.

Suggested References

El Assar, M., Angulo, J., & Rodríguez-Mañas, L. (2013). Oxidative stress and vascular inflammation in aging. *Free Radical Biology and Medicine, 65,* 380–401.

Good, P., Richard, R., Syrmis, W., Jenkins-Marsh, S., & Stephens, J. (2014). Medically assisted nutrition for adult palliative care patients. *Cochrane Database of Systematic Reviews.* (4). Art. No. CD006274.

Gorski, L. A., Hallock, D., Kuehn, S. C., Morris, P., Russell, J. M., & Skala, L. C. (2012). Recommendations for frequency of assessment of the short peripheral catheter site. *Journal of Infusion Nursing, 35*(5), 290–292. doi:10.1097/NAN.0b013e318267f636.

Gorski, L., Hadaway, L., Hagle, M., McGoldrick, M., Orr, M., & Doellman, D. (2016). Infusion therapy standards of practice. *Journal of Infusion Nursing, 39*(1S), 159.

Levant, S., Chari, K., & DeFrances, C. J. (2015). Hospitalizations for patients aged 85 and over in the United States, 2000–2010. *NCHS Data Brief, 182,* 1–8.

Li, H., Manwani, B., & Leng, S. X. (2014). Frailty, inflammation, and immunity. *Aging and Disease, 2*(6), 466–473.

Lochner, K. A. (2013). Prevalence of multiple chronic conditions among Medicare beneficiaries, United States, 2010. *Preventing Chronic Disease, 10,* E61.

McNichol, L., Lund, C., Rosen, T., & Gray, M. (2013). Medical adhesives and patient safety: State of the science: consensus statements for the assessment, prevention, and treatment of adhesive-related skin injuries. *Journal of Wound, Ostomy, and Continence Nursing, 40*(4), 365–380; quiz E361–362. doi:10.1097/WON.0b013e3182995516.

Phillips, L., & Gorski, L. (2014). *Manual of I.V. therapeutics* (6th ed.). Philadelphia, PA: FA Davis.

Weinstein, S. M., & Hagle, M. (2014). *Plumer's principles and practice of infusion therapy* (9th ed.). Philadelphia, PA: Wolters Kluwer Health.

Appendices

▮	**Practice makes perfect**	**416**
▮	**Checklist for prevention of central line-associated bloodstream infections**	**434**
▮	**Glossary**	**436**

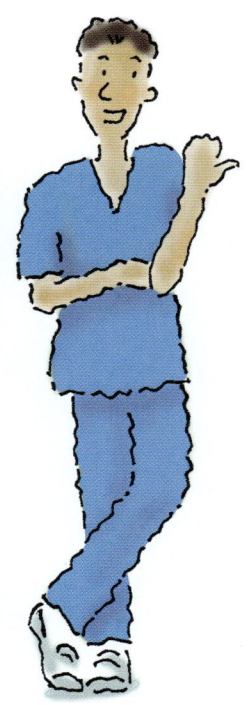

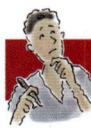

Practice makes perfect

1. An I.V. solution of dextrose 5% in half-normal saline solution is infusing on a postoperative patient. Which type of I.V. solution is the patient receiving?
    A. Isotonic
    B. Hypotonic
    C. Hypertonic
    D. Lactated

2. Thirst is caused by a decrease in intravascular volume triggered by receptors in the:
    A. hypothalamus.
    B. pituitary gland.
    C. adrenal gland.
    D. thyroid.

3. Which of the following electrolytes maintains cell electroneutrality?
    A. Sodium
    B. Magnesium
    C. Chloride
    D. Potassium

4. A 29-year-old patient with hepatitis is admitted to your unit with liver failure. Which type of I.V. solution may be difficult for the liver to metabolize?
    A. Lactated Ringer's solution
    B. Normal saline solution
    C. D_5W solution
    D. Parenteral nutrition

5. Which of the following statements about diffusion of solutes is accurate?
    A. They move from an area with a lower concentration to an area with a higher one.
    B. They ascend against the gradient of the concentration.
    C. They move from an area with a higher concentration to an area with a lower one.
    D. They move freely without regard to a gradient.

6. Fluid volume and concentration is regulated by the interaction of aldosterone and which other hormone?
    A. ADH
    B. TSH
    C. LSH
    D. FSH

7. Phosphorus is an electrolyte that's responsible for:
    A. maintaining cardiac muscle function.
    B. activating intracellular enzymes.
    C. maintaining serum osmolarity.
    D. maintaining bones and teeth.

8. A microdrip administration set delivers how many drops per milliliter?
    A. 10 gtt
    B. 20 gtt
    C. 60 gtt
    D. 80 gtt

9. Discharge is planned for your 47-year-old postoperative patient and you must remove the nontunneled CVAD from a subclavian site before discharge. Which patient position is required for this procedure?
    A. Sitting up in a chair
    B. Lying flat in the bed
    C. Lying on the side opposite the insertion site
    D. Lying in the bed with the head elevated 30 degrees

10. A 74-year-old patient is receiving an antibiotic through a secondary piggyback I.V. set on a gravity infusion. Which of the following devices prevents backflow of the secondary solution into the primary solution?
    A. Backcheck valve
    B. In-line filter
    C. Burette
    D. Volumetric pump

11. Your patient has a I.V. French PICC in the right upper arm and is receiving intermittent doses of Vancomycin every 12 hours. Immediately before starting the infusion, the most important step is to:
    A. observe the insertion site and ask the patient how it feels.
    B. connect the fluid container to a new administration set.
    C. set the rate of infusion on the infusion pump.
    D. assess patency by flushing with saline from a 10-mL syringe and aspirating for a blood return.

12. A 65-year-old patient with a history of abdominal aortic aneurysm resection and stage I.V. renal failure is admitted to the emergency department with dehydration. Which of the following conditions contraindicates insertion of an I.V. catheter into his arm?
    A. Dialysis fistula or graft
    B. Previous I.V. site
    C. Nondominant arm or hand
    D. Dominant arm or hand

13. Which layer of a vein acts to allow blood cells and platelets to flow smoothly?
   A. Tunica intima
   B. Tunica media
   C. Tunica adventitia
   D. Tunica externa

14. An 18-year-old patient is admitted to your unit with seizures, and the LIP orders the I.V. administration of phenytoin. He has an I.V. catheter in a vein of the antecubital fossa infusing dextrose 5% and 0.45% sodium chloride. Your plan for safe administration of phenytoin should include:
   A. use of an infusion pump to prevent infiltration.
   B. piggybacking the phenytoin to infuse through the infusing fluid.
   C. a new insertion site in the opposite forearm.
   D. ensuring that the fluid container is at least 4 feet above the venipuncture site.

15. What is the correct angle between the peripheral catheter and the skin for a peripheral venipuncture?
   A. 15- to 25-degree angle
   B. 30- to 40-degree angle
   C. 50- to 60-degree angle
   D. 70- to 80-degree angle

16. You are caring for a patient who underwent a left thoracotomy. He has I.V. fluids infusing through a CVAD in his right jugular vein. If the semipermeable transparent dressing remains intact, when should you change the dressing?
   A. Every shift
   B. Every day
   C. Every 2 days
   D. Every week

17. A 29-year-old patient is admitted to your unit after sustaining injuries in a motor vehicle accident. At the accident site, an 18-gauge catheter was inserted into the cephalic vein of his left lower forearm. When should this catheter be removed and another one inserted?
   A. When he complains of pain at the site
   B. At 72 hours
   C. At 96 hours
   D. As soon as the patient is stable

18. As you insert an I.V. catheter in your patient, he immediately complains of a sharp shock-like pain through his arm, most likely indicating:
   A. nerve damage.
   B. allergic reaction.
   C. systemic infection.
   D. infiltration.

19. A patient with acute pancreatitis requires a CVAD for parenteral nutrition administration. Which vein is the recommended tip location for this catheter?
    A. Lower superior vena cava
    B. Brachiocephalic vein
    C. Subclavian vein
    D. Internal jugular vein

20. A 29-year-old patient is admitted to your facility with penetrating injury to his foot from a metal object. After several days, he is not responding to the I.V. antibiotic and has an incision and drainage procedure with deep wound cultures. Three days later, wound cultures are positive for *Staphylococcus aureus* and a peripherally inserted central catheter (PICC) is inserted. One advantage of using a PICC is that it can be used:
    A. in patients with multiple previous venipunctures.
    B. in patients with scarring at the venipuncture site.
    C. to accomplish long-term access to central veins.
    D. without regard to the surgical site.

21. What is the maximum number of peripheral venipuncture attempts before collaboration with the LIP for a different type of vascular access?
    A. Six attempts by two clinicians
    B. Four attempts by two clinicians
    C. There is no limit
    D. Two attempts by two clinicians

22. Antineoplastic drugs are prepared:
    A. inside a biological safety cabinet by a pharmacist or nurse with special training.
    B. by the nurse at the patient's bedside after patient identification.
    C. in the medication room by the nurse.
    D. inside any type of laminar air flow workbench.

23. You assist the practitioner with insertion of a central venous access device and one of your primary tasks is:
    A. talking to the patient for distraction.
    B. choosing the insertion site.
    C. observing the entire procedure and completion of the checklist.
    D. flushing the catheter after it is inserted.

24. For a right or left subclavian vein insertion of a CVAD, in which position should the patient be placed?
    A. Semi-Fowler's
    B. Trendelenburg's
    C. Prone
    D. Left lateral

25. A 76-year-old male patient recovering from repair of a ruptured diverticulum has a CVAD in the right jugular vein with parenteral nutrition infusing. The dressing frequently becomes loose and has to be changed. What is the most appropriate action to take when applying the dressing?
    A. Angle the catheter along the length of the neck after shaving his beard.
    B. Loop the external catheter in a circle and secure it with sterile tape.
    C. Angle the external catheter toward the shoulder and use skin barrier solution.
    D. Use a gauze dressing and change it every 48 hours.

26. If the patient can't perform Valsalva's maneuver while you change the administration set or needleless connector of a CVAD, which of the following can serve as an alternative procedure?
    A. Ask the patient to perform pursed-lip breathing.
    B. Remove the cap during the inspiratory phase.
    C. Have the patient breathe normally.
    D. Clamp the external catheter and change the set or connector during the expiratory phase.

27. A 29-year-old patient who sustained a liver laceration in a motor vehicle accident has a CVAD recently inserted in the left subclavian vein. He calls you to his room with complaints of chest pain and shortness of breath. You note that he's cyanotic and diaphoretic. Which complication associated with CVAD insertion might this patient be experiencing?
    A. Pneumothorax
    B. Air embolism
    C. Thrombosis
    D. Fibrin sheath formation

28. A 37-year-old patient with acute leukemia has an implanted port in place. What type of needle should be used to access his implanted port?
    A. Winged infusion set
    B. Coring needle
    C. Noncoring safety needle
    D. Over-the-needle catheter

29. A 43-year-old patient with bladder cancer has an implanted port that will not produce a blood return on aspiration. When you flush with normal saline, she complains of a slight stinging sensation and you notice swelling in the subcutaneous tissue around the port. Which complication is she most likely experiencing?
    A. Fibrin sheath formation
    B. Chylothorax
    C. Thrombosis
    D. Infiltration

30. Which of the following are required when administering antineoplastic drugs? Check all that apply.
   A. Closed system drug transfer device
   B. Long-sleeved water-resistant gown with cuffs and a back closure
   C. Two pair of clean exam gloves
   D. Fit-tested respirator mask
   E. A paper gown commonly used for isolation patients
   F. Two pair of powder-free chemotherapy gloves
   G. Face shield or goggles

31. When administering a vesicant medication, you must check for a blood return:
   A. every hour during the infusion.
   B. before beginning the infusion.
   C. every 2 to 5 mL or every 5 to 10 minutes.
   D. every 15 mL or every 30 minutes.

32. Cytokine release syndrome is associated with:
   A. transfusion of packed red blood cells.
   B. cryoprecipitates and platelets.
   C. monoclonal antibodies.
   D. plasma proteins especially albumin.

33. The practitioner prescribes renal-dose dopamine for a patient with acute renal failure. To calculate the infusion rate, you must know the patient's weight in kilograms. Your patient weighs 186 lb. Which of the following operations will enable you to translate this weight to kilograms?
   A. Divide by 1.2
   B. Divide by 2.2
   C. Divide by 3.4
   D. Divide by 4.5

34. _____ is a common cause of skin damage in older adults that is prevented by using _____.
   A. Medical adhesive, skin barrier solution
   B. Bleeding, local pressure
   C. Infection, skin antiseptics
   D. Infection, gloves

35. You're infusing two antibiotics on a frail 92-year-old patient with very thin skin. Which techniques will reduce the risk for developing infiltration at the I.V. site?
   A. Site selection in the forearm and using a large gauge catheter
   B. Inserting a small gauge catheter in the forearm and using an engineered stabilization device
   C. Choosing a large vein of the antecubital fossa
   D. Infusion of all solutions through an infusion pump

36. An 82-year-old patient in a skilled nursing facility is dehydrated, has a history of heart failure, and very few venous access sites. A subcutaneous infusion of 5% dextrose and normal saline is prescribed. What is the maximum amount of fluid usually infused by this route in a 24-hour period?
   A. 500 mL
   B. 1,000 mL
   C. 1,500 mL
   D. 2,500 mL

37. What medication may be added to a subcutaneous infusion to increase its absorption?
   A. Gentamicin
   B. Cefazolin
   C. Alteplase
   D. Hyaluronidase

38. A patient is prescribed an I.V. antibiotic and I.V. fluids when admitted with a fever of unknown origin. You administer the antibiotic as a secondary piggyback infusion. The most accurate method of fluid flow control is:
   A. a roller clamp.
   B. an electronic infusion pump.
   C. a flow regulator.
   D. an elastomeric balloon pump.

39. A 2-year-old patient is receiving intermittent doses of cefazolin and tobramycin through a syringe pump. One advantage of using a syringe pump to administer medications is that it provides:
   A. the greatest control for large-volume infusions.
   B. the patient with control over his infusion.
   C. the greatest control for small-volume infusions.
   D. the greatest control for retrograde administration.

40. You received a report on a 65-year-old patient who recently underwent resection of an abdominal aortic aneurysm. The patient has lactated Ringer's solution infusing at 150 mL/hour. When you enter the patient's room to perform your assessment, you note that the patient is in respiratory distress. You check his blood pressure and find that it's elevated. You also note jugular vein distention. This patient is most likely experiencing:
   A. circulatory overload.
   B. hypersensitivity.
   C. systemic infection.
   D. a hemolytic reaction.

41. You note phlebitis at the I.V. site of a patient who has been receiving I.V. fluids for hydration over the past 3 days. The most appropriate nursing intervention is to:
  A. slow the infusion rate and contact the LIP.
  B. remove the catheter, apply warm compresses.
  C. apply a warm blanket to the extremity and continue to observe the site.
  D. apply a cold compress to the site and continue to monitor the patient complaints.

42. The most appropriate method for identifying healthy peripheral veins in all age groups is to:
  A. rely on use of a tourniquet.
  B. use the same finger to palpate for bouncy, resilient veins.
  C. see the vein as a blue line under the skin.
  D. apply heat to the extremity.

43. A patient is ordered a transfusion of 1 unit of packed red blood cells (RBCs) to treat a hemoglobin (Hb) level of 7.5 g/dl. As you administer the blood, you observe the patient closely, remembering that a hemolytic reaction can occur within:
  A. 5 minutes or 10 mL.
  B. 15 minutes or 50 mL.
  C. 30 minutes or 100 mL.
  D. 60 minutes or 250 mL.

44. A unit of "packed RBCs" is ordered for your 52-year-old patient. What is done to the unit of whole blood in the blood bank to create "packed RBCs"?
  A. Washing the blood to remove proteins
  B. Addition of a preservative solution
  C. Removal of 200 to 225 mL of plasma
  D. Addition of normal saline to the unit

45. An 88-year-old patient who underwent internal fixation of a fractured hip 3 days ago now has a hemoglobin level of 7.8 g/dl. The practitioner prescribes 2 units of packed red blood cells (RBCs) to run over 4 hours each. Before obtaining the unit of blood from the blood bank, you should:
  A. check the current I.V. site, prime the blood set, and piggyback it into the existing infusion.
  B. prime the blood set with normal saline solution and attach this set directly to the primary I.V. site after assessing it for complications.
  C. hang dextrose 5% in water as a piggyback infusion through a secondary I.V. set.
  D. check the size of the peripheral catheter ensuring that it is an 18 gauge.

46. You're administering a unit of packed red blood cells (RBCs) to a patient with excessive blood loss from a motor vehicle accident, but the infusion is running slowly. You need to use a pressure bag to speed up the rate. As you pump up the pressure bag, you should keep in mind that the cuff pressure should never exceed:
    A. 100 mm Hg.
    B. 150 mm Hg.
    C. 200 mm Hg.
    D. 300 mm Hg.

47. A patient with hemophilia A is admitted with bleeding after falling off his bicycle. Which factor, known as the *antihemophilic factor*, should be administered to this patient to control bleeding?
    A. Factor VII
    B. Factor VIII
    C. Factor IX
    D. Factor X

48. A 42-year-old patient with upper GI bleeding and a history of alcohol abuse has a hemoglobin level of 7.2 g/dl and 4 units of packed RBCs are ordered. After the third unit of blood is transfused, he complains of nausea, muscle cramps in his legs, and tingling in his fingers. This reaction is most likely:
    A. hypocalcemia from the citrate in the added preservative agents.
    B. hyperkalemia from hemolyzed red blood cells.
    C. transfusion-associated circulation overload
    D. hypothermia because of the cold blood

49. Which complication may occur as a result of the accumulation of an iron-containing pigment in a patient who received multiple transfusions?
    A. Hypothermia
    B. Potassium intoxication
    C. Hemosiderosis
    D. Hyperthermia

50. Which of the following types of drugs can cause necrosis to subcutaneous tissue surrounding the vein?
    A. Irritants
    B. Vesicants
    C. Nonvesicants
    D. Nonirritants

51. A patient who received her first dose of antineoplastic drugs 16 hours ago develops nausea. Which type of nausea occurs within the first 24 hours of treatment?
    A. Anticipatory
    B. Acute
    C. Delayed
    D. Intermittent

52. When carbohydrates, fats, and proteins are metabolized by the body, they produce:
    A. energy.
    B. lactose.
    C. cations.
    D. anions.

53. A nutrition solution that can safely be infused through a peripheral vein has:
    A. osmolarity less than 900 mOsm/L.
    B. total daily volume of less than 2 L.
    C. glucose content of more than 10%.
    D. osmolarity of 1,200 mOsm/L or less.

54. Anthropometric measurements for nutritional assessment include:
    A. height, weight, and midarm circumference.
    B. serum transferrin level and triglyceride levels.
    C. blood pressure, heart rate, and respiratory rate.
    D. hemoglobin and hematocrit.

55. The use of a 1.2-µm filter is indicated for:
    A. packed red blood cells and platelets.
    B. all I.V. medication.
    C. total nutrient admixture and all fat emulsion.
    D. all peripheral parenteral nutrition.

56. Biologic agents are made from:
    A. laboratory-created chemicals.
    B. chemicals found in living plants.
    C. blood components and bacteria and viruses.
    D. chemicals discovered in living animals.

57. Normal human immune response depends upon:
    A. white blood cells, cytokines, and immunoglobulins.
    B. red blood cells, platelets, and stem cells.
    C. bone marrow and white blood cells.
    D. the skin actin as a barrier and serum proteins.

58. You are starting peripheral I.V. therapy on a 3-year-old patient. In what order should you proceed with the following tasks?
    A. Select the catheter insertion site.
    B. Assemble and prepare supplies and equipment.
    C. Explain the procedure to the patient and family.
    D. Document catheter insertion and fluids and medications started.
    E. Check the LIP order.

59. Which type of biologic agents can be given by subcutaneous infusion?
    A. Immunoglobulins
    B. Interleukins
    C. Cytokines
    D. Colony-stimulating factors

60. Immunoglobulins are manufactured by:
    A. centrifuge of multiple units of packed RBCs.
    B. pooling proteins from 10 units of fresh frozen plasma.
    C. pooling 60,000 units of human plasma.
    D. allowing RBCs to settle from whole blood and drawing them off.

61. Which drug administration route is most effective for quickly achieving therapeutic levels?
    A. Subcutaneous
    B. Intramuscular (I.M.)
    C. Oral
    D. Intravenous (I.V.)

62. Which of the following are examples of a colloid solution?
    A. Albumin and dextran
    B. Ringer's lactate and normal saline
    C. Any dextrose solution
    D. Parenteral nutritional solution

63. An electronic infusion pump does NOT have alarms that will detect:
    A. air in the line.
    B. infiltration.
    C. occlusion.
    D. infusion complete.

64. Your patient is receiving a slow infusion of dopamine, a known vesicant medication, through a peripheral catheter and regulated on an infusion pump. To reduce the risk of extravasation, the I.V. catheter should be inserted in a:
    A. large vein of the forearm.
    B. large vein of the antecubital fossa.
    C. any vein of the hand.
    D. vein above the antecubital fossa.

65. You assess the peripheral site for the dopamine infusion and find there is no blood return when you aspirate from the catheter. Your first step is to:
    A. attempt slow aspiration with a smaller syringe.
    B. stop the infusion immediately.
    C. check the blood pressure and notify the LIP.
    D. ask the patient how the I.V. site feels.

66. Citrate toxicity is most likely to cause which imbalance?
    A. Hypercalcemia
    B. Hypocalcemia
    C. Potassium intoxication
    D. Hemosiderosis

67. How quickly can a transfusion reaction occur after the start of the infusion?
    A. 15 minutes
    B. 20 minutes
    C. 30 minutes
    D. 60 minutes

68. What is the smallest catheter size that can be used for transfusing blood?
    A. 18 gauge
    B. 20 gauge
    C. 22 gauge
    D. 24 gauge

69. Blood return should be:
    A. omitted from your assessment of a peripheral catheter because most will not produce blood upon aspiration.
    B. performed only when the patient complains of pain at the VAD site.
    C. aspirated from all CVADs at least daily.
    D. considered part of the assessment for all peripheral and central VADs before each infusion.

70. You notice that a patient who has been receiving an I.V. infusion of 5% dextrose and 0.45% sodium chloride is developing phlebitis at the I.V. insertion site. Which of the following nursing interventions should be implemented? Select all that apply in the correct sequence.
    A. Stop the infusion and remove the catheter.
    B. Apply warm compress.
    C. Apply ice packs.
    D. Assess for all signs and symptoms and assign a grade of phlebitis.
    E. If peripheral infusion is still needed, insert a new I.V. catheter at a new site.
    F. Raise the solution container.
    G. Assess oral intake and anticipated length of therapy remaining.
    H. Contact the LIP if your assessment indicates there could be a change in infusion needs.

71. You detect signs and symptoms of an acute transfusion reaction in a patient who has been receiving packed red blood cells (RBCs). Put the following nursing interventions in order of priority for treating this reaction.
    A. Infuse normal saline solution through a new administration set.
    B. Check vital signs including blood pressure, pulse, respirations, and temperature.
    C. Stop the transfusion.
    D. Notify the LIP.

72. To minimize the risk of a hemolytic reaction during a blood transfusion, recipient and donor blood must be thoroughly checked. Select all the facts that must be compared by two clinicians.
    A. Recipient name and identification number
    B. Recipient room number
    C. Blood component identification number
    D. Type and Rh of blood
    E. Hemoglobin and hematocrit
    F. Platelet count

Answers

1. C. Dextrose 5% in half-normal saline solution is a hypertonic I.V. solution.

2. A. Hypothalamus

3. D. Potassium maintains cell electroneutrality.

4. A. Lactated Ringer's solution should be avoided in patients with liver disease because the liver may not be able to metabolize the lactate contained in this solution.

5. C. In diffusion, solutes move from an area with a higher concentration to an area with a lower concentration.

6. A. Fluid volume and concentration is regulated by the interaction of two hormones: ADH and aldosterone.

7. D. Phosphorus is an electrolyte that's responsible for maintaining bones and teeth.

8. C. Microdrip tubing delivers 60 gtt/mL.

9. B. To prevent air embolism after the catheter is withdrawn from the vein, the patient must be lying flat so that the exit site is at or above the level of the heart.

10. A. A backcheck valve prevents backflow of the secondary solution into the primary solution.

11. D. Before each infusion, the VAD must be assessed for patency by flushing to observe for resistance and by aspirating for a blood return.

12. A. Never insert a catheter into the same arm where a dialysis fistula or graft is placed.

13. A. The tunica intima allows blood cells and platelets to flow smoothly.

14. C. Phenytoin is a vesicant and I.V. site in any joint should be avoided.

15. A. Place the bevel up and insert the catheter into the skin at a 15- to 25-degree angle to the vein.

16. D. Unless the dressing is compromised, a transparent semipermeable I.V. dressing should be changed weekly.

17. D. Any VAD inserted under emergent conditions do not allow for complete aseptic technique, and those catheters should be removed and a new one inserted as soon as the patient is stable.

18. A. Shock-like pain going in either direction on the arm indicates nerve damage due to direct needle to nerve contact and requires immediate removal of that catheter.

19. A. All CVADs should have the tip located in the lower segment of the superior vena cava near the junction with the right atrium.

20. C. A PICC provides long-term central venous access.

21. B. A maximum of 4 attempts, 2 each by 2 different clinicians. After this, a different plan for vascular access should be made which may include ultrasound-guided peripheral catheter, a midline or a PICC, or some other type of CVAD depending upon the complete assessment of the patient and needed infusion therapy.

22. A. A biological safety cabinet is required for preparing all antineoplastic agents and other hazardous drugs as this type of laminar air flow workbench has filtered air and special ventilation to prevent the preparer from contacting the drug.

23. C. During insertion of a central venous access device, the assistant observes every step and completes the checklist to ensure that all steps have been correctly performed. The assistant should be empowered to stop the procedure if a step is missed or contamination occurs.

24. B. The patient should be placed in Trendelenburg's position before insertion of a subclavian or internal jugular vein central venous access device. This position enlarges the veins but more importantly it aids in prevention of a venous air embolism.

25. C. Gently angle the catheter toward the shoulder to reduce the change of neck motion disturbing the dressing. Apply skin barrier solution to protect the skin integrity and to ensure that the dressing adheres better to the skin.

26. D. If the patient can't perform Valsalva's maneuver, close the clamp on the external catheter segment and replace the set or needleless connector during the expiratory phase of the respiratory cycle.

27. A. Chest pain, dyspnea, and cyanosis, along with decreased breath sounds on the affected side, may indicate pneumothorax, hemothorax, chylothorax, or hydrothorax.

28. C. To avoid damaging the port's silicone rubber septum, a noncoring needle should be used. To reduce accidental needlesticks when the needle is removed, that needle must have a safety mechanism on it.

29. D. Any type of discomfort and swelling of the subcutaneous tissue are signs of fluid leaking into the tissue. Since you are only injecting normal saline, this would be an infiltration. If the solution you administered was a vesicant, it would be an extravasation.

30. A, B, D, F, and G are all required for administration of antineoplastic drugs as they are considered to be hazardous.

31. C. When giving a vesicant medication by I.V. push, aspiration is required every 2 to 5 mL. When giving a vesicant by infusion, aspiration should be every 5 to 10 minutes.

32. C. Monoclonal antibodies are most frequently associated with cytokine release syndrome.

33. B. To convert a patient's body weight from pounds to kilograms, divide the number of pounds by 2.2 because 2.2 lb is equal to 1 kg.

34. A. Medical adhesives can cause skin damage in the older adult, and it is prevented by using skin barrier solution.

35. B. Small gauge catheters and an engineered stabilization device will reduce the risk of catheter movement, leading to infiltration.

36. C. 1,500 mL in a 24-hour period for most subcutaneous infusion sites.

37. D. Hyaluronidase is an enzyme that encourages subcutaneous fluid to move into the intravascular space.

38. B. An electronic infusion pump that has an accuracy rating of +/−5%.

39. C. An advantage of a syringe pump is that it provides the greatest control for small-volume infusions.

40. A. Jugular vein distention, respiratory distress, increased blood pressure, crackles, and positive fluid balance are signs of circulatory overload.

41. B. Remove the catheter and apply warm compresses.

42. B. Palpation with the same finger will encourage you to feel the resilience and bouncy feeling of the healthy vein.

43. B. A hemolytic reaction can occur with as little as 15 minutes or 50 mL infused.

44. C. Plasma is removed from the whole blood to make "packed red blood cells."

45. B. Blood can only be given in combination with normal saline. The blood administration set primed with normal saline should be connected to the primary I.V. catheter as piggybacking could involve contact with dextrose solution.

46. D. Don't allow the cuff to exceed 300 mm Hg because excessively high pressure can cause hemolysis and may damage the component container or rupture the blood bag.

47. B. Factor VIII, also referred to as *antihemophilic factor*, can be used to treat a patient with hemophilia A, to control bleeding associated with factor VIII deficiency, and to replace fibrinogen or factor VIII.

48. A. Signs and symptoms of hypocalcemia are produced because the citrate in the blood preservative solution binds to the serum calcium and reduces it.

49. C. Hemosiderosis is caused by accumulation of an iron-containing pigment called *hemosiderin* and may be associated with red blood cell destruction in a patient who has received many transfusions.

50. B. Vesicants can cause a reaction so severe that blisters form and tissue is damaged or destroyed.

51. B. Acute nausea and vomiting occur within the first 24 hours of treatment.

52. A. When carbohydrates, fats, and proteins are metabolized by the body, they produce energy.

53. A. Peripheral veins do not tolerate osmolarity of any infusing solution greater than 900 mOsm/L.

54. A. Height, weight, and midarm circumference are examples of anthropometric measurements.

55. C. A 1.2-μm filter is needed for infusion of all fat emulsion regardless of whether it is mixed in a total nutrient admixture or piggybacked into other nutrition solution.

56. C. Biological agents have this name because they are made from components of human blood or living bacteria or viruses.

57. A. WBC, cytokines, and immunoglobulins produce the immune response.

58. E, B, C, A, D. The correct sequence of events when initiating I.V. therapy in a 3-year-old is to first check the LIP order, assemble supplies needed and prepare equipment, then explain the procedure to the patient and family, select the site, and finally document the procedure.

59. A. Several brands of immunoglobulins can be infused into the subcutaneous area.

60. C. 60,000 units of human plasma are needed to manufacture a dose of immunoglobulin, thus requiring strict guidelines for collection of donated blood.

61. D. Unlike drugs that are administered orally, which take time to pass through and be absorbed by the GI system, drugs administered I.V. reach systemic circulation immediately. Because of the complexity of the musculoskeletal and integumentary systems, subcutaneous and I.M. drug administration absorption time may be slower.

62. A. Albumin and dextran are colloids, also known as plasma volume expanders.

63. B. Alarms on an electronic infusion pump will NOT detect an infiltration.

64. A. Veins of the forearm are naturally splinted by the bones of the arm and not effected by joint movement.

65. A. Changing to a smaller syringe for aspiration will produce less pressure and may yield a blood return. A larger syringe can be pulled harder and faster and this may occlude the backflow of blood.

66. B. Citrate, a preservative used in blood, binds with calcium, which causes a calcium deficiency (hypocalcemia).

67. A. Signs and symptoms of a transfusion reaction can appear within 15 minutes of the start of the transfusion. Assess and monitor the patient closely according to the patient's transfusion history and your facility's policy.

68. D. A 24-gauge catheter can be used for blood transfusion.

69. D. A blood return is a significant part of the complete assessment for patency on all VADs, both peripheral and central.

70. A, B, D, G, H, E. When phlebitis is suspected, the appropriate order of nursing interventions should be to stop the infusion, apply warm packs, and assign a grade based on the signs and symptoms. Then you should assess the oral intake and possible length of time the I.V. fluids will be needed and contact the LIP if your assessment indicates that the infusion therapy may require a different type of VAD or if it could be discontinued with adequate oral intake.

71. C, B, A, D. To remember the priority of nursing interventions for a transfusion reaction, think of the acronym SPIN: Stop the infusion, Pulse should be assessed, Infuse normal saline solution, and Notify the practitioner.

72. A, C, D. Comparison of all identification numbers for the patient, the unit of blood and the type of blood is required by two clinicians. Assessing lab data such as hemoglobin level, hematocrit, and platelet count are important tests for determining need for blood or blood plasma replacements, but they aren't indicators of compatibility.

Checklist for prevention of central line–associated bloodstream infections

Central Line Insertion Practices Adherence Monitoring

Page 1 of 2
*required for saving

Facility ID: _____	Event #: _____
*Patient ID: _____	Social Security #: ___ ___ ___ - ___ ___ - ___ ___ ___ ___
Secondary ID: _____	Medicare #: _____
Patient Name, Last: _____ First: _____	Middle: _____
*Gender: ☐ F ☐ M ☐ Other	*Date of Birth: ___/___/_____ (mm/dd/yyyy)
Ethnicity (specify): _____	Race (specify): _____

*Event Type: CLIP   *Location: _____   *Date of Insertion: ___/___/_____ (mm/dd/yyyy)

*Person recording insertion practice data: ☐ Inserter   ☐ Observer

Central line inserter ID: _____   Name, Last: _____   First: _____

*Occupation of inserter:

☐ Fellow   ☐ Medical student   ☐ Other student   ☐ Other medical staff
☐ Physician assistant   ☐ Attending physician   ☐ Intern/resident   ☐ Registered nurse
☐ Advanced practice nurse   ☐ Other (specify): _____

*Was inserter a member of PICC/IV Team?   ☐ Y   ☐ N

*Reason for insertion:

☐ New indication for central line (e.g., hemodynamic monitoring, fluid/medication administration, etc.)
☐ Replace malfunctioning central line
☐ Suspected central line-associated infection
☐ Other (specify): _____

If Suspected central line-associated infection, was the central line exchanged over a guidewire?   ☐ Y   ☐ N

*Inserter performed hand hygiene prior to central line insertion: ☐ Y   ☐ N   (if not observed directly, ask inserter)

*Maximal sterile barriers used: Mask ☐ Y ☐ N   Sterile gown ☐ Y ☐ N
                                  Large sterile drape ☐ Y ☐ N   Sterile gloves ☐ Y ☐ N   Cap ☐ Y ☐ N

*Skin preparation (check all that apply)   ☐ Chlorhexidine gluconate   ☐ Povidone iodine   ☐ Alcohol
                                           ☐ Other (specify): _____

If skin prep choice was <u>not</u> chlorhexidine, was there a contraindication to chlorhexidine?   ☐ Y   ☐ N   ☐ U

If there was a contraindication to chlorhexidine, indicate the type of contraindication:

☐ Patient is less than 2 months of age - chlorhexidine is to be used with caution in patients less than 2 months of age
☐ Patient has a documented/known allergy/reaction to CHG based products that would preclude its use
☐ Facility restrictions or safety concerns for CHG use in premature infants precludes its use

*Was skin prep agent completely dry at time of first skin puncture?   ☐ Y   ☐ N   (if not observed directly, ask inserter)

*Insertion site: ☐ Femoral   ☐ Jugular   ☐ Lower extremity   ☐ Scalp   ☐ Subclavian   ☐ Umbilical   ☐ Upper extremity

Antimicrobial coated catheter used: ☐ Y   ☐ N

Assurance of Confidentiality: The voluntarily provided information obtained in this surveillance system that would permit identification of any individual collected with a guarantee that it will be held in strict confidence, will be used only for the purposes stated, and will not otherwise be disclosed or released without the consent of the individual, or the institution in accordance with Sections 304, 306 and 308(d) of the Public Health Service Act (42 USC 242b, 242k, and 242m(d)). Public reporting burden of this collection of information is estimated to average 5 minutes per response, including the time for reviewing instructions, searching existing data sources, gathering and maintaining the data needed, and completing and reviewing the collection of information. An agency may not conduct or sponsor, and a

or any other aspect of this collection of information, including suggestions for reducing this burden to CDC, Reports Clearance Officer, 1600 Clifton Rd., MS D-74, Atlanta, GA 30333, ATTN: PRA (0920-0666).
CDC 57.125 (Front) Rev 5, v8.5

Central Line Insertion Practices Adherence Monitoring

*Central line catheter type:

- ☐ Non-tunneled (other than dialysis)
- ☐ Tunneled (other than dialysis)
- ☐ Dialysis non-tunneled
- ☐ Dialysis tunneled
- ☐ PICC
- ☐ Umbilical
- ☐ Other (specify): _____

("Other" should not specify brand names or number of lumens; most lines can be categorized accurately by selecting from options provided.)

*Did this insertion attempt result in a successful central line placement?   ☐ Y   ☐ N

Custom Fields

Label _____ ___/___/___

Label _____ ___/___/___

Comments

CDC 57.125 (Back) Rev 5, v8.5

Glossary

active transport: movement of solutes from an area of lower concentration to one of higher concentration (the solutes are said to move against the concentration gradient).

administration set: a set of plastic hollow tubing extending from the fluid container to the VAD hub; basic components include a spike, drip chamber, injection ports, male Luer-locking connection, and a roller clamp for manual flow control.

aerosolization: the process of dispersing small particles, usually in the form of a fine mist, into the air; a beneficial process for delivery of some medications but increases exposure to hazardous drugs not intended to be delivered by this method.

air embolism: a systemic complication of I.V. therapy that occurs when air is introduced into the venous system; signs and symptoms include respiratory distress, unequal breath sounds, weak pulse, increased central venous pressure, decreased blood pressure, and loss of consciousness.

albumin: a protein that can't pass through capillary walls and that draws water into the capillaries by osmosis.

aldosterone: a hormone secreted by the adrenal cortex that regulates sodium reabsorption by the kidneys (the renin-angiotensin system responds to decreased blood flow and decreased blood pressure to stimulate aldosterone secretion).

alopecia: hair loss that's partial or complete, local or general; with antineoplastic agents, it is caused by the destruction of rapidly dividing cells in the hair shaft or root.

anaphylactic reaction (anaphylaxis): severe allergic reaction that may include flushing, chills, anxiety, agitation, generalized itching, palpitations, paresthesia, throbbing in the ears, wheezing, coughing, seizures, and cardiac arrest; caused by release of histamine from mast cells and basophils.

anthropometry: an objective, noninvasive method of measuring overall body size, composition, and specific body parts that compares the patient's measurements with established standards (commonly used anthropometric measurements include height, weight, ideal body weight, body frame size, skinfold thickness, midarm circumference, and midarm muscle circumference).

antibody: an immunoglobulin molecule synthesized in response to a specific antigen.

antidiuretic hormone (ADH): a hormone produced in the hypothalamus and stored in the posterior pituitary gland that responds to osmolarity and blood pressure changes and also promotes water reabsorption by the kidneys.

antidote: a drug given to counteract the effects of another drug.

anti–free-flow device: a device built into the administration set used on an infusion pump; prevents inadvertent rapid infusion of fluids when the set is removed from the pump.

antigen: a foreign substance that can induce the formation of a corresponding antibody; subsequent exposure triggers an allergic reaction; also refers to naturally occurring antigens on the red blood cell used to identify blood type and does not provoke a reaction.

antineoplastic drugs: hazardous drugs used in precise doses to treat cancer; therapeutic action may or may not occur in a specific stage of the cell life cycle; may be commonly called "chemotherapy."

antiseptic agent: a solution that kills or inhibits the growth of organisms; applied to skin, wounds, or other tissue for infection prevention purposes.

arm board, also known as a hand board: a device used to stabilize joint motion when a peripheral I.V. cather must be placed in or near an area of joint flexion including the hand, wrist, antecubital fossa, or foot of an infant.

arteriovenous graft or fistula: a surgically created connection between an artery and vein for hemodialysis.

aseptic no touch technique: a framework of infection prevention practices that includes hand hygiene, appropriate use of gloves, maintenance of sterile components of administration sets and add-on devices (for example, areas originally under a cap), and appropriate methods to disinfect connection surfaces of needleless connectors.

aseptic technique: the major method of infection prevention when inserting all vascular access devices; requires absolute separation of sterile items from those that are not sterile and appropriate barrier precautions.

autoimmune disease: a variety of diseases characterized by inflammation where the immune system attacks healthy tissue.

backcheck valve: a device that stops flow from the primary fluid container, allowing a secondary piggybacked fluid to infuse; prevents backflow of a secondary solution into a primary administration set or fluid container; automatically opens to allow primary fluid flow after the secondary container is empty.

backpriming: the technique of allowing primary infusion fluids to backflow into an attached secondary set to wash residual fluid and air into the empty secondary container; a new secondary container with the next dose of medication is then attached and allowed to infuse. This method allows for repeated use of a single secondary set when all solutions are compatible, reducing the risk of contamination by frequent connection and disconnection of the secondary set.

bacteremia or bloodstream infection (BSI): the presence of bacteria in the bloodstream; signs and symptoms may range from none to those commonly associated with infection; may also lead to sepsis, a life-threatening condition.

beyond-use date (BUD): the date and time for disposal assigned when the drug is prepared for administration by opening packages and transferring to another container.

biologic therapy: agents created from human blood, bacteria, viruses, or other forms of biotechnology that stimulate, enhance, or suppress the human immune system; categorized in the same manner as naturally occurring cells of the immune system including interferons, interleukins, colony-stimulating factors, monoclonal antibodies, and immunoglobulins.

biological safety cabinet: an enclosed work space, with filtered air and special ventilation used for preparing hazardous drugs.

black box warning: the strictest warning placed in labeling of prescription drugs calling attention to a severe, life-threatening risk associated with the drug; FDA requires this information appear in a black box at the beginning of the document.

blood components: the individual components that make up whole blood and are available for transfusion therapy to correct specific blood deficiencies; includes packed red blood cells, fresh frozen plasma, platelets, cryoprecipitates, and granulocytes.

blood return: a significant component of a complete VAD assessment performed by aspirating from the VAD with an attached saline-filled syringe until blood appears in the external segment of the VAD; blood must be the color and consistency of whole blood; following this assessment, the blood is flushed back into the bloodstream without detaching the syringe.

blood type: a system for identifying the blood types using A, B, AB, and O; letters represent the presence of the antigens A, B, AB for both of these or O for neither that are carried on a person's red blood cells.

blood warmer: an electronic device with temperature control used to warm blood during massive or rapid transfusion.

body fluids: water and dissolved substances in the body (such as electrolytes) that help regulate body temperature, transport nutrients and gases throughout the body, carry wastes to excretion sites, and maintain cell shape.

body surface area: a person's size expressed in meter square (m^2) and based on accurate weight and height; used to calculate drug dosage.

bolus: rapid injection of a medication by manual push (over a few seconds or less than a minute) or rapid infusion of a specific amount of I.V. fluids (usually 15 to 30 minutes).

butterfly needle: common name for a metal needle with flexible wings and an attached extension set; most common use is for obtaining blood samples but may be used for a single medication injection.

cell cycle: the reproductive and resting phases through which every cell, normal and malignant, passes.

cellulitis: a bacterial infection of the skin and subcutaneous tissue; associated with VAD insertion when skin antisepsis is not adequate.

central vascular access device (CVAD): a catheter inserted through the veins of the upper extremity, subclavian, jugular, or femoral veins with the tip terminating in the superior vena cava or inferior vena cava near the cavoatrial junction; includes PICCs, nontunneled, tunneled cuffed, and implanted ports.

central venous pressure (CVP): an important indicator of circulatory function and the pumping ability of the right side of the heart; measured with a CVAD whose tip is placed at or near the right atrium.

chylothorax: puncture of a lymph node with leakage of lymph fluid.

circulatory overload: a large volume of fluid that the heart is incapable of pumping through the circulatory system; includes neck vein engorgement, respiratory distress, increased blood pressure, and crackles in the lungs.

closed system drug transfer (CSDT) device: a device used to administer hazardous drugs, which prevents environmental contamination from entering the solution and the escape of solution from the infusion system.

colloid osmotic pressure: the pulling force of proteins that draws fluid into the intravascular space.

compatibility in fluids and medications: the capability of the drug, diluent, and fluid container to be used successfully together without problems of adsorption, precipitate formation, or other physical and chemical changes to the solution.

compatibility in transfusion therapy: typing and cross-matching the donor and recipient blood to minimize the risk of a hemolytic reaction (the most important compatibility tests include ABO blood typing, Rh typing, cross-matching, direct antiglobulin test, and antibody screening test).

competency: the individual clinician's ability to perform job-related activities, usually assessed by the integration of activities in the work environment.

complement system: proteins found in the bloodstream that augments antibodies and other cells in removing organisms and damaged cells.

compounding: the act of combining, mixing, or altering ingredients of a drug; a process performed in the pharmacy meeting strict requirements from the United States Pharmacopeia.

continuous infusion: administration of infusion fluid constantly over a prolonged period through a peripheral or central vascular access device; used for medication infusion when a constant infusion is required to achieve therapeutic blood levels (for example, dopamine, heparin, epinephrine).

cyclic parenteral nutrition: delivery of the entire volume of daily nutrition solution during a limited number of hours, usually overnight, allowing the patient to be free from infusion during the daytime.

cytokine release syndrome (CRS): a reaction occurring during the infusion of biologic agents characterized by fever, chills, nausea, vomiting, hypotension, headache, and dyspnea.

cytokines: small proteins released by cells that allow communication between cells; includes interferon, interleukins, tumor necrosis factor, colony-stimulating factors, and chemokines.

cytotoxic therapy: destroys cancer cells or makes it difficult for cancer cells to grow and reproduce.

DEHP (Di[2-ethylhexyl] phthalate): a chemical used to make polyvinyl chloride soft and flexible but may leach into some solutions posing a risk to some patients.

diffusion: movement of solutes from an area of higher concentration to one of lower concentration by passive transport (a fluid movement process that requires no energy).

diluent: a liquid used to reconstitute I.V. drugs originally supplied in powder form; includes normal saline solution, sterile water for injection, dextrose 5% in water.

disinfectant: antimicrobial agents applied to surfaces of inanimate objects that kills all microorganisms except spores.

dislodgment: partial or complete inadvertent removal of a VAD; for a CVAD, this may result in suboptimal tip location requiring further assessment; see tip migration also.

distal: located away from the center of the body; usually refers to the patient's body; however, some product instructions for use are written using the design engineer as the reference point, resulting in the opposite location in the patient.

elastomeric balloon pump: a mechanical flow control device consisting of a balloon inside a hard plastic shell with a microbore infusion set attached; flow rate is controlled by the size of the opening where the set attaches to the balloon and infusion pressure is generated by the collapsing balloon.

electrolytes: salts and minerals that carry an electrical charge when dissolved in body fluids; necessary for the process of fluid balance and normal cell functioning; major electrolytes include sodium, potassium, calcium, chloride, phosphate, and magnesium.

expiration date: the date assigned by the manufacturer on the original and unopened drug packaging, identifying when the drug must be discarded.

extension set: tubing sets available in a variety of configurations including single or multiple lumens, microbore tubing, needleless injection ports, and slide clamp; placed between the I.V. administration set and the VAD hub to add more length, add additional injection ports, or provide a connection away from the VAD hub to reduce hub manipulation; required to have Luer-locking connections.

extracellular fluid (ECF): any fluid in the body that isn't contained inside the cells, including interstitial, intravascular, and transcellular fluids.

extravasation: infiltration or escape of vesicant fluids or medications into the tissue surrounding the vein resulting in tissue damage, which can include necrotic ulcers and nerve injury.

fat emulsion: in parenteral nutrition, a concentrated source of energy from a fat source and an emulsifying system: prevents or corrects fatty acid deficiencies; also known as lipids.

flare reaction: an inflammatory response to infusion of an irritant; a local venous response with or without accompanying visible signs; the patient may complain of burning, pain, aching along the vein, or itching; redness may appear surrounding the venipuncture site or along the vein path.

flow rate control devices: manual, mechanical, or electronic devices used to regulate the flow of fluid from the fluid container to the VAD; see flow regulator, roller clamp, elastomeric balloon pump, infusion pump.

flow regulator: a manual device integral to or added to an I.V. administration set used to control flow rate by adjusting a dial to the required milliliters per hour; accuracy is equal to a roller clamp and counting drops is required.

fluid balance: constant and approximately equal distribution of fluids between the intracellular and extracellular fluid compartments.

fluid container: a glass bottle, plastic bag, or syringe used to hold any infusion fluid.

fluid movement: the process that helps regulate fluid and electrolyte balance between the major fluid compartments and transports nutrients, waste products, and other substances into and out of cells, organs, and systems.

flushing: the process of manually injecting normal saline solution into the VAD directly or an injection port on the I.V. administration set for the purposes of assessing VAD functionality, clearing the locking solution left from the previous medication dose, or preventing contact between incompatible medications.

French scale: a system for labeling the diameter of a CVAD, measurement is obtained in millimeters and multiplied by 3 (for example, 9 French would have a diameter of 3 mm).

gauge: diameter of a needle or catheter with smaller numbers indicating a larger size.

gluconeogenesis: the conversion of noncarbohydrates such as protein into glucose for energy when the body's energy needs are not met.

glycogenolysis: in metabolism, the mobilization and conversion of glycogen to glucose in the body.

guidewire: a long flexible wire device advanced through a vein to guide VAD insertion.

hazardous drugs: drugs known to cause harm including changes in genetic materials, fetal defects, alternation in fertility, and cancer; all preparation and administration of drugs in this category requires specific methods for safe handling.

hematocrit: the percentage of red blood cells in whole blood.

hematoma: bruising resulting from bleeding in a specific area; symptoms include a raised dark area with accompanying tenderness; may appear at a venipuncture site during VAD insertion or removal when appropriate methods (that is, manual pressure) are not used to achieve hemostasis.

hemolytic reaction: a life-threatening reaction to blood transfusion that occurs as a result of incompatible ABO or Rh blood.

hemosiderosis: a form of iron overload that can be caused by frequent or multiple transfusions.

hemothorax: bleeding into the pleural cavity, a complication of CVAD insertion; treated with the insertion of a chest tube for draining blood.

heparin: an anticoagulant that prevents thrombi from growing larger but does not directly remove it.

human leukocyte antigen (HLA): antigen that's essential to immunity; part of the histocompatibility system, which controls compatibility between transplant or transfusion recipients and donors (generally, the closer the HLA match between donor and recipient, the less likely the tissue or organ will be rejected).

hydrothorax: infusion of a solution into the pleural cavity, a complication of CVAD insertion.

hyperglycemia: high blood glucose; a possible complication of parenteral nutrition.

hyperosmolar hyperglycemic state: a complication of parenteral nutrition caused by excessively high glucose levels resulting in dehydration, electrolyte imbalances, and coma.

hypersensitivity: a set of five types of reactions caused by the immune system, which includes allergy and anaphylaxis.

hypertonic solution: a solution with osmolarity (concentration) greater than 375 mOsm/L; includes dextrose 5% in 0.45% sodium chloride, dextrose 5% in 0.9% sodium chloride, and dextrose 5% in lactated Ringer's solution.

hypocalcemia: calcium deficiency; signs and symptoms include tingling in the fingers, muscle cramps, nausea, vomiting, hypotension, cardiac arrhythmias, and seizures.

hypoglycemia: low blood glucose; a possible complication of parenteral nutrition; signs and symptoms include sweating, shaking, and irritability.

hypokalemia: low blood potassium; signs and symptoms include muscle weakness, paralysis, paresthesia, and arrhythmias.

hypomagnesemia: low blood magnesium; patient may complain of tingling around the mouth or paresthesia in the fingers and may show signs of mental changes, hyperreflexia, tetany, and arrhythmias.

hypophosphatemia: low blood phosphates; patient may be irritable or weak and may have paresthesia; in extreme cases, coma and cardiac arrest can occur.

hypotonic solution: a solution with osmolarity (concentration) less than 250 mOsm/L; includes 0.45% sodium chloride, 0.33% sodium chloride, and dextrose 2.5% in water.

hypovolemic shock: shock due to loss of systemic volume; caused by internal bleeding, hemorrhage, or sepsis; signs and symptoms include increased heart rate, decreased blood pressure, mental confusion, and cool, clammy skin.

I.V. push: manual injection of a small quantity of medication by attaching a fluid-filled syringe and slowly pushing the medication into the infusion system.

immune response: the body's mechanism of defense that recognizes foreign substances (antigens) and provides a physical or chemical barrier to them or produces an antibody to the invader.

immunocompromise: having an impaired immune system, increasing the risk of infection; caused by many disease or injury states and aging.

immunodeficiency diseases: diseases characterized by missing or improperly functioning components of the immune system.

immunoglobulins: five antibodies (IgG, IgM, IgA, IgD, and IgE) manufactured by plasma cells as part of the immune system.

immunotherapy: methods and agents that create a hostile environment for the existence or growth of cancer in the body.

implanted port: a CVAD used when infusion needs are infrequent but long term; composed of a port body placed into a surgically created pocket under the skin and the attached catheter that is tunneled through subcutaneous tissue to either subclavian or internal jugular veins; the catheter tip should be placed in the lower superior vena cava near the cavoatrial junction; accessed with a specially designed, noncoring needle; may be placed into an artery, epidural space, peritoneum, or pericardial or pleural cavity.

incompatibility: an unwanted outcome when I.V. fluids or drugs are mixed together; includes physical and chemical changes to the solution.

independent double check: the process used before administration of designated I.V. drugs and procedures requiring two clinicians to perform separate dosage calculations and assessment of dilution, rate of administration or infusion pump settings; after independent assessments, comparison of results should verify accuracy.

inferior vena cava: a central vein that carries blood returning from the lower body back to the right atrium.

infiltration: escape of infusing solution or nonvesicant medications from the vein into surrounding tissues; tissue damage can occur from a large quantity of fluid that leads to compartment syndrome.

informed consent: voluntary agreement to a procedure or treatment following a thorough educational process resulting in knowledge and understanding of relevant information.

infusion pump: a device controlled by electricity or batteries that regulates the flow of I.V. solutions and drugs and provides the greatest level of flow rate accuracy; may be a large pole-mounted device or a small ambulatory device.

inline filter: a filter in the administration set that removes organisms, particulate matter, and air from the infusing fluids.

intermittent infusion: administration of a medication at set intervals for a shorter infusion period; includes manual injection, secondary piggyback into a continuous infusion or directly attached to the VAD hub.

interstitial fluid (ISF): extracellular fluid that bathes all cells in the body.

intracellular fluid (ICF): fluid that's contained inside the cells of the body.

intraosseous (IO) infusion: fluids, medication, or blood infused through a metal needle placed through a puncture site into the medullary cavity of a bone; used during emergency situations when a peripheral I.V. catheter cannot be rapidly inserted; may remain in place for only 24 hours.

intrathecal: within the spinal canal or brain, under the arachnoid membrane.

irritant: an agent that can produce burning, stinging, and pain due to irritation to the internal lining of the vein wall; may or may not produce external signs of inflammation (for example, redness, edema).

isotonic solution: a solution with osmolarity ranging from 250 to 375 mOsm/L, similar to intravascular fluids; includes lactated Ringer's solution and 0.9% sodium chloride solution.

licensed independent practitioner (LIP): any individual permitted by law and the organization's policy to provide care and services without direction or supervision; usually includes physicians, physician assistants, and advanced practice registered nurses depending upon state laws.

lipid emulsion: a solution of fats and an emulsifying system used as a major source of calories in parenteral nutrition, also called fat emulsion.

locking: the process of instilling a specific solution into the lumen of a VAD to reduce the risk of thrombotic lumen occlusion or to prevent or treat VAD-associated bloodstream infection; locking solutions include normal saline, heparin lock 10 units/mL, antibiotic and antiseptic solutions alone or in combination.

lock-out interval: a time set on a patient-controlled analgesia device during which the device can't be activated.

Luer-lock: the standard method of connecting all components of an infusion system together (that is, administration set, extension set, filters, VAD hub); composed of a plastic male tube inserted into the female opening with a collar that rotates to lock the two pieces together; national standards of practice requires the use of Luer-locking connections on all infusion systems to prevent accidental disconnection and associated complications such as venous air embolism.

lymphedema: swelling occurring in an extremity commonly caused by removal or surgical procedures to lymph nodes.

medical adhesive–related skin injury (MARSI): many forms of skin injury caused by the adhesive attaching more firmly to the skin surface than the skin cells are attached to each other; includes skin stripping, tears, irritant contact dermatitis, allergic dermatitis, skin maceration, and folliculitis.

micronutrients: in parenteral nutrition solutions, used to promote normal metabolism; also called *trace elements*; includes zinc, copper, chromium, iodide, selenium, and manganese.

midline catheter: a catheter inserted into the peripheral veins of the upper arm in adults with the tip lying level with the axilla or armpit; tip location should not be placed in the shoulder; tip location lies in a peripheral vein and should not be confused with a CVAD.

migration: movement of the tip of a CVAD from the original location into another vein; common locations for tip migration include the internal jugular or contralateral subclavian vein; there is no change in the external catheter length.

milliequivalents: the measurement of the chemical combining power of ions.

millimole: the atomic weight of a substance measured in grams.

mucositis: inflammation of the mucous membranes.

myelosuppression: the interference with and suppression of the blood-forming stem cells in the bone marrow; a possible complication of antineoplastic agents.

nadir: the lowest point in some series of measurements, such as white blood cell, hemoglobin, or platelet levels.

necrosis: tissue death.

needleless connector: a safety device placed on a VAD hub or injection site of an administration set used to allow connection of other administration sets and syringes without the use of needles; their use is required by OSHA in the United States to prevent accidental needlestick injuries and the risk of transmission of bloodborne diseases.

noncoring needle: a special needle with an angled or deflected point used to access an implanted port; tip deflection slices the septum on entry rather than coring it as a conventional needle does; also includes an attached extension set and a safety mechanism to house the needle upon removal.

nontunneled catheter: type of CVAD placed by a venipuncture made directly through the skin; insertion sites include the upper extremity, jugular, subclavian, and femoral sites in adults.

nutritional assessment: assessment of the relationship between nutrients consumed and energy expended, especially when illness or surgery compromises a patient's intake or alters his metabolic requirements; includes a dietary history, physical assessment, anthropometric measurements, and diagnostic tests.

occlusion: blockage that prevents the ability to infuse fluids or flush a VAD due to the accumulation of thrombus, fibrin, drug precipitates, or fat emulsion inside the VAD lumen; may be due to thrombosis inside the vein at or near the catheter tip; identifying the location of the occlusion cannot be done by clinical assessment alone.

osmolality: the concentration of a solution measured by weight and expressed as milliosmols per kilogram.

osmolarity: the concentration of a solution expressed in milliosmols of solute per liter of solution.

osmosis: the passive transport of fluid across a membrane from an area of lower concentration to one of higher concentration that stops when the solute concentrations are equal.

over-the-needle catheter: the most commonly used device for peripheral I.V. therapy, which consists of a plastic catheter, a metal needle (stylet), and a safety mechanism to prevent accidental needlesticks; the needle is removed during insertion, leaving the plastic catheter in place.

parenteral nutrition: provision of all nutritional needs by I.V. infusion through a CVAD when the patient cannot or should not eat; solutions include a patient-specific formula of protein, carbohydrates, fat emulsion, vitamins, and micronutrients; solutions with lower osmolarity meeting partial nutrition needs may be infused through peripheral veins.

parenteral: any route other than the GI tract by which drugs, nutrients, or other solutions may enter the body (for example, I.V., I.M., or subcutaneously).

Paresthesia: pain or other abnormal sensation such as tingling or an electrical shock-like feeling caused by nerve damage including direct needle to nerve contact and compression from fluid or blood in the tissue.

particulate matter: undissolved drug particles or precipitate, rubber stopper cores, glass particles, and plastic pieces found as very small unwanted components of infusion fluids or medications.

passive transport: fluid movement that requires no energy and in which solutes move from an area of higher concentration to one of lower concentration (this change is called *moving down the concentration gradient* and results in an equal distribution of solutes).

patency: the state of being freely open; a patent VAD will easily yield a blood return that is the color and consistency of whole blood and does not offer any resistance to a manual push of normal saline using a 10-mL size syringe.

patient-controlled analgesia (PCA): a pain management method that allows the patient to control I.V. delivery of an analgesic such as morphine to maintain therapeutic blood levels; employs a specialized infusion pump with a timing unit that delivers a single dose on demand.

peripheral parenteral nutrition (PPN): the delivery of nutrients meeting partial nutritional needs into a peripheral vein; formulation contains less dextrose, and the maximum osmolarity is recommended to not exceed 900 mOsm/L.

peripherally inserted central catheter (PICC): a central venous access device that's inserted through a vein of the upper extremity with the tip located in the superior vena cava at or near the cavoatrial junction; in pediatric patients, it may be inserted through veins of the lower extremities with the tip terminating in the inferior vena cava above the diaphragm; indicated for patients needing long term (that is, several weeks to months) of infusion therapy.

phlebitis: inflammation of the vein at or near the catheter site; a common complication of I.V. therapy; signs and symptoms include pain, redness (erythema) at the site and along the vein, edema, increased warmth at the site, induration, or hardness on palpation; caused by mechanical, chemical, and bacterial factors.

piggyback infusion: addition of a secondary I.V. administration set to an injection site on the primary I.V. set for the purpose of giving a compatible medication or solution.

plasma: the liquid component of blood, which makes up about half of the total blood volume.

platelets: cellular elements of blood that are infused to prevent or control bleeding; may be depleted in patients with hematologic disease or those receiving antineoplastic therapy.

pneumothorax: air in the pleural cavity; a complication of CVAD placement; signs and symptoms include chest pain, dyspnea, cyanosis, or decreased or absent breath sounds on the affected side (a thoracotomy should be performed and a chest tube inserted if pneumothorax is severe enough for intervention).

policy: the nonmodifiable written and approved rules of an organization; changes require official review and revision.

potassium intoxication: an increase in potassium levels after a transfusion that occurs because of blood cell maturation in stored blood components.

power injectable: the ability of a VAD or attached extension set or add-on devices to tolerate the pressure needed for rapid contrast injection during certain radiology procedures; all devices used for injection of contrast under pressure must be labeled as power injectable.

procedure: the step-by-step process required to accomplish a task or intervention.

protocol: a written description of components that address clinical decision-making for specific patient care issues (for example, preferred methods for giving a specific drug).

proximal: located near the center of the body, the opposite of distal.

refeeding syndrome: excessive provision of oral, enteral, or parenteral nutrition characterized by fluid and electrolyte imbalances.

rhesus (Rh) system: in blood physiology, a major blood antigen system that is expressed by the presence (Rh positive) or absence (Rh negative) of the D antigen.

roller clamp: a device used to manually regulate fluid flow; consists of a plastic housing that contains a round device that exerts pressure against the plastic tubing of the I.V. administration set; use requires manually counting drops and rolling the device to increase or decrease the flow rate; accuracy rating is usually ±25% and requires frequent assessment.

sarcopenia: loss of skeletal muscle mass and strength; a precursor to frailty in older adults.

sclerosis: the hardening of a tissue or vessel.

secondary set: a short I.V. set attached to the primary I.V. set; used for the administration of I.V. medication, also called *piggyback infusion set*.

sepsis: an overwhelming immune response to bacterial infection producing systemic inflammation and has the potential to cause damage to multiple vital organs.

site protectors: a ventilated plastic dome device placed over the VAD site to provide protection; used in pediatrics and others with any form of confusion.

skin barrier solution: a solution applied to the skin to add a protective layer between the skin and adhesive products.

"smart" pumps: an electronic infusion pump containing software that allows each organization to enter a drug library with set parameters for concentrations, dose limits, and advisory information.

speed shock: shock caused by too-rapid administration of an I.V. drug.

stability: the ability of a pharmacological preparation to maintain its strength and purity during storage, preparation, and administration.

stabilization device: an engineered device designed to secure and stabilize a VAD and prevent movement that leads to complications.

standard of care: statements about what the patient experience should be or the expected outcome of care.

standard of practice: statements about the acceptable level of performance for the clinician.

sterile: free from living organisms.

stomatitis: inflammation of the mouth usually associated with antineoplastic agents.

subcutaneous infusion: infusion of fluids and certain medications into the tissue underneath the skin.

superior vena cava: a large diameter central vein returning blood from the head, neck, and arms into the right atrium.

syringe pump: a type of infusion pump accommodating syringes of various sizes; used for giving small-volume intermittent I.V. medications or those requiring very slow infusion rates.

thrombocytopenia: blood platelet depletion.

thrombophlebitis: inflammation of the vein with formation of a blood clot.

thrombosis: the development of a thrombus (blood clot).

total nutrient admixture (TNA): mixture of all parenteral nutrition components in a single, 3-L bag; also called *3:1 solution* (protein, carbohydrates, and fat).

tourniquet: wide soft rubber band that encircles a limb and traps blood in the veins by applying enough pressure to impede the venous flow; use must be dedicated to a single patient only.

toxicity: the quality of being poisonous.

transcellular fluids: a form of extracellular fluid that includes cerebrospinal fluid, lymph, and fluids in such spaces as the pleural and abdominal cavities.

transfusion reaction: adverse reaction to blood transfusion, the most severe of which is a hemolytic reaction, which destroys red blood cells and may become life threatening; signs include fever, chills, rigors, headache, and nausea.

transfusion trigger: a hemoglobulin level and other conditions set by a organization's blood committee that would determine the clinical appropriateness of giving blood.

transparent semipermeable dressing: a plastic film with an adhesive backing placed over an insertion site and allows visibility of the site and surrounding area.

treatment cycle: a course of medications, usually antineoplastic or biologic agents used to treat cancer, given on a regular basis (that is, every 3 to 4 weeks).

Trendelenburg's position: position in which the head is low and the body and legs are on an inclined plane; used for CVAD insertion in the jugular and subclavian veins to distend veins and reduce the risk of venous air embolism.

tumor resistance: the ability of a tumor to withstand the effects of antineoplastic agents, either initially during treatment or developed after treatment.

tunneled cuffed CVAD: central venous catheter with a cuff encircling the catheter; a portion of the catheter containing the cuff is placed in a subcutaneous tunnel between the skin exit site and the vein entrance site; subcutaneous tissue grows into the cuff to anchor the catheter; indicated when infusion needs are frequent and long term (that is, several months to years); requires surgical insertion and resection of the cuff for removal.

universal donor: a person with group O negative blood, which lacks both A, B, and D antigens and can be transfused in limited amounts in an emergency to any patient, regardless of the recipient's blood type with little risk of adverse reaction.

universal recipient: a person with AB blood type, which may receive A, B, AB, or O blood; if Rh negative, only Rh-negative blood of any ABO type can be used; if Rh positive, either negative or positive blood can be used.

urticaria: a vascular reaction of the skin characterized by the eruption of hives and severe itching.

Valsalva's maneuver: a maneuver involving forced exhalation that a patient can perform to help prevent air embolism when a CVAD is opened to change the I.V. set or needleless connector.

vascular access device (VAD): any catheter designed for insertion into a vein or artery including all peripherally and centrally inserted devices.

vasoconstriction: narrowing of the lumen of a blood vessel.

vasovagal reaction: an involuntary reaction of the nervous system with a slow heart rate, blood vessel dilation, and hypotension causing fainting.

vesicant: an agent that can cause blisters, ulceration, and necrosis of tissue if it leaks from the vein into the tissue surrounding the vein.

visualization technologies: visible light, near-infrared light, and ultrasound devices used to visualize veins, greatly enhancing the success of finding veins and inserting VADs with the minimum number of attempts.

winged infusion set: see butterfly needle.

Y-site: an injection port on an I.V. administration set that allows separate or simultaneous infusion of two compatible solutions.

Index

A

Abatacept (Orencia), 316t
Abciximab (ReoPro), 316t
ABO system, 245–248
    antigens in, 245, 245t
    blood groups in, 245t, 246t
    blood type compatibility, 246–247, 248t
    human leukocyte antigen, 248
    plasma antibodies, 247
    Rh system, 245–246
Abraxane, 295t
Absorption, effective, I.V. drug therapy and, 199
Accessory cephalic vein as venipuncture site, 65, 67t
Acetone, 336t
Actinomycin D, 275
Active transport, fluid movement and, 11, 12t
Acute extravascular hemolytic transfusion reactions, 260t
Acute intravascular hemolytic transfusion reactions, 260t
Acute lymphocytic leukemia, antineoplastic protocol, 277t
Acute myelogenous leukemia, 275
Adalimumab, 319
Additives in parenteral nutrition solutions, 338
Add-on devices, 28–29, 28i, 29i, 58
Adhesive removers, in older adults, 408
Administration set(s), 26–27, 26i, 27i
    attaching I.V. container to, 60–61
    changing, 63, 64t, 102, 103
    as pediatric infusion therapy equipment, 384
    priming, 61–62
    types of, 56–58, 56i, 57i
Adoptive immunotherapy. *See* Passive immunotherapy
Ado-trastuzumab, 313
Ado-trastuzumab emtansine (Kadcyla), 316t
Adriamycin (doxorubicin), 278t, 279t
Adult nomogram, 210
Adverse effects
    anemia, 300t
    leukopenia, 300t
    long-term effects, 299, 301
    short-term effects
        diarrhea, 299
        hair loss (alopecia), 298–299, 300t
        myelosuppression, 299
        nausea and vomiting, 297–298
        stomatitis, 299
    thrombocytopenia, 300t
Aging
    fluid balance and, 395, 396–397t
    in older adults, 390
    physiologic changes of, 391–395
    skin effects, 392i
Air embolism
    as CV therapy complication, 164–165t, 169–170
    with peripheral cathetar, 106
    prevention, 150
    systemic complications, 105
Albumin, 242, 335
Albumin transfusion in pediatric patient, 366t
Aldesleukin, 314
Aldosterone, fluid regulation and, 6
Alemtuzumab (Campath), 316t
Alkyl sulfonates, 274
Alkylating agents, 288t, 295t
    antineoplastic therapy, 274
    DNA-binding vesicant drugs, 288t
    Hodgkin's disease, 301
    irritants, 288t
    malignant lymphomas, 301
    myeloma, 301
Allergic dermatitis, 399
Allergic reaction(s)
    as I.V. therapy complication, 113t
    as pediatric infusion therapy complication, 379–380
Allergic transfusion reactions, 259, 261t
Altretamine, 274
American Society of Health-System Pharmacists, 279
Amino acids as parenteral nutrition element, 336
AML. *See* Acute myelogenous leukemia
Anaphylaxis, 322
Anaphylaxis transfusion reactions, 262t
Antecubital veins, 371
    as CV insertion site, 138
Anthracenedione, 295t
Anthracyclines, 275, 288t
Anthropometric measurements, 333–334
    interpreting, 334t
    taking, 334i
Antibodies, 308–309
Antibodies, ABO system and, 247, 247t
Antidiuretic hormone, fluid regulation and, 6
Antiemetics, 400
Antigen(s), 306, 391
    in ABO system, 245
    in Rh system, 245–246
Antihemophiliac factors, 242
Antimetabolites, 274–275, 288t
Antimicrobial properties, CV access device, 125–126
Antineoplastic protocols, 276, 277–278t
Antineoplastic spill kit, 285, 286t
Antineoplastic therapy
    administration, 269
    advantages, 269
    alkylating agents, 274
    antimetabolites, 274–275
    antitumor antibiotics, 275
    biological agents, 273
    cell cycle, 270–273
    cell reproduction, 273
    complications
        extravasation, 293–294, 295t
        hypersensitivity or anaphylactic reaction, 296–297, 296t
        irritant or flare reaction, 293
        long-term adverse effects, 299, 301
        management, 300t
        short-term adverse effects, 297–299
    corticosteroids, 276
    drug administration
        completion process, 292
        electronic infusion pump, 290
        investigating infiltration and extravasation, 290, 291

Notes: Page numbers followed by i refers to an illustration; t refers to table.

Antineoplastic therapy (*continued*)
    preadministration check, 287–289
    reducing extravasation risks, 291t
    small ambulatory infusion pumps, 290
    variations, 290
  drug preparation, 280
  equipment preparation
    air protection, 281, 281i
    gloves, 282–283
    goggles, 281, 282t
    gowns, 281
    items, 281, 282t
    protective clothing, 282, 283i
    safety measures, 283–286
  guidelines, 279–280
  with hazardous drugs, 279
  healthy cells, 270
  miscellaneous antineoplastic agents, 276
  multitasking drugs, 276
  plant alkaloids, 275–276
  preparation, 278–279
  protection, 279
  protective measures, 280
  sample antineoplastic protocols, 276, 277–278t
  selection process, 272
    determining tumor response, 273t
    second-or third-line antineoplastic agents, 272
    treatment cycles, 272
  targeted therapies, 273
  teaching and documentation, 301
  topoisomerase inhibitors, 275
Antithrombotic properties, CV access device, 125–126
Antitumor antibiotics, 295t
  antineoplastic therapy, 275
Arboviruses transmission as transfusion risk, 243
Arterial puncture as CV therapy complication, 167
Asparaginase, 278t
Authorized agent-controlled analgesia, 227
Autoimmune disorders, biologic therapy
  immunosuppressants, 311–312
  inflammation, 311
Axillary vein, as CV insertion site, 135

B

B lymphocytes, 307
Babeoisis, 244
Bacteremia, as I.V. therapy complication, 111t
Bacterial contamination as transfusion reaction cause, 218t, 220-22, 259t, 263t
Bacterial phlebitis, 169
Basilic vein
  as CV insertion site, 123i, 135t, 138
  as venipuncture site, 65, 67t
Basiliximab (Simulect), 316t
Basophils, 307
Belimumab (Benlysta), 316t
Bendamustine, 273
Bevacizumab (Avastin), 316t
Biologic therapy
  administration, 319–320
  antibodies, 308–309
  autoimmune disorders, 311–312
  clinical indications, 309–311
  colony-stimulating factors
    side effects, 321
    types of, 314–315, 315t
  cytokines, 307–308
  definition, 305
  immune system, 305–307
  immunodeficiency diseases, 312
  immunoglobulins, 308–309
    side effects, 321
    types of, 317–318
  interferons
    side effects, 321
    types of, 314
  interleukins
    side effects, 321
    types of, 314
  managing infusion reactions, 321–322
  monoclonal antibodies
    side effects, 321
    types of, 315–317, 316–317t
  patient assessment, 318–319
  patient education, 322–323
  white blood cells, 307
Biological safety cabinet, 281
Bladder cancer, 277t
Bleeding as PICC therapy complicationl, 169
Bleeding tendencies as multiple-transfusion complication, 265t

Bleomycin, 275, 279t, 288t
Blood. *See also* Blood administration; Transfusion therapy
  ABO system and, 245–248, 245–248t
  components of, 239–244, 240–241t
  HLA system and, 248, 248t
  oxygen-carrying capacity of, 239
  recipient-donor compatibility and, 244–248, 245–248t
  Rh system and, 245–246
  typing and crossmatching, 245
Blood administration
  cellular elements used in, 20
  infusion therapy and, 20
  pediatric guidelines for, 365, 366–367t
  purpose of, 20
Blood component administration, 20
Blood filters, 251
Blood sample collection
  during CV therapy, 132, 145, 156, 157
  from implanted port, 183
  during infusion therapy, 98
Blood warmer, 253
Bloodstream infection (BSI), as I.V. therapy complication, 106, 111t
Body fluid
  composition of, 3
  daily gains and losses of, 5i
  deficit, identifying, 7t
  distribution of, 3, 3i
  excess, identifying, 7t
  functions of, 3–7
  movement of, 11–15
  percentage of, in total body weight, 3
  regulation of, 6
Bolus injection, 201
Bortezomib (Velcade), 276
Brachial vein, as CV insertion site, 135t, 138
Breast cancer, 277t
Brentuximab vedotin (Adcetris), 313, 316t
Broviac catheter, 382
Busulfan, 274
Butterfly needles. *See* Winged infusion needles

C

Cabazitaxel, 273
CACI. *See* Compounding aseptic containment isolator

Notes: Page numbers followed by i refers to an illustration; t refers to table.

Calcium, 9t
Cancer, biologic therapy for
   cytotoxic therapy, 311
   direct and indirect, 309–310
   immunotherapy, 310–311
Capecitabine (Xeloda), 274
Capillary exchange, 14i
Capillary filtration, fluid movement and, 14
Capillary reabsorption, fluid movement and, 14
Carboplatin, 274, 288t
Cardiovascular system, age-related changes in, 393–394
Carmustine, 288t
Carmustine (BCNU), 274
Catheter dislodgment, as PN complication, 350
Catheter gauges, 77t
Catheter-related complications of PN, 350, 351t
CD. *See* Clusters of differentiation
Cell cycle
   beneficial damage, 271
   collateral cost calculation, 272
   cycle-nonspecific, 270, 272
   cycle-specific, 270, 272
   different site/take action, 272
   five phases, 270, 271t
Cell membrane permeability, 12
Cellular elements of blood, 239. *See also* Transfusion therapy
   indications for transfusing, 240–241t
   types of, 239
Cellulitis, as I.V. therapy complication, 108t
Central vascular access devices
   parenteral nutrition through, 328
   in pediatric infusion therapy
      care of, 381
      implanted ports, 382
      nontunneled catheters, 381
      peripherally inserted central catheters, 382–383
      tunneled cuffed catheters, 382
      types, 381
Central vein, 21–22
Central venous access devices, 20, 22, 119–188, 289
   benefits of, 120
   characteristics
      antimicrobial properties, 125–126
      antithrombotic properties, 125–126
      catheter materials, 124
      integral valves, 125, 125i
      nonstaggered exits, 126
      power injection, 124
      sizes, 124
      staggered lumen exits, 125, 125i
   complications of, 120, 163–170, 164–167t
   discontinuing, 170–171
   documenting, 147, 156
   implanted ports for, 172–188, 173i, 175i, 179i, 180i, 185–187t (*See also* Implanted ports)
   indications for, 119
   inserting catheter for, 144–145
   managing problems in, 158–160, 161–162t
   monitoring patient for complications of, 145–146
   obtaining blood sample during, 132–133
   pathways for, 123i
   patient teaching for, 139–141
   planning, 122–123
   positioning patient for, 143–144
   preparing equipment for, 141–143
   preparing insertion site for, 144
   removing, 133–134, 172
   routine care for, 147–158, 149i
      dressings change, 148–149
      fluid containers and administration sets, changing, 149–152
      flushing and locking, 152–154
      integrity check, 155
      needleless connectors changing, 154–155
      secondary piggyback sets, 156
   selecting insertion site for, 134–138, 135t
      concerns related to, 138–139
   special-needs patients and, 162–163
   syringe sizes, 133
   transfusing blood products through, 250
   types of catheters for, 126–132, 129–131t
   venous circulation and, 120–122, 121i
Central venous therapy
   preparation, 134–143
   veins used for, 23i
Cephalic veins
   as CV insertion site, 135t, 138
   as venipuncture site, 65, 67t
Cervical cancer, 277t
Cetuximab (Erbitux), 316t
Chagas's disease, 244
Chemical phlebitis, 169
Chemokines, 308
Chlorambucil, 274
Chloride, 9t
Chylothorax as CV therapy complication, 164t
Circulatory overload
   infusion fluid and medications complications, 234t
   as I.V. therapy complication, 112t
Cisplatin, 274, 278t, 279t, 288t
Citrate toxicity as multiple-transfusion complication, 264t
Class II Biological Safety Cabinet, 279
Clofarabine, 273
Closed system drug transfer device, 284, 285
Clusters of differentiation, 315
CMV transmission as transfusion risk, 243
Colloid osmotic pressure, 13, 15
Colloid solutions, 193, 196t
Colony-stimulating factors, 308, 314–315, 315t, 319
   agents, action and indications, 315t
   cytokines, 308
   side effects, 321
   stem cell production, 315
Competency, 43–44
Compounding aseptic containment isolator, 281
Compounding sterile medication, 201–204, 203i
Connective tissue, age-related changes in, 391–392
Continuous infusion, 22, 24, 32, 200–201
   administering, with implanted port, 178, 183
   backpriming medications, 220–221
   converting, to intermittent infusion, 94, 95i
   infusion fluids, 193, 194
   piggybacking medications, 218–219
Continuous PN delivery, 340
   switching from, to cyclic delivery, 341

Notes: Page numbers followed by i refers to an illustration; t refers to table.

Corticosteroids, 276, 322, 400
C-reactive protein, 395
Creatinine height index, 335t
Crohn's disease, 311
CRP. *See* C-reactive protein
CRS. *See* Cytokine release syndrome
Cryoprecipitate as plasma product for transfusion, 241t, 248t
Crystalloids, 193, 196t
CSDT devive. *See* Closed system drug transfer device
CSFs. *See* Colony-stimulating factors
CV therapy. *See* Central venous therapy
CVAD. *See* Central venous access devices
Cycle-nonspecific antineoplastic drug, 272
Cyclic delivery, 341
    switching from continuous delivery to, 340
Cyclophosphamide, 274, 278t, 279t, 288t
Cytarabine (Ara-C), 274, 288t
Cytokine release syndrome, 322
Cytokine storm. *See* Cytokine release syndrome
Cytokines, 395
    chemokines, 308
    colony-stimulating factors, 308
    interferon, 308
    interleukins, 308
    tumor necrosis factor, 308
Cytotoxic T cells, 307
Cytotoxic therapy, 311

D

Dacarbazine, 278t, 279t, 288t
Daclizumab (Zinbryta), 316t
Dactinomycin (actinomycin D, Cosmegen), 288t, 295t
Daily fluid gains and losses, 5i
Daunorubicin, 275, 278t, 288t
Daunorubicin (Cerubidine), 295t
Decitabine, 273
Deferoxamine mesylate, 400
Dehydration
    correlating severity of, with clinical status, 359, 360i
    preventing, in older adults, 394
Delayed extravascular hemolysis, 261, 261t
Delivery methods, 22–25

Devastating effect, antineoplastic drug treatment, 301
Dexamethasone (Decadron), 232, 276, 279t
Dexrazoxane (Totect), 295t
Dextrose as parenteral nutrition element, 336
Diarrhea, 299
    as chemotherapy adverse effect, 253
Dietary history, 333
Diffusion, fluid movement and, 12t
Diphenhydramine, 322
Direct injection, 24–25
Discontinuation of infusion therapy, documenting, 46
Disease transmission as transfusion risk, 242–244, 263t
Disease-related malnutrition
    with inflammation, 330–331
    without inflammation, 332
Docetaxel (taxotere), 276, 288t, 295t
Documentation
    of CV access device, 147, 156
    of implanted port infusions, 183
    of infusion therapy, 44–46
    of I.V. therapy, 410
    of noncoring needle removal, 188
    in older adults, 410
    of venipuncture, 98–99
Donor-recipient compatibility, testing for, 244–248, 245–248t
Dorsal venous network, 65, 68t
    as venipuncture site, 66, 68t
Dosage calculation, 209
    for adult patients, 209, 210i
    for pediatric patients, 210i
Doxorubicin (Adriamycin), 275, 278t, 288t, 295t
Dressing
    changing, 100–102
        in CV therapy, 148, 149i, 150–151
    how to label, 45
    transparent, applying, 91i
    transparent semipermeable, applying, 97, 97i
Drug administration
    infusion therapy and, 19–20
    in pediatric patient, 368

E

Ears, age-related changes in, 393
Ebola virus transmission as transfusion risk, 244

Eculizumab (Soliris), 316t
EID. *See* Electronic infusion devices
Elastomeric balloon pump, 35
Electrolytes, 8, 9–10t
    balance of, 10–11
    as parenteral nutrition elements, 338
Electronic infusion devices, 24, 33, 36, 37, 61, 384
Electronic infusion pump, 197, 216–217, 252
Eosinophils, 307
Epinephrine, 322
Epirubicin (ellence), 275, 278t, 288t, 295t
Epothilones, 276
Eribulin, 273
Essential nutrients, parenteral nutrition and, 326
Estramustine (emcyt), 276
Etanercept, 319
Ethylenimines, 274
Etoposide (VP-16), 275, 278t, 279t, 288t
External jugular vein as CV insertion site, 135t, 138
Extracellular fluid, 4
    distribution of, 3i
    electrolyte components of, 11
Extravasation
    as implanted port complication, 186t
    as infusion fluids and medication complication, 197, 231
    as I.V. therapy complication, 105, 107–108t
    management guidelines, 295t
    as pediatric infusion therapy complication, 376–378
    as PN complication, 350
Eyes, age-related changes in, 392–393

F

Facility policy related to infusion therapy, 43–44
Factor VIII concentrate as plasma product for transfusion, 367t
    in pediatric patient, 365, 367t
Fats as parenteral nutrition element, 336. *See also* Lipid emulsions
Febrile transfusion reactions, 253, 259
Federal regulations related to infusion therapy, 40–41
Femoral veins as CV insertion sites, 136–137
Filgrastim, 279t

Notes: Page numbers followed by i refers to an illustration; t refers to table.

Filters, infusion medications, 217
First-pass metabolism, 199
Flow rate, infusion fluids, 195, 197–198, 198t
Floxuridine, 274
Fludarabine, 274, 288t
Fluid. *See* Body fluid
Fluid and electrolyte imbalances
　correcting, 15–19, 16i–19i
　identifying, 7t
　in pediatric patient, 363, 364i
Fluid delivery systems for pediatric patient, 380–384, 383i. *See also* Pediatric infusion therapy
Fluid overload as pediatric infusion therapy complication, 378–379
Fluid volume deficit
　in older adults, 395, 396t
　in pediatric patient, 364t
Fluid volume excess in older adults, 396t
Fluid volume status, assessing, in older adults, 397
Fluorouracil, 278t
5-fluorouracil, 274, 288t
Flushing
　of access device, 152–154
　of implanted port, 182–183
Folliculitis, 399
Food intake, decreased, nutritional deficiencies and, 329
Frailty, older adults in, 391
Fresh frozen plasma as plasma product
　for transfusion, 241t
　in pediatric patient, 366t

G

3 G's, 283
Gastric cancer, 277t
Gastrointestinal system, age-related changes in, 394–395
Gemcitabine (Gemzar), 274, 288t
Glass bottle, attaching, to administration set, 60
Gluconeogenesis, 330
Glucose balance, 339
　PPN and, 347
Glycerized red cells transfusion, 241t
Glycogenolysis, 330
Granulocyte transfusion, indications for, 241t, 248t, 256. *See also* Transfusion therapy

H

Hair, age-related changes in, 392
Hair loss (alopecia), 298–299, 300t
Haloperidol, 400
Hearing, age-related changes in, 393
Helper T cells, 307
Hematocrit, nutritional status and, 335t
Hematology, age-related changes in, 395
Hematoma as I.V. therapy complication, 109t
Hematopoietic growth factors, 314
Hemoglobin, nutritional status and, 335t
Hemolytic transfusion reaction, 245
Hemosiderosis as multiple-transfusion complication, 259t, 264t
Hemothorax as CV therapy complication, 164t
Heparin, 24, 183, 208, 337, 338
Hepatitis transmission as transfusion risk, 243
Hexamethylmelamine, 274
Hickman catheter, 341
HIV transmission as transfusion risk, 243
HLA blood group, 248, 248t
Home therapy patient
　CV therapy considerations for, 162
　implanted port considerations for, 184
Hospital-acquired anemia, 158
Hyaluronidase, 295t
Hydrocortisone, 337
Hydrostatic pressure, 13, 15
Hydrothorax as CV therapy complication, 164t
Hydroxydoxorubicin, 278t
Hydroxyurea, 274
Hyperammonemia, with metabolic alkalosis as multiple-transfusion complication, 265t
Hypercalcemia, signs and symptoms of, 9t
Hyperchloremia, signs and symptoms of, 9t
Hyperglycemia as PN complication, 351t, 352
Hyperkalemia
　as multiple-transfusion complication, 265t
　in older adults, 397t
　in pediatric patient, 364t
　as PN complication, 351t, 352
　sins and symptoms of, 9t
Hypermagnesemia, signs and symptoms of, 10t

Hypernatremia
　in older adults, 396t
　in pediatric patient, 364t
　signs and symptoms of, 9t
Hyperosmolar hyperglycemic state as PN complication, 351t, 352
Hyperphosphatemia, signs and symptoms of, 10t
Hypersensitivity as infusion fluids and medication complication, 232–233, 233t
Hypersensitivity or anaphylactic reaction, 296–297, 296t
Hypertonic solutions, 17–18, 17i, 18i, 194–195, 196t
Hypervolemia in older adults, 396t
Hypocalcemia
　as multiple-transfusion complication, 264t
　as PN complication, 351t, 352
　signs and symptoms of, 9t
Hypochloremia, signs and symptoms of, 9t
Hypokalemia
　with metabolic alkalosis as multiple-transfusion complication, 264t
　in older adults, 397t
　in pediatric patient, 364t
　as PN complication, 351t, 352
　signs and symptoms of, 9t
Hypomagnesemia
　as PN complication, 351t, 352
　signs and symptoms of, 10t
Hyponatremia
　in older adults, 396t
　in pediatric patient, 364t
　signs and symptoms of, 9t
Hypophosphatemia
　as PN complication, 351t, 352
　signs and symptoms of, 10t
Hypothermia as multiple-transfusion complication, 253, 263t
Hypotonic solution(s), 17i, 18–19, 19i, 195, 196t
Hypovolemia
　in older adults, 396t
　in pediatric patient, 364t

I

Ibritumomab tiuxetan (Zevalin), 316t
Idarubicin (Idamycin), 275, 288t, 295t
Idiosyncratic reaction, infusion fluids and medication and, 232

Notes: Page numbers followed by i refers to an illustration; t refers to table.

450 Index

IFN. *See* Interferon
Ifosfamide, 274, 288t
Ig therapy. *See* Immunoglobulins (Ig) therapy
ILs. *See* Interleukins
Immediate hypersensitivity, 296t
Immune globulin, 242
Immune system
    adaptive/acquired immunity, 306
    age-related changes in, 395
    defense lines, 306
    innate/nonspecific immunity, 306
    transfusion reaction, 258, 259t
Immunodeficiency diseases, 312
Immunoglobulins, 317–318
    clinical use, 317
    Ig intravenous, 318
    IgA, 309
    IgD, 309
    IgE, 309
    IgG, 308
    IgM, 308
    preparation, 317
    side effects, 321
Immunoglobulins (Ig) therapy, 312
Immunotherapy, 305, 310–311
Impaired ventilation, older adults, 393
Implanted ports, 130–132, 131t
    administering continuous infusion using, 180i, 182
    administering infusion using, 178–181, 179i, 180i
        giving injections and infusions, 181
        preparing equipment for, 178
        preparing site for, 178–180, 179i, 180i
    blood sample collection from, 157, 183
    comparing, with long-term CV catheters, 130, 131t
    complications of, 186–187t
    discontinuing, 187–188
    documenting, 188
    documenting infusions using, 183
    flushing, 182–183
    giving bolus injection through, 201
    indications for, 172–173
    insertion of, 176–177
        monitoring patient for, 177
        preparing patient for, 176–177
    managing problems with, 185t
    noncoring needles for, 175, 175i
    postoperative care for, 177
    on punctures and patients, 173–174, 173i
    removing needle from, 188
    reservoir for, 174
    special precautions for, 184
Implanted ports, CVAD, in pediatric patient, 382
Incompatibility of I.V. drugs, 207t
    chemical, 208
    physical, 207t, 208
    therapeutic, 208
Infection
    local
        as CV therapy complication, 166t
        as implanted port complication, 186t
        as pediatric infusion therapy complication, 379
    prevention, 93–94
    reducing risk of, in TPN, 27
    systemic, as CV therapy complication, 166–167t
Infection as transfusion reaction cause, 263t
Infiltration
    as I.V. drug therapy complication, 231
    as I.V. therapy complication, 105, 107t
    as pediatric infusion therapy complication, 379
Infiltration scale, as pediatric infusion therapy complication, 377t
Inflammaging, 390–391
Inflammation, older adults in, 390–391
Inflammatory bowel diseases, 311
Infliximab (Remicade), 317t
Infusion flow rates, 32–39
    calculating, gravity, 33, 34i
    regulating, 34–37, 35i, 36i
Infusion fluids
    continuous infusion, 193, 194
    documenting, 235
    flow rate, 195, 197–198, 198t
    hypertonic solution, 194–195, 196t
    hypotonic solution, 195, 196t
    indications for, 193
    intermittent infusion, 193
    isotonic solutions, 194, 196t
    managing complications, 231, 234t
Infusion medications, 198–199
    administering of, 216–218
    adverse events
        adverse drug reaction, 232
        hypersensitivity, 232–233, 233t
        side effects, 232
    calculating dosages for, 209–210
    continuous infusion, 200–201, 218–221
    documenting, 235
    effective absorption, 199
    high-risk, 208–209
    identifying and reducing risks, 200
    intermittent infusion, 200–201
    issues
        compatibility, 205–207, 207t
        compounding sterile medication, 201–204, 203i
        incompatibilities, 208
        stability, 204–205
    liquid drugs, 214–216, 215i
    locked VAD, 221, 224–225
    managing complications, 231, 234t
    patient-controlled analgesia and
        advantages, 226
        complications of, 230
        components of order for, 227
        disadvantages, 226–227
        managing therapy with, 228–229
        patient teaching, 230–231
        pumps, 227–228
    preparation, 210–216
        liquid form, reconstituting, 214–216, 215i
        powdered drugs, reconstituting, 212–214
        safety considerations for, 211–212
    primary intermittent medication, 222–223
    selecting equipment, 216
Infusion Nurses Society, 279
Infusion Nursing Standards of Practice, 42
Infusion order, how to read, 37, 38
Infusion pump
    alarms, 63
    monitoring, 62–63
    setting up, 62–63
Infusion therapy, 389–412. *See also* Aging, physiologic changes of; Older adults
    administration sets for, 26–32, 26i–31i
    benefits of, 2
    for blood administration, 20
    for blood component administration, 20

Notes: Page numbers followed by i refers to an illustration; t refers to table.

correcting imbalances with, 15–19, 16i–19i
definition, 1–2
delivery methods for, 22–25
documenting, 44–46
for drug administration, 19–20
facility policy and, 43–44
fluid and electrolyte balance and, 3, 6, 7, 10–15
infusion flow rates for, 32–39, 34i–36i, 38i
for parenteral nutrition, 20
patient teaching for, 47–49
professional and legal standards for, 40
risks of, 2
veins used in, 23i
Infusion therapy flow sheet, 45–46
Initiating infusion therapy, documenting, 44–45
In-line filters, 29–30, 30i, 59, 62
Innate immunity, 391
Insulin, 205, 208, 338, 400
Insulin requirements, PPN and, 348. *See also* Glucose balance
Intake and output sheets, 46
Interferon, 308, 314, 319
  alpha-, 314
  beta-, 314
  cytokines, 308
  gamma-, 314
  side effects, 321
Interleukins, 308, 314, 319
  cytokines, 308
  melanoma, 314
  renal cell carcinoma, 314
  rheumatoid arthritis, 314
  side effects, 321
Intermittent infusion, 22, 24
  converting to, from continuous infusion, 94, 95i
  with saline lock, 78, 94
Intermittent infusion device, 94–95
  benefits of, 94
  flushing, 94
  purpose of, 94
Internal jugular vein as CV insertion site, 123i, 135t, 136, 137
Interstitial fluid, 4
  distribution of, 3i
Intracellular fluid, 4
  distribution of, 3i

electrolyte components of, 11
Intraosseous (IO) access device, 74–75, 75i
Intraosseous infusion, 21, 199
  pediatric patient and, 383, 383i
Intraspinal infusion, 21
Intravascular fluid, 4
  distribution of, 3i
Intravenous bag
  adding drug to, 212
  attaching, to administration set, 61
  how to label, 46
Intravenous bolus, 22
Intravenous catheter, changing, 103–104
Intravenous clamps, 38, 38i
Intravenous drug therapy
  for drug administration, in pediatric patient, 368
  special-needs patients and, 368
Intravenous fat emulsion, 327
Intravenous infusion
  device insertion
    direct approach, 404
    indirect approach, 404–405
  dressing, 405
  securing VAD in, 405
  selecting site for, 402–403
  site preparation, 404
  site visualization, 406
  skin barrier solution, 405
  vein palpation, 403
Intravenous solution
  changing, 102, 148
  inspecting, 59–60
  preparing, 60
  types of, 16–19, 16i–19i
Ions, 8
Ipilimumab (Yervoy), 317t
Irinotecan (CPT-11), 275, 288t
Irritant contact dermatitis, 399
Irritants, 287, 288t
Isotonic solutions, 16, 16i, 17i, 194, 196
IVFE. *See* Intravenous fat emulsion
Ixabepilone (Ixempra), 276

L

Lactated Ringer's, 251
Laryngeal cancer, 277t
Lawsuits involving I.V. therapy, 48–49
Leukocyte-poor red blood cell transfusion, indications for, 251. *See also* Transfusion therapy

Leukocytes. *See* White blood cells
Licensed independent practitioner, 342, 348
Lidocaine, administering, for venipuncture, 83, 84, 84i
LIP. *See* Licensed independent practitioner
Lipid emulsions, 340
  adverse reactions to, 348
  clearance rate of, 348
  complications of, 353
  safe administration of, 344
Liquid form, reconstituting, 214–216, 215i
Liver dysfunction as PN complication, 351t, 352
Local anesthetic, administering, for venipuncture, 83–84, 84i
Local site infection, as I.V. therapy complication, 108t
Lomustine, 274
Lung cancer
  non-small, 278t
  small cell, 277t
Lymphocytes, 307
Lymphoma
  Hodgkin's disease, 278t
  malignant, 278t
  non-Hodgkin's, 277t

M

mAbs. *See* Monoclonal antibodies
Macrodrip administration set, 34i
Magnesium, 10t
Maintenance of infusion therapy, documenting, 45–46
Malnutrition
  clinical outcomes, 330
  DRM with inflammation, 330–331
  DRM without inflammation, 332
  in hospitalized patients, 332
  related conditions, 331–332
  without disease, 332
Malposition disposition, 170
Manual disinfection, 31
Material Safety Data Sheets, 314
MCC. *See* Multiple chronic conditions
Mechanical phlebitis, 169
Mechlorethamine, 274
Mechlorethamine hydrochloride (Mustargen), 295t
Median antebrachial vein as venipuncture site, 65, 67t

Notes: Page numbers followed by i refers to an illustration; t refers to table.

Index

Median basilic vein as venipuncture site, 65, 67t, 68t
Median cephalic vein as venipuncture site, 65, 67t
Median cubital vein
    as CV insertion site, 135t
    as venipuncture site, 65, 68t
Medicaid, federal-state requirements for, 41
Medical adhesive–related skin injury (MARSI), 398–399
Medicare, reimbursement claims and, 41
Melanoma, 277t
Melphalan, 274, 288t
Mental capacity changes in older adults, patient teaching and, 409
6-mercaptopurine, 274
Metabolic acidosis as PN complication, 351t, 352
Metabolic complications of PN, 351t, 352–353
Metabolic needs, increased, nutritional deficiencies and, 329
Metacarpal veins as venipuncture sites, 65, 67t
Metered chamber sets. *See* Volume-control sets
Methotrexate, 232, 275, 278t, 288t
Methylprednisolone (Solu-Medrol), 276
Microaggregate filter, 251
Microdrip administration set, 34i
Micronutrient deficiency, 331
Micronutrients as parenteral nutrition elements, 338
Midarm circumference, measuring, 334i
Midarm muscle circumference, measuring, 334i
Midazolam, 400
Midline catheters, 73–74, 74i
Minerals as parenteral nutrition elements, 338
Minocycline, 125
Mitomycin (Mutamycin), 295t
Mitomycin-C, 275, 288t
Mitotic inhibitors, 275
Mitoxantrone (Novantrone), 275, 295t
Monoclonal antibodies, 310, 312, 315–317, 316–317t, 319
    agents, 316–317t
    clusters of differentiation, 315
    effectiveness, 316
    side effects, 321

Monocytes, 307
Morphine, 21
Multiple chronic conditions, 389–390
Multiple myeloma, 278t
Multiple sclerosis, 311
Muromonab-CD3 (Orthoclone), 317t
Myelosuppression, 299

N

Nails, age-related changes in, 392
Naloxone, 230
Narcotics, 208
Natalizumab (Tysabri), 317t
National Institute for Occupational Safety and Health, 313
Natural killer (NK) cells, 307
Nausea
    acute, 298
    anticipatory pattern, 297–298
    delayed, 298
Needle gauges, 77t
Needleless connectors, 30–32, 31i, 94, 154–155
Nelarabine, 273
Nerve injury, as I.V. therapy complication, 110t
Neutrophils, 307
Nitrogen mustards, 274
Nitroglycerin, 205
Nitrosoureas, 274
Noncoring needles, 175, 175i
    removing, 188
Nonhemolytic febrile reaction, 253, 259, 261t
Nonimmune hemolysis, 261, 261t
Nonimmune system, transfusion reaction, 259, 259t
Nonspecific active methods, 310
Nontunneled CVAD, 126–127, 129t, 381
Nonvesicants, 287, 288t
Nurse practice acts (NPA), 41
Nutrition disorders, 330–332
Nutrition, poor, signs of, 333
Nutritional assessment, 332–336
Nutritional deficiency(ies), 329–332
    diagnostic studies to detect, 335, 335–336t

O

Occlusions, 159–160
    as I.V. therapy complication, 109t
    managing, 160

Occupational Safety and Health Administration, 279
Ofatumumab (Arzerra), 317t
OIRD. *See* Opioid-induced respiratory depression
Older adults. *See also* Infusion therapy
    age groups, example of, 389
    age-related changes in, 391–395
    assessing fluid volume status in, 397
    fluid and electrolyte imbalances in, 395, 396–397t
    life expectancy, 389
    MCC, 389–390
    modifications, 390
    parenteral nutrition and, 350
    transfusion considerations for, 258
Omacetaxine, 273
Oncology Nursing Society, 279
Oncotic pressure, 13, 15
Oncovin (vincristine), 278t, 279t
OPAL, 114
Opioid-induced respiratory depression, 226
Opioids, 400
Osmolality, 6
Osmolarity, 6, 15
Osmosis, fluid movement and, 13
Over-the-needle catheter, 72–73, 76i
Oxaliplatin, 274, 288t
Oxygen affinity for hemoglobin, increased, as multiple-transfusion complication, 263t

P

Packed red blood cell transfusion. *See also* Transfusion therapy
    indications for, 240t, 250
    in pediatric patient, 365, 366t
Paclitaxel (Taxol), 276, 279t, 288t, 295t
Pain, as PICC therapy complication, 169
Panitumumab (Vectibix), 313, 317t
Parenteral nutrition, 326–354. *See also* Peripheral parenteral nutrition
    additives for, 338
    administering, 340–348
    benefits of, 327
    checking order for, 343
    complications of, 350–354, 351t
    conditions that necessitate, 326
    discontinuing, 354
    essential nutrients and, 326
    indications, 329

Notes: Page numbers followed by i refers to an illustration; t refers to table.

infusion methods for, 328
infusion therapy and, 20
initiating infusion of, 343
maintaining infusion of, 344–345
for pediatric patient, 367
preparing equipment for, 342–343
preparing patient for, 341–342
reducing infection risk in, 345
risks and disadvantages of, 327, 328
safe administration of lipid emulsions in, 344
solutions for, 336–340
    elements in, 327, 336–338, 337t
special considerations for
    in older adult patients, 350
    in pediatric patient, 349
special-needs patients and, 349–350
switching from continuous, to cyclic, 341
types of delivery for, 340
Passive disinfection, 31
Passive immunotherapy, 310
Passive transport, fluid movement and, 11, 12t
Patient assessment, biologic therapy for, 318–319
Patient education, biologic therapy for, 322–323
Patient teaching, 47–49
    about peripheral I.V. therapy, 55
    for CV therapy, 139–141
    for implanted port, 176–177
    for I.V. therapy, 409
    for patient-controlled analgesia, 230–231
Patient-controlled analgesia
    advantages, 226
    complications of, 230
    components of order for, 227
    disadvantages, 226–227
    managing therapy with, 228–229
    patient teaching, 230–231
    pumps, 227–228
    risks of, 225–226
Pediatric infusion therapy, 357–384
    administer, 369
    administration sets, 384
    assessment of, 375–376
    calculating fluid maintenance and replacement needs for, 360–362, 361i–362i

complications of, 376–378
CVAD
    care of, 381
    implanted ports, 382
    nontunneled catheters, 381
    peripherally inserted central catheters, 382–383
    tunneled cuffed catheters, 382
    types, 381
electronic infusion devices/pumps, 384
growth and developmental stages, 357–359t
inserting catheter for, 373
management, 375–376
preparing to insert catheter for, 371–373
reasons for providing, 359–360, 363, 364t, 365, 366–367t
securing site of, 373–375, 374i–375i
selecting catheter site for, 369–370
    in children over age 1, 371
    neonates and infants, 370–371
Pediatric patient. See also Pediatric infusion therapy
alternate fluid delivery systems for, 380–384, 383i
calculating dosages for, 210i
fluid and electrolyte imbalances in, 363, 364i
implanted port considerations for, 184
intraosseous infusion and, 383, 383i
parenteral nutrition and, 349–350
transfusion considerations for, 257–258
Pemetrexed (Alimta), 275
Peripheral infusion therapy
    I.V. therapy (See Peripheral I.V. therapy)
    veins used for, 23i
Peripheral I.V. therapy, 53–115
    advantages of, 54
    adverse effects of, 54
    complications of, 104–106, 107–113t, 113–114
    discontinuing, 115
    documenting venipuncture for, 98–99
    patient teaching for, 55
    performing venipuncture for, 78–99, 84i, 86i, 87i, 89t, 91–93i, 95i, 97i
    preparing equipment for, 59–63
    preparing patient for, 55–56
    routine care for, 100–104

    selecting equipment for, 56–59, 56i, 57i
    selecting insertion site for, 63–69, 66i, 67–68t
    selecting venous access device for, 71–78, 73–75i, 76t, 77t
    uses for, 54
Peripheral parenteral nutrition, 328
    administering, 346
    checking order for, 347
    complications of, 353–354
    discontinuing, 354
    indications for, 329, 337t
    initiating infusion of, 347
    insulin dosage adjustment and, 348
    maintaining infusion of, 347–348
    monitoring, 347
    preparing equipment for, 347
    preparing patient for, 346
    solutions for, 337t, 340
    special consideration for, in older adult patients, 350
Peripheral vascular access device, 20
Peripheral vein, 21–22. See also Peripheral I.V. therapy
Peripheral veins as CV insertion sites, 137–138
Peripheral venous catheter, transfusing blood products through, 250
Peripherally inserted central catheter, 40, 127–128, 129t, 250, 382–383
    advantages of, 127
    complications specific to, 168–170
    indications for, 127–128
    insertion site selection, 134–135, 135t, 138–139
        axillary vein, 136
        femoral veins, 136–137
        internal jugular vein, 136
        peripheral veins, 137–138
        subclavian vein, 136
    pediatric patient and, 382–383
Pertuzumab (Perjeta), 313, 317t
Phlebitis
    bacterial, as PICC therapy complication, 169
    as infusion fluids and medication complication, 231
    as I.V. therapy complication, 105–106, 107t
    mechanical, as PICC therapy complication, 169
    as PN complication, 350

Notes: Page numbers followed by i refers to an illustration; t refers to table.

Phosphate concentrations, 208
Phosphorus, 10t
Physical assessment, 333
    for nutritional problems, 333, 334i
Physical incompatibility, 208
PICC. *See* Peripherally inserted central catheter
Piggybacking medications, 218–219. *See also* Intermittent infusion
Plant alkaloids, 295t
    antineoplastic therapy, 275–276
Plasma antibodies, 247
Plasma transfusion, 20
Platelet transfusion
    indications for, 241t, 248t, 251 (*See also* Transfusion therapy)
    in pediatric patient, 367t
Platinol (cisplatin), 279t
Platinum drugs, 274
PN. *See* Parenteral nutrition
Pneumothorax
    as CV theapy complication, 163, 164t
    as PN complication, 350
Polyurethane, 124
Posttransfusion purpura transfusion reactions, 262t
Potassium, 9t
Potassium chloride, 208
Powdered drugs, reconstituting, 212–214
PPN. *See* Peripheral parenteral nutrition
Pralatrexate, 273
Preadministration check
    confirmation, 287
    order of drugs, 287
    patient's blood count, 287
    preventing errors, 287, 291t
    tissue damage, risks of, 287, 288t
    VAD patency, assessment of, 289–290
    vascular access, 288–289
    verification, 287
Prealbumin level, nutritional status and, 336t
Prednisone, 276, 278t
Primary infusion administration sets, 56, 56i
    priming, 61–62
Procarbazine, 279t
Professional organizations, 42
Proleukin, 314
Promethazine, 208
Prostate cancer, 277t

Protein-calorie deficiencies, effects of, 330
Psoriasis, 311
Psoriatic arthritis, 311
Pulmonary edema, as I.V. therapy complication, 112t
Pumps, 35–36
Purinethol (mercaptopurine), 278t
Push injection, 22, 24–25
PVAD. *See* Peripheral vascular access device

R

Raltitrexed, 288t
Rapid response, I.V. medications and, 199
Raxibacumab (ABthrax), 317t
Recombinant interleukin-2, 314
Red man syndrome, 232
Refeeding syndrome, 331
Replacement therapy in pediatric patient, 362–369
    calculating maintenance and fluid requirements in, 361i–362i
    calculating percentage of fluid loss in, 363i
Respiratory system, age-related changes in, 393
Response evaluation criteria in solid tumors, 273t
Rh system, 245–246
    antigens in, 245–246
    blood groups in, 245
    factor incompatibility in, 245–246
Rheumatoid arthritis, 311
Rifampin, 125
Ringer's lactate, 205
Rituximab (Rituxan), 317t
RMS. *See* Red man syndrome
Romidepsin, 273
Routine care, 147–158, 149i
    for CV therapy
        dressings change, 148–149
        fluid containers and administration sets, changing, 149–152
        flushing and locking, 152–154
        integrity check, 155
        needleless connectors changing, 154–155
        secondary piggyback sets, 156
    for implanted port, 184
    for peripheral I.V. therapy, 100–104

S

Safety measures
    accidental exposure, 284
    antineoplastic spill kit, 285, 286t
    closed system drug transfer device, 285
    protective gear, 284
    safety precautions, 284–285
    transport, 285
Saline lock, intermittent infusion with, 78, 94. *See also* Intermittent infusion device
Sample antineoplastic protocols, 276, 277–278t
Saphenous vein as venipuncture site, 65
Scalp veins as venipuncture site, 370, 371i
Secondary/piggyback administration sets, 57, 57i, 58
    priming, 62
Sedatives, 400
Sensory losses in older adults, patient teaching and, 409–410
Sepsis, 168
Serum albumin level, nutritional status and, 335t
Serum transferrin level, nutritional status and, 335t
Serum triglycerides, nutritional status and, 335t
Silicone, 124
Skin
    age-related changes in, 391–392, 392i
    anatomy of, 70i
    antisepsis, 401
    integrity, 91, 398
    medical adhesive–related skin injury, 398–399
    paper tape, 398
    plastic-perforated tape, 398
    silicone tapes and dressings, 398
    stripping or pulling, 399
    tear or complete separation, 399
    venous access devices, 398
Skin barrier solution in older adults, securing VAD and, 405
Skin breakdown as implanted port complication, 178
Skin maceration, 399
Sodium, 9t
Sodium thiosulfate, 295t
Sodium-potassium pump, 11

Notes: Page numbers followed by i refers to an illustration; t refers to table.

Solutes in body fluid, 3
3:1 solution, 339
Solution container, 56
    attaching, to administration set, 60–61
    inspecting, 59–60
    labeling, 216
Speed shock
    as infusion fluid and medications complication, 234t
    as I.V. therapy complication, 112t
State practice acts, 41
Steroids, 276
Stomatitis, 299
Streptozocin, 274
Stretch net for securing venous access device, 98
Subclavian vein as CV insertion site, 123i, 135t, 136
Subcutaneous access device, 75–76, 75i
Subcutaneous infusion, 21
    site assessment and rotation, 402
    site preparation, 401
    site selection, 401
    subcutaneous device, 401
Syringe pump, 26, 33, 369, 384
Systemic complications, CV therapy, 163

T

Targeted therapies, 273
Taxanes, 276, 288t, 295t
Taxol (paclitaxel), 278t
Taxotere (docetaxel), 278t
Temozolomide (Temodar), 274
Teniposide, 275
Testicular cancer, 278t
The Institute for Safe Medication Practices, 43
The Joint Commission, 42
Thiotepa, 274, 288t
Thirst mechanism, 6
Thrombolytic agents, 208
Thrombophlebitis
    as I.V. therapy complication, 105–106, 107t
    as PN complication, 350
Thrombosis
    as CV therapy complication, 195t
    as I.V. therapy complication, 107t
    as PN complication, 350
TILs. See Tumor-infiltrating lymphocytes
Time tape, 40i

Tissue damage, risks of, 287, 288t
Titration, accurate, I.V. drug therapy and, 147
Tocilizumab (Actemra), 317t
Topoisomerase I inhibitors, 275
Topoisomerase II inhibitor, 275
Topotecan, 275
Total lymphocyte count, nutritional status and, 336t
Total nutrient admixture, 339
Total parenteral nutrition, 328
Total protein screen, nutritional status and, 336t
Tourniquet, applying, 80–81, 96
TRALI. See Transfusion-related acute lung injury
Transcellular fluid, 4
Transdermal analgesic cream, administering, for venipuncture, 386
Transdermal anesthetic cream, 83–84
Transferrin, 335
Transfusion associated graft vs. host disease, 262t
Transfusion reactions
    signs and symptoms of, 260–261t
    types of, 258–259, 259t
Transfusion therapy, 238–265. See also Blood; specific blood products
    ABO system, 245–248, 245–248t
    actions to avoid during, 256
    administration for, 249
    administration set, 251–253, 252i
    allogenic blood, 242
    autologous, 242
    blood components, 239–244, 240–241t
    compatibility, 244–245
    complications of, 258–265, 260–265t
    documenting, 257
    initiating, 254–256, 254–256i
    monitoring, 257
    for older adults, 258
    patient identification, 249–250
    for pediatric patient, 257–258, 365, 366–367t
    premedication and vital signs, 253
    protection from exposure during, 244
    purpose of, 238–239
    risks of, 242–244
    selecting equipment for, 250
    signs and symptoms of reaction to, 260–265t
    terminating, 258

Transfusion-associated circulatory overload, 258, 264t
Transfusion-related acute lung injury, 262t
Transparent semipermeable membrane dressing, 91, 91i, 92, 97, 97i
Transport mechanisms, fluid movement, 12t
Transthyretin, 336t
Transthyretin level, nutritional status and, 336t
Trastuzumab (Herceptin), 317t
Traumatic complications, CV therapy, 163
Triazines, 274
Triceps skinfold thickness, measuring, 334i
Triglyceride levels, 335
Tumor cell modulation, 311
Tumor necrosis factor, 308
Tumor-infiltrating lymphocytes, 311
Tunneled cuffed CVAD, 128, 130t
    comparing, with implanted ports, 130, 131t
    in pediatric patient, 382
Typing and cross-matching blood, 244–245

U

Ulcerative colitis, 311
Umbilical vessel catheter, as pediatric patient and, 383–384
United States Pharmcopeial Convention (USP) Standards, 279
Universal donor, 247
Universal recipient, 247
Urine ketone bodies, 336t
U.S. Pharmacopeia, 313

V

VAD. See Vascular access device
Vancomycin, 133, 232
Vascular access device, 2, 21, 22, 33
Vascular access methods, for pediatric patient, 380–384. See also Pediatric infusion therapy
Vasovagal reaction, as I.V. therapy complication, 111t
Vein
    anatomy of, 70i
    dilating, for venipuncture, 80–81
Vein preservation, biologic agents, 320

Notes: Page numbers followed by i refers to an illustration; t refers to table.

Vein thrombosis, as implanted port complication, 187t
Venipuncture
  dilating vein for, 80–81
  documenting, 98–99
  local anesthetic for, 83–84, 84i, 372
  patient assessment, 79
  patient education, 79
  patient identification, 79
  performing, 87–94, 91i, 92i, 93i
  preparing site, 85, 86i
  selecting site for, 63–69, 66i, 67–68t
    guidelines for, 69
    skin and vein anatomy and, 70i
  stabilizing vein for, 86, 89i
Venous access device
  adaptation of, for intermittent infusion, 78
  advancing, 89–94
  inserting, 87–89
  safety, 71–78, 73–75i, 76i, 77t
  selection of, 71–78
  stable and secure, 91, 91i
  types of, 76, 76i
Venous air embolism, as I.V. therapy complication, 106, 112t
Venous circulation, CVAD and, 120–122, 121i
Venous spasm, as I.V. therapy complication, 109t
Vesicant drug, 287, 288t, 295t
Vinblastine (Velban), 276, 278t, 279t, 288t, 295t
Vinca alkaloids, 276, 288t
Vincristine (Oncovin), 276, 278t, 279t, 288t, 295t
Vinorelbine (Navelbine), 276, 288t, 295t
Vision, age-related changes in, 392–393
Vitamins as parenteral nutrition elements, 338
Volume-control sets, 57, 57i, 58
Vomiting
  acute, 298
  anticipatory pattern, 297–298
  delayed, 298
Vorinostat, 273

W

Water as parenteral nutrition element, 338
White blood cells, 307. *See also* Transfusion therapy
  indications for transfusion of, 248
Whole blood transfusion, 20. *See also* Transfusion therapy
  indications for, 240, 241–242t, 248t
  in pediatric patient, 365, 366t
Winged infusion needles, 73, 89
Winged-set type infusion set, 73, 76, 76i, 89

Z

Ziv-aflibercept, 313
Zoonotic diseases, 243–244

Notes: Page numbers followed by i refers to an illustration; t refers to table.